Praise for *Ayurveda Lifestyle Wisdom*

"Acharya Shunya is one of the extraordinary teachers of the living, embodied wisdom of Ayurveda. She transmits it through the roots of her family lineage as well as throughout *Ayurveda Lifestyle Wisdom*. She is a model of how to access the healing power of nature within."

SHIVA REA
author of *Tending the Heart Fire*

"*Ayurveda Lifestyle Wisdom* is a valuable companion for those wishing to understand and apply holistic concepts of health and healing to real-life challenges. You will find many pearls of wisdom that will inspire you to a mindful and positive lifestyle."

SUHAS KSHIRSAGAR
BAMS MD (Ayurveda), and author of *The Hot Belly Diet*

"Acharya Shunya has gifted all of us with her story of learning Vedic wisdom from her grandfather, Baba, as a very young girl. Baba's timeless wisdom is woven throughout *Ayurveda Lifestyle Wisdom* as Shunya teaches us all the pearls of Ayurveda, Baba through Acharya, and now to us."

JOHN DOUILLARD
author of *Eat Wheat; Body, Mind, and Sport;* and *The 3-Season Diet*

"Shunya offers us a path that integrates body with mind and spirit, showing us the secrets of Ayurvedic daily practice, self-care, and much more. This is a book to cherish, consult often, and use throughout your life."

SALLY KEMPTON
author of *Awakening Shakti* and *Meditation for the Love of It*

"Acharya Shunya shares with us a prescription to optimize our health in a clear and straightforward fashion, giving each of us the power to change our lives."

JAMES R. DOTY, MD
clinical professor of neurosurgery and director at the Center for Compassion and Altruism Research and Education, Stanford University School of Medicine

"*Ayurveda Lifestyle Wisdom* rings out like a temple bell and shines like the sun at dawn. A healing balm for our distracted lives, it offers us easy-to-implement, practical Ayurvedic guidance for healthy living every day. It boldly inspires us to claim our inherent healing power and shows us how to do it. You won't want to put this book down, and fortunately, we don't have to because its wisdom continues to whisper in our inner ear, like Acharya Shunya's beloved Baba: 'Your life is sacred; remember, you can live that way.'"

YOGACHARYA ELLEN GRACE O'BRIAN
spiritual director at the Center for Spiritual Enlightenment and author of *Living the Eternal Way: Spiritual Meaning and Practice for Daily Life*

"Reading this book is an enchantment. This is a rare and refreshing appearance of the heart and soul of Ayurveda, alongside the body of wisdom in a modern lifestyle book. Enough story to relate easily and enough tools to transform your experience of life, and finally, finally, a book on Ayurveda that speaks to all the parts of us."

SIVA MOHAN, MD
founder of AyurvedaBySiva.com, founder of Veda MeLA, and board member of the California Association of Ayurvedic Medicine

"*Ayurveda Lifestyle Wisdom* is a poetic and inspiring journey through the joy of life deeply rooted in a millennia-long tradition. With Ayurveda and the way Shunya explains it, life is an art, a wisdom, and the embodiment of a tradition going far back in time. Acharya Shunya brings that tradition back to life in the twenty-first century."

ALAIN TOUWAIDE, PHD
cofounder and scientific director at the Institute for the Preservation of Medical Traditions

"*Ayurveda Lifestyle Wisdom* is the ultimate practical guide that promises to reconnect you to the fundamental truth of your spiritual nature and the divine cosmic laws of balance, rhythm, seasonal detox, and so much more. Shunya's deep-seated knowledge about Ayurveda, and her compassionate and warmhearted writing gave me the confidence to try her suggestions about losing weight and getting better sleep and eliminating heartburn. It all worked—when nothing else would!"

MEG JORDAN, PHD
chair of the Department of Integrative Health and Human Sexuality, California Institute of Integral Studies

"With this highly readable and eminently practical book, Acharya Shunya illuminates Ayurveda in all its fullness—not just a collection of remedies for preventing and treating disease, but a holistic system that draws from its venerable sister sciences, yoga and Vedanta, to address all facets of human life. Every household should own a copy."

PHILIP GOLDBERG
author of *American Veda: From Emerson and the Beatles to Yoga and Meditation, How Indian Spirituality Changed the West*

"A beautifully written book that offers a unique perspective of the simple and effective diet and lifestyle changes from Ayurveda that you can make to achieve better health."

DIANA I. LURIE, PHD
professor of neuropharmacology at the University of Montana and editor-in-chief of the *Ayurveda Journal of Health*

"*Ayurveda Lifestyle Wisdom* encourages us to explore all aspects of our lives as they contribute to health. Acharya Shunya's explanations are comprehensive, clear, passionate, and often poetic. They offer us opportunities to reconsider assumptions of what we consider 'normal' in our daily lives and show us how to gradually achieve health-enhancing change."

RICKI POLLYCOVE, MD
author of *The Pocket Guide to Bioidentical Hormones*

"Acharya Shunya, a well-respected Ayurvedic teacher and practitioner, acquired this authentic knowledge from her grandfather and guru shri Baba, distilled it through her personal experience and practice, and observed the transformative effect of this knowledge. Now she shares that eternal knowledge through this book with stories and examples that are easy to follow and put into practice. This book serves as an invaluable resource for anyone who is embarking on a journey to restore vibrant health, and as a source of inspiration to those who have already embarked on that transformative journey."

DHAVAL DHRU, MD
Ayurveda chair at Bastyr University and president of the board of the National Ayurvedic Medical Association

"I love how Shunya weaves together easy-to-understand, health-focused practices that are deeply rooted in ethical and socially responsible interventions, which are good for both our inner health and outer relationships. This is a must-read that belongs in every home and on the reading table of everyone who wants to lead a natural, healthy, and happy life."

RICHARD MILLER, PHD
author of *iRest Meditation: Restorative Practices for Health, Resiliency, and Well-Being*

"Acharya Shunya takes you home in this fascinating, detailed guide to proactive health practices through the principles of Ayurveda. She conveys profound, time-proven knowledge in this passionate, step-by-step guide that can be easily embraced by all, at any age, for a life of balance, order, rhythm, and harmony."

PETER Z. WASOWSKI
founder and CEO of Vasper Systems, NASA Ames Research Park

"*Ayurveda Lifestyle Wisdom* offers a way of living that promotes continued well-being for those who are healthy and a path back to health for those who have been unwell. Acharya Shunya skillfully guides the reader in incorporating these time-tested health practices to create a balanced state of natural resiliency."

ANAND DHRUVA, MD
associate professor of medicine at the University of California San Francisco Osher Center for Integrative Medicine

"This is a masterpiece book that should be an essential for every Ayurvedic practitioner, health care professionals, and all the patients with chronic diseases, who will find themselves coming back to the text time and time again for deeper study and practice."

DILIP SARKAR, MD
president of the International Association of Yoga Therapists (IAYT)

"A unique and profound guide to healing as well as the art balancing life energies, this book presents an elegant and practical approach to health and well-being appropriate for anyone."

JAMES KELLEHER
cofounder of the American Council of Vedic Astrology and author of *Path of Light: Volumes I and II*

"*Ayurveda Lifestyle Wisdom* is a pleasure to read and inspiring in its mission to provide the tools with which we can reclaim our lives. The book highlights a spiritually and ecologically conscious, ethically grounded, health-centered rather than disease-focused Ayurvedic method, with extensive information and pragmatic instructions that make it easy to follow the counsel within."

RITA D. SHERMA, PHD
chair of hindu studies at the Graduate Theological Union, Berkeley, and editor-in-chief of the *International Journal of Dharma Studies*

"Have you ever wondered what you would have learned if you were raised by an Ayurvedic guru? Acharya Shunya shares her experience in growing up in family of Ayurvedic sages and carrying on the healing traditions in the United States. She shares her best family stories, recipes, and authentic Ayurvedic lifestyle wisdom in her book, which is sure to become a classic of students of Ayurveda around our Earth."

CATE STILLMAN
founder of Yogahealer.com and
author of *Body Thrive*

"*Ayurveda Lifestyle Wisdom* by Acharya Shunya beautifully unfolds the ancient Ayurvedic wisdom in an experiential manner relevant to our contemporary lifestyles."

YOGINI SHAMBHAVI DEVI
co-director of the American Institute of
Vedic Studies in Santa Fe and author of
Yogini: Unfolding the Goddess Within

"In this gorgeous book, Acharya Shunya combines stories of the lessons she learned from her family with her years of experience training students and coaching clients. The combinations of stories, recipes, practices, and rituals is a superb addition to the bookshelf of any seeker. Acharya Shunya offers the advice of a trusted sister, whose dedication to Ayurveda shines through every page."

FELICIA TOMASKO
editor-in-chief of *LA Yoga* magazine
and president of the Bliss Network

AYURVEDA
Lifestyle Wisdom

AYURVEDA
Lifestyle Wisdom

A Complete Prescription to Optimize Your Health,
Prevent Disease, and Live with Vitality and Joy

ACHARYA SHUNYA

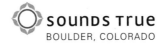

sounds true
BOULDER, COLORADO

Sounds True
Boulder, CO 80306

This work is solely for personal growth and education. It should not be treated as a
substitute for professional assistance or medical advice. Any attempt to diagnose or
treat an illness should be done under the direction of a health care professional. The
application of protocols and information in this book is the choice of each reader, who
assumes full responsibility for his or her understandings, interpretations, and results.
Should the reader have any questions concerning the appropriateness of any procedure
or preparation mentioned, the author and publisher strongly suggest consulting a
professional health care advisor. The author and publisher assume no responsibility for
the actions or choices of any reader.

Published 2017

Cover design by Jennifer Miles
Book design by Beth Skelley

Cover image © Gita Kulinitch Studio, Shutterstock.com
Illustrations by Lisa Kerans

Printed in Canada

Library of Congress Cataloging-in-Publication Data
Names: Acharya Shunya, author.
Title: Ayurveda lifestyle wisdom : a complete prescription to optimize your health,
    prevent disease, and live with vitality and joy / By Acharya Shunya.
Description: Boulder, Colorado : Sounds True, 2017. |
    Includes bibliographical references and index.
Identifiers: LCCN 2016026178 (print) | LCCN 2016046320 (ebook) |
    ISBN 9781622038275 (pbk.) | ISBN 9781622038282 (Ebook) |
    ISBN 9781622038282 (ebook)
Subjects: LCSH: Medicine, Ayurvedic. | Medicine, Ayurvedic—Religious aspects.
Classification: LCC R605 .A25 2017 (print) | LCC R605 (ebook) |
    DDC 615.5/38—dc23
LC record available at https://lccn.loc.gov/2016026178

10 9 8 7 6 5 4 3 2 1

To my guru, my grandfather, my Baba,

For transmitting to me his lived wisdom with such grace and compassion.

Baba planted the spiritual seed of who I am today.

To my mentors, my mother and father,

Due to their trust in my inherent capacities and calling,

My seed blossomed into who I am today.

To my companion, my husband,

Through him, I understood the purpose of soul collaborations.

My seed strengthened into who I am today.

To my shishyas, my beautiful students,

Through their dedicated living of my teachings,

The seed of my knowledge shall live on tomorrow.

This book is for you.

CONTENTS

FOREWORD BY DR. DAVID FRAWLEY

Acharya Shunya is a dynamic and original teacher in the Vedic tradition, well trained on many levels of study with great traditional teachers and her own extensive personal practice. I have watched her teaching and healing center develop and flower over the years according to her consistent attention, dedicated efforts, and long-term vision.

Acharya Shunya's motivating ideal is of a global Vedic education, arising from a firm foundation of right living according to Ayurveda, which she is developing in Vedika Global, her organization and school. She shares this Ayurvedic basis for developing our higher potentials in life in her book, *Ayurveda Lifestyle Wisdom*.

Ayurveda is not just another system of disease treatment, but rests upon a profound inner science of positive health and natural living. It shows us how to harmonize ourselves with the greater universe within and around us, with all its secret powers and divine blessings. Ayurveda's concern is not simply with the treatment of disease but with optimal well-being for body, mind, and consciousness extending from every cell of our body into the Infinite.

We can compare the modern medical doctor with the fireman who puts out a fire in a house, namely the fire of disease in the house of the body. An Ayurvedic practitioner does not merely take such a defensive role; he or she teaches you how to build a fireproof house in the beginning and maintain it over the full course of your life. This constructive and creative lifestyle foundation of Ayurveda is both protective and transformational.

Ayurveda teaches us how to promote and nourish optimal well-being, not simply how to destroy pathogens. It helps us awaken our own inspiration to higher living, not simply offering us drugs to sedate us. Acharya Shunya shows us this detailed Ayurvedic blueprint to build a healthy, creative, and conscious way of life, from right diet and exercise to right thinking and meditation.

Acharya Shunya teaches us how to determine our unique Ayurveda lifestyle and align it with the forces of nature as they are specially arrayed and rhythmically changing within us. Ayurveda's view of the three doshic types is unique, powerful, and without parallel in the main medical systems available today.

Ayurveda's system of right living and behavioral medicine is vast, multileveled, and encompasses not just our physical reality but our subtle energy system and deeper thought patterns. Ayurveda is a medicine of the universal life which is enduring, not simply a passing fad or a temporary phase in the development of medical science. It represents both the wisdom of the past and the future evolution of consciousness for our species in our perennial quest for lasting happiness and truth. *Ayurveda Lifestyle Wisdom* clearly and consistently guides us in this direction.

In my own work with Ayurveda, I have emphasized Ayurveda relative to the mind, our behavior, and our daily activity. I think this is the most important aspect of Ayurveda, though its ability to treat specific diseases, particularly of a severe nature, has its compelling value as well.

Ayurveda increases both physical and psychological immunity, promoting longevity for both the body as a whole and for the mind, brain, and nervous system. As we realize that well-being is a function of how we live, we will come to better appreciate Ayurveda's great contribution to world health.

Ayurveda takes the wisdom of yoga and its philosophy of the unity of existence and unfolds it relative to both physical and psychological health and disease. It is the medical side of yogic thought and healing that many are seeking today. As such, it naturally leads us to the practice of yoga and meditation such as Shunya explores.

Acharya Shunya is one of the pioneers in the growing field of Ayurveda in the West. Her book fills an important place in our appreciation and application of Ayurveda in our daily lives, providing many simple prescriptions to help us take control of our own health and happiness.

Ayurveda helps us reclaim our lives and shows us how to live our lives as a great adventure in consciousness open to the flow of divine grace. Acharya Shunya provides important guidance and practical tools to do this. I welcome her addition to the growing literature on Ayurveda and look forward to her future contributions.

PREFACE

Every book accomplishes its own spiritual journey before being born, and this one is no different. Join me in an inspiring transformative voyage to abiding health.

This book has the potential to change your state of health for the better—permanently. Health is not just a possibility that you might achieve. It is a reality, an underlying natural state of being. Health will manifest once you begin to live in alignment with Nature's intelligence. This is the promise of Ayurveda, India's five-thousand-year-old system of health and healing.

When I was growing up in India, I witnessed a spiritual master, my grandfather, whom I addressed as Baba, remind the diseased and the suffering of their abidingly healthy nature. He taught them simple ways to align with Nature on a daily basis, and enigmatically, this ignited powerful healing of body, mind, and soul. While there wasn't a focus on the symptoms of disease per se, I saw cancers disappear, ulcers heal, and chronic depressions lift.

I think I had rationalized that these "miracles" were possible because my teacher was a spiritually realized being. Clearly, my guru's spiritual presence was undeniable. But as I grew up and observed more, I recognized that Baba's skills in transmitting a highly rational science of Ayurveda lifestyle were also a key factor. I am so glad that my teacher imparted to me his spiritual conviction along with his scientific knowledge, which includes Ayurveda's lifestyle wisdom. His teachings and his blessings have taken the form of this book so that more and more people can discover the truth of health for themselves.

Reading and implementing the lessons in this book can be a rite of transition, from a life lived routinely or unmindfully, to masterful living, encompassing the freedom that comes from embracing health consciousness, self-determination, and Nature's blessings to proactively influence the course of your health and well-being. Health alone will completely undo the paradigm of disease permanently.

Ayurveda proposes two methodologies toward approaching health. The first is preventive and promotive. It proposes protecting and enhancing health with a set of lifestyle practices. This is the "wisdom" approach of evoking inner health, known as *swasthya-raksha* in Sanskrit. It incorporates at every step lessons from the spiritual sister sciences of yoga and Vedanta.

The second methodology is "restorative." It includes disease management using herbal drugs, body treatments, and even surgery (though surgery is no longer an active modality in Ayurveda today). This methodology is known as *vikara prashamana* in Sanskrit. Both approaches are equally valid, at appropriate junctures.

However, we must not quit evoking health at any point of time. If disease management via drugs is taken up without a parallel investment in a healthy lifestyle, the body becomes a battleground all too quickly. There is a wellspring of power within us, a spiritual truth, that we must honor; and we never give away our power to any disease, just because we have a scary-sounding condition with a grim prognosis. In fact, it is now more than ever that we must activate our latent health response through a scientific lifestyle that is in sync with Nature's laws. If you are consuming Eastern or Western drugs, a healthy Ayurveda-inspired lifestyle in conjunction will expedite recovery and additionally facilitate well-being.

Your body is remarkably wise and possesses self-repair mechanisms. "*Trust it some more, and help it heal itself,*" Baba explained to me. Besides, Ayurveda lifestyle is often enough in and of itself to activate the dormant "health response."

And at the least, lifestyle is like evocative art; it suffuses our consciousness with all-new possibilities of being and becoming. A lifestyle that makes us feel fulfilled and optimistic at some level will positively impact our beliefs and feelings about our universe and ourselves. Sometimes you will find that you are smiling through the day, and for no particular reason.

When we examine Ayurveda's source literature, spanning from the Vedas (4500 BCE) all the way to the sixteenth century (that is, texts progressing from the remote past onward), it was lifestyle wisdom that occupied the central stage. Disease management gained increasing priority in the later texts. In fact, this is how the sages who gave us the ancient Vedas and original spiritual sciences of Ayurveda, yoga, Vedanta, meditation, sacred art, architecture, music, and dance lived! They boldly cultivated radiant health day by day as an expression of their god consciousness. They were not living in constant fear of disease. They thought health, lived health, and enjoyed health. It is no wonder that their ancient teachings offer original wisdom that holds the potential of making our entire planet healthy today. Even if disease came to the wise seers (as decay is part of the natural order), they

would heal it (or accept it) with grace and beauty, without collapsing their entire consciousness into a "broken-shattered" mode.

Unfortunately, many Ayurveda practitioners today choose to "fix" disease and eschew time-consuming patient education on lifestyle. At times, the practitioners possess academic knowledge of lifestyle principles but not a lived knowledge borne from personal experience, and hence, they are very much bound in "disease consciousness" themselves, often harboring negative outcome beliefs, which invariably reduce the chances of recovery. They are also quick to prescribe herbal drugs. For example, instead of elucidating the lifestyle wisdom pertaining to healthy sleep, far too often the endangered herb *Nardostachys jatamansi* is prescribed for insomnia. I call this a "prescriptive" model of Ayurveda, very similar to the Western medical approach that matches drugs with symptoms but does not care to address the underlying life (style) issue. It encourages dependency on drugs, not self-reliance through leading a balanced life, which is greater than any drug. I personally stay away from this mode of Ayurveda.

This book, instead, restores the wisdom teachings on lifestyle to their rightful place and shines the light on health. This book will thereby empower ordinary people, you and me, because lifestyle sets us free to craft our own health, in our own homes, on our own terms.

My Experiments with Evoking the Health Response

My guru imprinted my soul with a spiritual seed of relentless conviction in the self-healing and self-repairing mechanisms of the living body. My entire life and message as a spiritual teacher revolve around this power, which is inherently spiritual. My own journey with a genetic disorder that confines many people to wheelchairs (yet, has spared me) and my ability to cheerfully withstand the severe aftermath of a traumatic neck injury—without painkillers or surgery, with hope to heal fully one day and courage to continue undeterred with my life mission, in spite of everything—has strengthened my belief that deliberate and unhurried self-loving lifestyle practices synced with Nature awaken health as well as personal power and courage.

The same idea has been confirmed again and again, not only in my personal life and private practice, but on a larger scale through public teachings, community education, and wellness initiatives undertaken in California since 2007 through my not-for-profit Vedika Global, a foundation for the living wisdom of Ayurveda, yoga, and Vedanta.

To confirm my learned belief that a health response can be evoked through lifestyle implementation alone, I experimented for over a decade by creating several drug-free lifestyle courses (taught by my well-trained graduates and myself) and lifestyle clinics in California overseen by my school's graduates. In both, I deliberately bypass the paradigm of disease management and, instead, focus on evoking health of body and mind through lifestyle teachings plus personal empowerment through connecting with a disease-free, ageless higher Self as the underlying reality.

Anyone, of any age and any constitution, whether healthy or sick, was welcome to sign up. Participants were as young as ten years old and also as old as eighty! And what did I find? They all got better! Within a matter of weeks, both course and clinic participants started reporting increased well-being. Some even shared their latest blood test results or other clinical findings—unsolicited by us—to rejoice in their newfound health parameters.

Many of them were shocked, too. What was going on? How was health sneaking up on them so quickly, merely through education in a health-evoking lifestyle and healthy beliefs, in spite of years of ill health and after their doctors had given up on them, or worse, when they had given up on themselves?

While their actual results were based on length and commitment of engagement with lifestyle practices, there was not a single participant who reported a deterioration of health.

Countless individuals with beginning, chronic, or advanced disorders were reclaiming health and well-being, simply by implementing lifestyle changes impacting core personal areas of food (*ahara*), rest and sleep (*nidra*), and sexual and behavioral self-regulation (*brahmacharya* and *sadvritta*) in the overall context of prescribed daily regimen (*dinacharya*) and seasonal regimen (*ritucharya*). Lifestyle practices even improved the well-being of people with terminal diseases, and some reported outliving their prognosis or at least feeling more at peace until the last day. It was uncanny and incredible.

By shining the light on health and consciousness, the miracles I witnessed with my guru Baba, in his lifetime, had now begun to accrue around my initiatives with health versus disease. This was a powerful reinforcement of my own belief systems.

I was convinced that I was onto something and that perhaps a scalable clinical as well as educational self-help model could be crafted from my spiritually anchored lifestyle teachings that evoke the health response. Perhaps it was time to simply stop overly focusing on disease anyway. Is counteracting disease with herbs (versus synthetically designed drugs) still battling it anyway, keeping us locked in disease consciousness? Are we merely changing our doctors from Western medicine to Eastern medicine providers, but each time getting locked up all over again in disease-combating dogmatic belief systems, prescriptions, and protocols? Are we scaring ourselves again and again (with disease), forgetful of our natural inheritance, which is health?

Are we panicking and creating more work for ourselves in medicine instead of simply realigning the quality of our lives with lifestyle adjustments? Have we generated a tremendous number of myths around disease, and its heavy-duty management, instead of evoking the sweet song of health from the truth and light sourced within?

I am all for modern medical intervention, when necessary. I also advocate no single approach, as a judicious integration is the wisest way. However, I do wonder if we need a greater, or at least parallel, focus on a healthy lifestyle, which will greatly support us in overcoming disease by evoking a health response from within. Is it time to begin a new narrative after all?

Further—and this pertains especially to those who have an intrinsic belief in naturally sourced drugs as an alternative to pharmaceuticals—an important question to ask is whether we are overmedicating ourselves, simply because the medicine in question is from a plant source and not created in a laboratory. Should a natural drug be the end of our quest for health? Are we settling for less?

These were some of the questions that were arising in my mind. Sadly, the bane of reductionism is so pervasive that it has also quietly crept into the domains of spiritualized systems like Ayurveda. Instead of being seen as a health-promoting system, more and

more, Ayurveda is taught, practiced, and promoted worldwide as a complementary system of disease management. Herbs are safer than prescriptive drugs; we know that (although some will even question that), yet all drugs mask the body's self-regenerating mechanism to an extent; hence, I believe that herbs must be prescribed as an exception, or in advanced conditions only, and never without accompanying lifestyle restoration teaching.

According to the Botanical Survey of India, 93 percent of Ayurveda medicinal plants are endangered today.[1] Even so, unfettered export by India and import and consumption worldwide burgeons. Patent wars on Ayurveda botanicals are being fought in multiple courts, and the bulk of claims are filed right here in the United States (including battles over neem and turmeric). Now, almost every drug company on the planet wants to cash in on Ayurveda's ancient pharmacopedic wisdom. Shockingly, all institutions of Ayurveda education in India, and more and more now emerging worldwide, continue to impart a medical paradigm focused around these disappearing herbs, blissfully ignoring the magnitude of the environmental problem.

When it came to using plant-based medicines, my teacher modeled an ultraconservative, almost reverential, approach. I too prefer utilizing spice- and food-based home remedies or employing garden herbs that we can grow in our own homes in a relatively short time. I also consider it my responsibility to screen for botanicals that are not endangered before utilizing them myself or prescribing them to others. This is vastly preferred to consuming and prescribing wild-grown herbs—some of which take decades to grow and ripen.

Are we ultimately expecting our environment to foot the bill of natural medicine?

We still have time to put aside our fallacious notions about disease.

This book fills a gap in promoting a spiritualized and health-focused, environmentally sound, ethically rooted Ayurveda lifestyle so that more and more people can adopt these practices in their lives along with a sense of *dharma*, or social responsibility, toward our planet and its environment.

Conceivably, what I am sharing through this book is the best-kept secret of humanity, and this information will help many more people reclaim sound health. Ayurveda's lifestyle wisdom is tried and tested and is, above all, an economical solution to the epidemic of wide-ranging lifestyle disorders like hypertension, diabetes, dyslipidemia, obesity, cardiovascular disease, and psychological/stress-induced disorders, including depression, that humanity is facing today.

I am glad I followed my inner voice to expect the miracle of health, no matter how poor the prognosis may be. The thank-you cards, letters of acknowledgment, tears of joy, and flowers of gratitude are countless and still arriving. And don't just take my word for it. Read comments and stories of transformation from course and clinic participants throughout this book.

Healthy Lifestyle Triggers Genetic Changes—A Clinical Study

You can understand how pleased I was to confirm that what I learned from my teacher has an echo in the science of epigenetics, according to which, our genes are not fixed but fluid, and our environment—composed of our daily food, habits, thoughts, quality of relationships, and daily self-care routine—impacts our genes, both positively and negatively. This rang a bell

with me right away, explaining why I did not manifest gross physical disability in spite of a genetic predisposition. My Ayurveda lifestyle and positive health outcome belief were perhaps my best allies in this journey.

A study by Dr. Dean Ornish, published in *Proceedings of the National Academy of Sciences*, sheds more light on the far-reaching health benefits reaped by my course and clinic participants from apparently minor lifestyle variations.[2] As reported by Reuters: "In a small study, the researchers tracked thirty men with low-risk prostate cancer who underwent three months of major lifestyle changes. As expected, they lost weight, lowered their blood pressure, and saw other health improvements. But the researchers found more profound changes when they compared prostate biopsies taken before and after the lifestyle changes. After the three months, the men had changes in activity in about 500 genes—including 48 that were turned on and 453 genes that were turned off. The activity of disease-preventing genes increased while a number of disease-promoting genes, including those involved in prostate cancer and breast cancer, shut down."[3]

While we cannot literally amend our genes, a change this dramatic is possible when we positively modify our lifestyle.

Karma and Continuation of a Spiritual Legacy

And finally, I should tell you, I did not simply wake up one morning and decide that I was going to be a champion of Ayurveda's lifestyle wisdom. I believe it was my karma or my spiritual destiny that decided, even before I was born, that I would indeed write the first book (an authoritative bible of sorts) on Ayurveda lifestyle wisdom. No other books (in any language) address Ayurveda's lifestyle teachings in this depth, along with the spiritual, philosophical, and scientific context and step-by-step instruction.

I am one of the fortunate teachers born into a family of teachers with an uninterrupted educational lineage, a family that has lived as well as transmitted this ancient wisdom for untold years in the plains of northern India. I have not only mastered the knowledge academically, I have also lived it.

As for the word *lineage*, it sounds mystical these days, but the idea is common enough in India where, for centuries, sacred and healing knowledge was carefully passed on from mentor to disciple in the rarefied environment of a special family-style school called *gurukulam*. Here, Vedic education was imparted to the student for a minimum of twelve years. I studied for fourteen, along with regular schooling, and

graduated as an *acharya*, which means "a master spiritual teacher of lived Vedic knowledge who teaches not only by word, but through role modeling by behavior." My education was rigorous, to say the least, yet spiritually charged and always experiential.

When I was growing up in India, living and learning this knowledge in the family of my teacher, I had no idea that one day I would be writing this book for a world audience. And yet, this is what has happened. This is less a testimony of my life journey and more of a shout-out for Ayurveda. What is the truth cannot be kept under wraps for long. More and more people are seeking Ayurveda's lifestyle and benefiting from its transformative wisdom.

I hope this wisdom will change your life for the better too, as it did mine. But first, you have to believe that anything is possible.

Shunya

INTRODUCTION

The Art of Ayurveda Lifestyle

I didn't realize how sick I was until I got healthy." At twenty-two, Brittany Barrett was taking eighteen pills a day—prescription medications from physicians who told her there wasn't much they could do about her pain and nothing they could do to cure her illness. She had been diagnosed with ulcerative colitis. "My body was literally eating holes into itself," she said, "and my life felt like it was on hold. I had moved back in with my parents. There were times when I had to remain close to a bathroom. It was devastating. I tried to keep a positive attitude, but I was numb. I was depressed. I went to support groups, but that made me even more depressed."

After just a year, this San Francisco Bay Area resident became free from the condition that had once plagued her. She healed herself through the Ayurveda system of health and healing, which is India's traditional and time-proven method to establish physical, mental, and spiritual well-being. It is a way of eating, a way of living, a way of approaching life itself—and it is inherently medicinal.

I have been imparting Ayurveda lifestyle wisdom for the last twenty-five years, and I am grateful that I have lived the principles outlined in this book since birth. My teacher, my guru, was my grandfather, Baba Ayodhya Nath, a renowned Vedic teacher and healer of his time, and the line of wisdom bearers in my family goes back uncountable generations, all the way back to the holy *Rig-Veda,* the oldest wisdom scripture, originating in India. When I was nine, my guru formally initiated me into rigorous study of the Veda, along with three important bodies of knowledge that originate from the singular Veda: namely, Ayurveda for abiding health, yoga for a pure mind, and Vedanta for elevation of spiritual consciousness.

I now impart this same timeless and transformative wisdom through a traditional schooling format called the gurukulam, in which the authentic teachings—derived from original ancient texts as well as instruction from my guru (my grandfather) and our uninterrupted lineage dating back several thousand years in India—come alive through embodied and experiential education, including lifestyle, well-being, cooking, diet, healing, god-consciousness, meditation, and yoga. My students feel uplifted, peaceful, balanced, happier, healthier, blessed, confident, and on the path to self-mastery. But perhaps even more important, students feel part of an ancient tradition and trusted lineage in which they feel held—and at home.

I will never forget the evening when, giving a talk on the fundamentals of Ayurveda lifestyle wisdom at a Bay Area bookstore, I found myself watching an exceptionally beautiful young woman in the front row who sat staring at me with tears running down her face. I could see that she was taking in every word. Afterward, Brittany Barrett introduced herself and said,

"You've changed my life. I'm going to pursue my health because you have inspired me." What had ignited her was the message that her body was not broken, but rather that an ailing body is out of balance, and whatever it is about the body that's out of balance can be brought back *into* balance. It was quite a different message than the one this troubled young woman had been hearing for years from Western medicine!

Britt was touched by my talk, and I too was touched—by the strength of her intention. That night, I dreamt of this young woman. In my dream, I took her hand and led her back home to the sacred town of Ayodhya in Uttar Pradesh, India. It was here that I learned the Ayurvedic principles I teach. The dream turned out to be somewhat prophetic because Britt did, indeed, follow me—not to India, but into an exploration of Ayurveda.

A few weeks later, Britt registered for a three-day retreat on getting in touch with one's inner *shakti*, or "spiritual power." Making such a connection within oneself is fundamental to Ayurveda. Though at this particular retreat I didn't lecture on Ayurvedic dietary recommendations, I do always make certain that retreat participants eat correctly by providing healthy, balanced meals cooked from fresh foods appropriate to the season. I hadn't reckoned, however, that participants might show up with their own food! This is exactly what Britt did, following her ideas, gleaned misinformation, about what she "needed" to eat to address her digestive problems. She sat down at the dinner table, telling other participants, "Oh, your food looks so good! It's too bad I have to eat this," and unpacking a meal of raw fruit and yogurt.

It's a funny thing about food misconceptions. In the West, yogurt, with its live cultures, is often seen as a miracle food, and fresh fruit is thought to be as pure as water itself. This is not, however, the case. I discuss this in much greater detail in later chapters, but for now, I will simply point out—as one of my senior students did that day to Britt—that fruit and dairy are an incompatible food combination and, taken together, are quite difficult for the body to digest.

At the time, Britt thought, *These ladies are really nice, but they don't know what they're talking about!* It was, of course, Britt herself who didn't know. And how could she? Her medical doctors had told her that her diet made no difference in ulcerative colitis; she need only continue taking her eighteen daily pills. To her credit, Britt saw the inherent fallacy in this—how could food be unrelated to digestion!—and so she explored the diets she found in the media. This was how she'd found my lecture in that bookstore.

Britt walked away from the retreat with a list of five things she was to do daily:

1. Wake up early each morning at a set time.

2. Have an altar in her room and put fresh flowers on it every day.

3. Every morning, meditate on her healing for fifteen minutes.

4. Stop eating (or minimize her consumption of) harmful foods—toxin-generating foods, such as yogurt, cheese, processed foods, and cold foods like raw salads.

5. Eat beneficial foods such as mung lentils, or green gram; homemade Ayurvedic buttermilk; clarified butter,

or *ghee* (Ayurvedic clarified butter); and good spices like turmeric, cumin, fennel, and ginger.

These lifestyle and dietary principles, especially numbers 4 and 5, are discussed in detail in later chapters, but this simple list was enough for Britt to work with. And work with it she did. Every day she went down this list, and before long she noticed that her bowels were less erratic and that her mood was beginning to elevate.

I feel this kind of transformation is a testimony to the power of Ayurveda. With just a few lifestyle changes, instrumented daily, the body becomes strong enough to begin healing itself. This is because Ayurveda principles and foods work with—and never against—the body's innate intelligence.

Recognizing the undeniable improvement in her health from following five simple precepts, Britt signed up for the beginner's self-care course at my school, Vedika Global. I designed this course with people like Britt in mind, to help them awaken to health. Students learn the basics of Ayurveda lifestyle under the direction of experts. Students are given the fundamentals to support a healthy lifestyle and eating habits. In addition to going over theory, in every class they also cook healthy foods, timeless recipes that heal each time they are consumed. Learning these skills, students are then able to awaken their own self-healing. Britt, as it turned out, was inspired to study further.

By the end of her first year of study with me, Britt's ulcerative colitis virtually disappeared, and she was completely symptom-free. She was also able to wean herself off prescription antidepressants she had been taking since she was sixteen years old, and you can imagine how proud she felt about being free from those chains!

What had begun as a year of self-healing was transformed into an unquenchable thirst for knowledge of this magical science! Britt then completed a three-year practitioner-level training with me, and since 2012 she has been attending to clients herself, offering them advice and giving to them a list of five daily directions that is quite similar to the one she received herself.

The profoundly personal and deeply enriching style of my traditional gurukulam's training (a spiritually transformative educational process based on the ancient Vedas) immediately and irrefutably deepens self-awareness. Britt's journey went beyond academics into real life, into a living, breathing immersion in Ayurveda lifestyle wisdom under my watchful eye, and this built profound confidence in her. Step by step, Britt transformed her health, and as she did this, she matured emotionally and spiritually until she was prepared to give back to society. Today, she is featured on popular blog sites and in magazines and is in the process of launching a television show on healing with food. Moving from desolation to hope, from isolation to connection, Britt has become a light for her community in her own unique way, and Ayurveda lifestyle wisdom has successfully anchored her at every step. Seeing my student give from the fund of knowledge she has received makes my heart overflow with gratitude. I bow again and again to the great sages, the *rishis*, who selflessly granted us this invaluable knowledge of Ayurveda. I thank my primary teacher, my guru Baba Ayodhya Nath, who passed this treasure on to me, precisely and without shortcuts, along with the certainty that health of body, mind, and soul is our inherent state, that it is our human birthright.

In the final analysis, Nature is the grandest of all teachers. It is Nature herself who beckons us to come home to her by following Ayurvedic lifestyle practices, which are nothing other than manifestations of natural laws of the cosmos. Ayurvedic wisdom reminds us that our entire life is an opportunity to make the natural yet discriminating choices that will bring us into balance and reclaim the deep spiritual harmony that lies within us.

Let us explore the living wisdom and Ayurvedic lifestyle practices that changed the life of this young woman. Perhaps you, too, can benefit from adopting an Ayurveda lifestyle!

Ayurveda: A Path to Self-Fulfillment

It is said that some five thousand years ago, India was home to the spiritually evolved beings who were the rishis, or sages, of Ayurveda. After a prolonged spiritual quest and untold years of meditation, these great souls elevated their consciousness to the point that they could receive the special healing wisdom that is known as Ayurveda. This Sanskrit word translates as "the knowledge of life."

To rid ourselves of the suffering that afflicts body, mind, and soul, we do not require specialized technology to combat disease (and "dis-ease"). What we need is an affirmative knowledge of life and how to lead it in such a way that in each moment we experience being in alignment with Nature, which is both our source and destination.

Thus, Ayurveda is a science of conscious living that originated in ancient India, that flourishes today in modern India, and that extends its influence worldwide. Ayurveda teaches a lifestyle that, when lived, prevents disease and optimizes health and well-being.

Ayurveda addresses body, mind, and spirit in one sweep. It restores hope and wholeness in a gentle and constructive fashion. Rather than struggling with disease, Ayurveda opens us to our own natural wholeness. Ayurvedic principles remind us that we are self-healing creatures and that we can maintain—or regain—good health by choosing healing foods, a balanced lifestyle, and inner calm.

The Gateways of Positive Change

Ayurveda is the recorded insights of visionary, spiritually inspired, out-of-the-box scientists, the rishis, who were keenly in dialogue with the transcendental realities of life. You could say that these sages were the original researchers who discovered Ayurveda and advanced its use among the rest of humanity.

Ayurveda's sages observed Nature deeply, meditating on her rhythmic changes—the days, the seasons, the phases of life in birth, aging, and death. They concluded that while change is the essence of life, it is possible to adapt to these changes artfully and, by so doing, to reap abiding health. Balance in our adaption to change means health, and the lack of balance translates as ill health. These teachings became encoded over time in the great science of Ayurveda.

The natural wisdom that humanity once possessed when we all lived close to Nature has been collectively forgotten. This is not anybody's fault, as such. The urbanization of our natural landscapes has forced on us forgetfulness and alienation from Nature. For this, humanity pays a large price. Thankfully, however, Ayurveda reminds us that we have nothing to fear, for there is no such thing as a permanent damage. As long as we are alive, we can embrace new beliefs that spawn fresh choices and reap new fruits. New beginnings are the essence of life.

In fact, Ayurveda reassures us that these changes in Nature are actually gateways, lending opportunity for a deeper communion with the essence of life and abiding health, which is our true nature. To pass through these gateways, however, requires life wisdom and alignment with Nature. The sages, therefore, teach humanity perhaps its first lesson on how to navigate Nature through an artfully lived lifestyle, first and foremost.

Wellness Encompasses Both the Material and the Spiritual

The *Rig-Veda*, the oldest of India's scriptures and the source book of the Indian worldview, declares, "The truth is one: the wise call it by many names."[1]

This is a greatly liberal perspective. Truth, precisely because it is truth, need not be artificially broken up into realms of existence and operation—one truth for the external world, which is the territory of the scientist, and one truth for the internal world, which is the focus for the mystic. Rather, truth is one, indivisible and nonnegotiable, and the living being is a perfect meeting ground of the material and the spiritual dimensions of truth. In Ayurveda, this truth is known as *satyam*.

Consequently, Ayurveda is a unique medical science that is beyond the limitations of scientific or physical realism (materialism), which claims that only matter is real and that all else is imagination. Nor is Ayurveda limited to spiritual idealism. It is, rather, a judicious mix of the material and the spiritual in terms of both relevant levels of understanding and of healing. Ayurveda offers a highly creative and original understanding of the human plane of existence and its challenges to health from the perspective of both the material and the spiritual.

This is why Ayurveda does not force us to box ourselves into being either 100 percent spiritual entities or 100 percent material entities. Ayurveda accommodates both paradigms in recognition of our inherent multidimensional existence. This position is mature, to say the least, and five thousand years ahead of its time. Transcending opinions and differences, it offers the benefit of inclusiveness to us all. While the sages of Ayurveda were deeply spiritual, they were also dedicated to scientific rigor and methodology. And this is how the sages were able to glean the highest transcendental truth that lies both within and beyond the world of matter.

Ayurveda is both a gentle, nurturing, mothering, healing art—a way of living in alignment with Nature and with humankind's spiritual essence—and an efficient, matter-of-fact, methodical way of correcting, balancing, and fixing health through the protection of good health and the prevention and management of disease. Ayurveda goes beyond dogma to recognize and highlight the fact that life cannot be understood by only one set of mechanisms or theories. Thus, Ayurveda accommodates a variety of designs and wellness strategies.

Learning the Old but Ever-New Principles of Ayurveda

Ayurveda's fundamental principles have stood the test of time. They are in as much use today in the twenty-first century as they were in ancient times. The survival of Ayurveda is a living testimony to the accomplishments of its scientist sages. Ayurvedic concepts have delivered consistent, and at times astonishing, results over time. This book weaves these same eternal principles through lifestyle teachings. The practices you encounter in this book have stood the test of time. They were valid then, they are valid today, and they will be valid tomorrow.

I am fortunate to have studied with a modern-day sage of Ayurveda, my guru, my grandfather and teacher, Baba Ayodhya Nath, whom I simply refer to as Baba. It is a generic name, spoken affectionately, in the same way that in the West we might call someone Grandpa. Baba is also the title used all over India to address holy people. Perhaps these mystics, sages, and seers are known as baba because they are collectively regarded as India's spiritual elders.

Baba was born in 1900 in northern India, into the family of a renowned Hindu saint and yogi with an uninterrupted lineage going back untold years. Baba overcame early childhood disease and went on to live ninety remarkably healthy years, impacting his community with his spiritual radiance, charismatic leadership, profound Vedic knowledge, and social service. In my formative years, I lived with my Baba and our extended family in our large ancestral home, built by Baba's great-grandfather in the holy city of Ayodhya in northern India, renowned because King Ram, who was considered an avatar of Lord Vishnu, was born there, according to the ancient Hindu epic Ramayana. So it is a pilgrimage town for millions still today.

Over the years, Baba bestowed on me the spiritual wisdom of the Vedas and began my initiation into the transformative wisdom of the related Upanishads and the Bhagavad Gita, two of the most sacred Vedic texts expounding a rare, universal spiritual philosophy (known as Adwaita Vedanta) teaching self-actualization (*dharma*) as well as Self-realization (*mukti*), which is the same as God realization (*moksha*). His teachings of Ayurveda were truly classical, based on core texts, hands-on, practical yet poetic, and sublime at the same time. Baba's

fierce, unflinching belief in the living body's inherent intelligence to heal itself (with the help of Mother Nature) became my core belief system too. To this day, I may look at a dying person, and instead of feeling dismayed, I connect with what is vital and amazing in that being, even in that terminal stage. And often enough, the so-called "medical miracles" begin to transpire too. Baba told me, *"Never lose hope, as hopelessness is the disease that precedes all symptoms."*

Baba's out-of-the-box personality, calm presence, continuous state of god consciousness, and profound teachings impacted my soul in deeper ways than I could have been aware of at that young age. My essential education happened through observation of a spiritually realized being. I watched how Baba faced the ups and downs of his own life—and how he chose to respond to them from a place of inner restfulness cultivated through a committed art of living inspired by Ayurveda. I listened to Baba's wise words even before I could fully understand them. It has taken me the rest of my life to comprehend and integrate the impact of the valuable gift of the knowledge Baba imparted to my soul. My body and mind were those of a child, but my soul was apparently ready to receive this wisdom. As a result, my life today as an educator and leader in Ayurveda revolves around the paradigm-shifting conversations I had with my Baba.

I believe the direct teacher-student relationship is special and potentially superior to any academic, test- and degree-based system for spiritualized sciences, like Ayurveda, yoga, and Vedanta. This personalized process of training creates the meticulous transfer of knowledge, experience, and expertise—the central matters on which wisdom is founded—that cannot be imparted except through a kind of apprenticeship, face-to-face, knee-to-knee, as has been impressed on my soul by decades of learning from my guru, Baba.

This was the main way Vedic knowledge was transmitted from the beginning of Indian civilization until the social, political, and educational structures started disintegrating with multiple invasions and finally Muslim rule beginning in the twelfth century. Next, colonization attempts by the Portuguese and French, and finally imposition of British imperial rule starting in 1857 all but destroyed this indigenous and highly spiritualized process of education. I am so fortunate that I got to study in one of the few remaining grassroots institutes of such rarefied education. So the gurukulam process is the old way, not a new way of education, just not so common nowadays.

I know Baba's soul guides me intimately as I write this book. I will be communicating his profound teachings on lifestyle to you through these pages. Throughout, I share some of my conversations with Baba—and my own first glimpses of Ayurvedic principles, which I received in the traditional way, sitting at the feet of a master.

 One night, as Baba and I sat inside watching the monsoon rains pouring down, he said, "Shunya, within your body lies buried the rare and potent ability to regenerate." That year, the monsoon came after a tremendous delay. Everything had dried up in northern India. Even our favorite river, the vast Sarayu that flowed through town, was so shallow that my older cousins would wade almost all the way across to the other side. On this night, the heavens had unexpectedly obliged us, and we listened to the rain pound down almost violently, as if making up for lost time. The sky lit up dramatically with lightning bolts that sparked across the horizon. Ominous and gigantic cloud masses were bursting with deafening explosions above our house.

In my hometown, whenever the thunderclouds bellowed, we children cried out too, beckoning each other to splash in the puddles and streaking through the narrow streets yelling, *"Baarish aayi! Baarish aayi!"* ("Here come the rains!"), as if our neighbors might somehow miss the spectacle of this huge rainstorm without our calling it to their attention.

Peacocks, who lived by the hundreds in this river town, would spread their beautiful feathers majestically on the rooftops and riverbanks, performing an ethereal dance in the rain that, each year, held us spellbound. That night, I confess, I was a bit overcome by Nature's sound and fury. I wondered how our family's cow, Nandini, was doing in the lightning. The cowshed was warm and dry, but would all of this sound frighten her? Should I make her come sit by Baba too? She was only two years old, after all, and I was eight, so like any older sister, I often worried about her.

Later that evening, Baba told me about the powerful storm gods, the unstoppable spirits that "empty the udders of the sky" and bring life-giving rain to the earth. Known in the Vedas as the *Maruts*, these subtle forces know intimately the powerful medicinal herbs that grow on high mountaintops or deep inside the belly of overflowing rivers. "We refer to such extraordinary elements and phenomena of Nature as *devas* or *devata*." By this, he was saying that they are gods or godly.

"Why is this meaningful?" Baba asked in the way that he did when he fully intended to supply the answer from some Vedic text. He then did so: "By knowing one handful of earth, all earthen articles become known. The Veda reveals to us that one Ultimate Reality, Brahman, pure divine consciousness, is the substratum of all beings, all worlds, and all gods—and having known that, nothing else remains to be known. To a mind that has been initiated into this macro-understanding of divinity, the various forms of Nature—the five elements (ether, fire, air, water, earth) as well as the stars, sun, moon, clouds, rain, lightning, storms, rivers, mountains, planets, and, of course, our beloved mother planet Earth—are all revealed to be identical with the common truth of our existence. Truly, these are illumined forms within the common web of divine consciousness."

"See Shunya," he said, "how the Veda has given us the original vision of oneness even amid the plurality of our experiences. There is neither a multiplicity nor hierarchy of gods. There is merely the recognition of oneness and sacredness everywhere."

I liked his message that we live in a world charged with devas. Even if I did not have the words to express my Baba's teachings that night as the Maruts drenched my home, my Baba was putting into words my own spiritual intuition. He gave expression to the experience of sacredness in every nook and cranny of our existence. I had felt this all along, even though I wouldn't be able to express it in words until many years later.

Every morning, I enjoyed wading into River Sarayu. "She is my very absolute favorite devi," I had concluded in my eight-year-old heart. There was also our aged Peepal tree, which is also renowned as the Bodhi tree, under which Gautama Buddha had gained enlightenment. Every morning, my mother would chant a special Vedic hymn, the Aswatha Vriksha Stotram, to this most sacred tree of Hindus, evoking its myriad blessings. I was told that my numerous sage ancestors, beginning with Rishi Vashishtha from Ayodhya, had meditated under its deep foliage, and we always approached it with the words, *Vriksha rajaya namaha*, meaning, "I bow to the deva of trees." Besides, that was my favorite tree to climb. In fact, my own list of devas was endless. I was grateful for and reassured by these devas and my feeling of connectedness with everything.

Amid dramatic lightning, and our evocative conversation on gods and goddesses, we sat in serenity sipping a warm drink made with Nandini's fresh milk. My mother added saffron, turmeric, and other herbs according to my Baba's medicinal recipe. Baba continued talking in his quiet and deeply reassuring voice—both his voice and his words taking away my fear of the thunderclouds. He explained that although they are fierce and often their will is almost demonic, the Maruts are actually divine healers. What they do benefits all that live on Earth. Human beings, animals, and plants would all wither and die if the Maruts did not force the clouds to release, drenching our planet with life-giving moisture. "See Shunya," Baba said, "soon all will be green, juicy, and filled with sap."

As Baba described Nature's "divine healers," a wave of joy arose in my heart, along with a desire to thank the loudly bellowing Maruts, but the hot-spiced milk flooding my mouth made me gulp instead. I kept quiet, listening to Baba. In my child's mind, I did not know if it was story time or teaching time, as they were often one and the same with my Baba. I just knew it was something important, something I would need to tell the whole world about one day.

He spoke then about how our barren and dried-out Earth, exhausted from the burning heat of a parched summer, was being restored to a moist and green abundance. I knew that tomorrow, on my walk to school, I would find tiny flowers and grasses and herbs that had not been there the day before. Overnight, a bleak landscape would have burst into life and colorful splendor.

And it did. For the rains are messengers of life and the promise of continuity, herbs, fertility, abundant crops, health, and happiness to all. The circle of healing always continues. It will not be stopped.

"As human beings," Baba said, "we too can be rejuvenated. We need to mindfully apply God's special ingredients." By this, my grandfather meant the special foods and herbs that have but one dharma (purpose), and that is to rejuvenate. As the rains rejuvenate the Earth, any part of the body treated by these sacred and natural medicines can become rejuvenated. We will be bursting with health, in all its awesomeness, in the same way the Earth bursts forth with new life when there is rain. This is a natural law. ✒

So on that stormy night so long ago, Baba taught me about a grand state of health that is entirely possible for each human being. If we honor and anticipate this extraordinary state of health, we will manifest it. Our own natural health is so much more than the absence of disease sought by Western medicine. It is an abundant, fruitful, flourishing, and overflowing state of well-being.

Never underestimate the physical body. It holds the great power that lies latent inside you, there for you to discover and to own. When you are unwell, never look at your disease alone, become weary in heart and spirit, and give up. Know that your body is a field of healing potential. Your body too is like the Earth, where seeds of health lie dormant, patiently waiting for rain. Much like monsoon flowers, your body simply waits for you to give it just a little bit of love, and the invisible potential will actualize into blossoms of health. Recognize the amazing regenerative power of your body, a power that exists in all of its tissues and in each and every cell. Given half a chance—with the right nutrition and positive living conditions—the body wants to self-heal.

Death is certain, but as I teach my students, disease is optional. We are not born inadequate; we are perfect as we are, by design. Life is not tomorrow or yesterday; life is today, here and now in the choices we make in the present moment. This realization is most important. This one shift in our consciousness, from fighting disease to evaluating our lifestyle choices today, can lead us to the magical fruit of true and abiding well-being from within.

The power to self-transform at every level—body, mind, and soul—is the promise of Ayurveda. The sages who crafted Ayurveda were consumed with the notion of exploring the body's natural intelligence, its inherent immunity to the wear and tear of living. When we consciously cultivate good health through mindful lifestyle practices and rejuvenating food and medicine, our bodies can become transformed. We can manifest a state of health that is vibrant with ease, energy, and flow. This is Ayurveda.

Ayurveda Defined

The term *Ayurveda* is self-defined. *Ayu* refers to "life" and *veda* refers to "knowledge." It is "knowledge of life" as a whole that Ayurveda elaborates, and through its name, Ayurveda's wide scope as a science becomes clear. Hence, Ayurveda should not be seen as merely another natural system of "fighting" disease. Rejecting a disease-based mind-set, Ayurveda promotes vigorous and joyful health consciousness, first and foremost, by enriching the quality of our lives. Ayurveda does this by asking us to choose measures that promote our well-being, such as consuming a pure, fresh, cooked diet and adopting daily and seasonal rituals. A renowned Ayurvedic sage known as Rishi Sushruta or Sage Sushruta, who is thought to have lived in the first to second centuries, is considered the father of holistic surgery in Ayurveda, along with being the author of one of the most important treatises on this subject. He has provided a wonderful definition of health that demonstrates this ancient modality's truly expansive vision. According to Sage Sushruta, a healthy person is one who enjoys balance in the fundamental physiological factors—including the three *doshas* (*vata*, *pitta*, and *kapha*, which I will discuss in depth)—as well as steadiness in the digestive and metabolic processes, firmness of the biological tissues, and efficiency in the excretion process. When such a person's faculties of sense perception, mind, and intellect are in harmony with the inner Self, known as *Atman*, then *swastha*, or the optimal state of health, is achieved.[2]

Thus, in Ayurveda, health is a state of well-being due to a balance of the physical body, the senses, psyche, and the spirit. Ayurveda's definition of health—perhaps the oldest definition of health we have from a systematic medical paradigm—goes well beyond the scope of Western medicine's definition of health as "the absence of disease."

The World Health Organization (WHO) takes this Western definition further: "Health is a state of complete physical, mental, and social well-being and not merely the absence of disease or infirmity."[3] Yet WHO has yet to include the spiritual dimension, and so Ayurveda's definition is more expansive.

Ayurvedic medicine approaches the health of human beings in all of our many dimensions: not only in body and mind but also in soul. Through Ayurveda, we can hope to gain health and well-being in all our complexity: physical (*sharirika*), mental (*manasika*), sensorial (*airndrika*), social (*samajika*), and of course spiritual (*adhyatmika*).

In Ayurveda, all of our experiences are valid, each and every one of them. In Ayurveda, we are not dismembered organs, structures, and functions. We are more than our parts; we are whole. We are in all, and all is in us. And these are not just my words; these are the teachings of ancient sages of Ayurveda.

Today, there is considerable rhetoric about the value of perceiving, diagnosing, and treating patients holistically, yet thousands of years ago, Ayurveda forwarded a wholly practical and usable system to implement these holistic ideals

in health, including health's interconnecting links with environment, society, and culture.

Let me give you an example. A man named Duncan came to Vedika Global looking for freedom from the symptoms he was suffering from—and found instead swastha, a state of deep health marked by inner freedom and fulfillment, an experience so intense and joyful that he exclaimed, "I feel like a billion dollars!" Do your visits to medical doctors' offices leave you exclaiming with this kind of joy?

FEELING LIKE A BILLION DOLLARS WITH AYURVEDA!

Duncan came to Vedika Global for a basic course on Ayurvedic self-care for beginners. That was four years ago. In the intervening time, he has come back twice to take the same course. I asked him why, and he grinned. "I come back for the food," he said.

He was joking. Though he obviously loved the food, Duncan was taking in much more from our classes than just good food. This sixty-eight-year-old man was a true seeker, actively exploring modalities for his own healing. Five years prior, he had been leading a full and creative life, giving no thought at all to the health of his body. Duncan had a degree in psychology and a three-decade career in data processing. In his spare time, he volunteered at his child's school and took classes at dozens of colleges, finally earning a master's degree in creation spirituality. He was in the process of constructing his "dream home" on a hilltop, surrounded by twenty-five acres of green beauty, when he fell from the roof and his life changed dramatically.

Surgery helped him walk without a cane, and a bouquet of complementary modalities—trigger point therapy, myofascial tissue release, acupuncture, chiropractic, and a great deal of therapeutic massage—almost eliminated the remaining aches and pains.

Then, in the following year, Duncan discovered Ayurveda, and as his health awakened from within, one by one his remaining physical problems were resolved. Initially, just eating Ayurvedic cooking four nights a week—two at Vedika Global and two with another student who made him *khichadi* (a dish made from rice and lentils)—led to his losing ten pounds of extra weight in the first few months "without even trying!" And he didn't feel as if he were sacrificing anything on those "healthy" nights; he found the food delicious and satisfying.

By the end of his first two-month course, a post-nasal condition was gone, a troublesome itchy cyst disappeared, and a lifelong issue with constipation was resolved. Also, after learning the Ayurvedic approach to hydration—a few sips of water when thirsty, not forcing down eight cups of water a day—he no longer needed to urinate every two hours through the night. And with the Ayurvedic guidance on easing into sleep, he now fell asleep much more readily. While he had been getting as few as four restless hours of sleep each night, he was now sleeping soundly for six or seven, and when he was awake, Duncan was "on the go." He said, "When I discovered Ayurveda, I told myself, 'I feel like a million dollars!' After eight months as a student, I now feel like a billion dollars!"

In the longer term, the help Duncan received from Ayurveda was truly priceless. At age sixty, he had begun taking pharmaceuticals to deal with moderately rising blood pressure and experienced the negative effect these drugs have on the bladder. Now, because he paid attention to when he woke up and went to bed,

gave himself a daily oil massage, and followed a simple Ayurvedic diet, Duncan was able to successfully eliminate all pharmaceuticals from his daily regime. Recently, his lab tests were the best they had been in five years. He wrote in a blog, "One of my goals now is to live healthy, happy, and pain-free for thirty more years, on top of my own mountain in my little RV, surrounded by trees, peace, and quiet, and incredible views of nature. Thank you, Ayurveda, for making me believe this is possible!"

The Original Green Medicine

As a canonized system of thought, Ayurveda recognizes one fundamental truth: *The closer we are to Nature and her ways, the healthier we will be. The farther we wander away from Nature, the more we will suffer.* The Ayurvedic sages recommend conscious living by aligning our inner nature (the microcosm) with external Nature (the macrocosm). This is why, in Ayurveda, the individual and his or her larger environment—which is societal, interpersonal, climatic, and also geographic—are seen as intimately intertwined. The quality of our lives is not an afterthought that has a casual impact on our health; it is the most important aspect of our health.

Accordingly, Ayurveda reintroduces humanity to natural laws, so we can appreciate the fact that our inner nature is really one and the same with outer Nature. Learning and experiencing this essential unity, we begin to relax at our deepest level. Rather than struggling against Nature's laws consciously or unconsciously, we start to actively cooperate with Nature.

This is really all we have to do. When we simply stop our battle and allow Nature to take over, abiding health reasserts its presence along with all its attending comfort, relief, and joy. It's as simple as that. Hence, this book on Ayurveda is all about reacquainting us with natural laws and rhythms. These teachings of health are codified as the lifestyle teachings of Ayurveda.

Cultivating Peace Before Health

Ayurveda demonstrates how to cultivate peace with our physical, psychological, and spiritual dimensions of existence. In the peaceful garden of Ayurveda, health awaits us quietly and with none of the attending drama of insurance companies, drugs with side effects, and forbiddingly high-risk experimental surgeries. Inside the peaceful garden of Ayurveda, the flower of health awakens naturally, breathes the air that is peaceful, absorbs the warmth and radiance of a natural sun, sips the water that rests on its petals, and thrusts its roots deeper into the Earth. Ayurveda reminds us that health is not the source of well-being; well-being is the source of health.

Since the body itself manifests from the laws of Nature, then the body is nourished by Nature's own loving, caring, and eternally peaceful helpers:

- Cultivated sacred and inspiring space to dwell in with cleanliness and purity

- Fresh air breathed in deeply, with joy and recognition of its presence in our being as our life force

- Adequate sunlight, whose sacred radiance enlivens both body and mind

- Pure drinking water that nurtures our being and quenches physical and metaphorical desires

- Peace with Mother Earth and peace with her environment, who is our first mother and life sustainer

- Organic, seasonally appropriate foods, cooked with love and the spices that sustain us

- Exercise that recharges us and infuses us with vitality

- Sexuality that fills us with pleasure and laughter

- Sleep that nurtures us in the lap of the divine Mother

- And finally, in a mind tranquil from the rest, meditation that takes us back to our spiritual center

With all of these helpers at our service, we experience total health.

How profound are the insights of Ayurveda, existing thousands of years and declaring that a body well rested, well fed, comfortable in its natural rhythms, and supported by peaceful contemplation will rejuvenate itself, again and again. This is the promise of Ayurveda.

Fortunately for us, the sages did not copyright the health-empowering wisdom or claim that this knowledge is meant only for people who look or worship like they did. Instead, they acknowledged eloquently the existence of collective suffering and, with benevolent compassion, professed that Ayurveda is universal knowledge to be rid of this suffering. Ayurveda is, then, a noble gift for all humanity, and it will remain relevant in every era and applicable for all of life—including plants and animals.

Ayurveda attempts not to eradicate disease but to enhance our inborn immunity and strength so that we can withstand disease and always enjoy good health. Ayurveda is a way of leading a wholesome life, a path of mindful living by which we become masters of our own destiny and meet with satisfaction our life goals, including those of abundance, pleasures, self-actualization, and self-realization. Ayurveda not only gives us back our right to earthly health and well-being, but also gives us opportunities to connect with our transcendent spiritual essence. The best part of all is that this path to health is extremely economical: you can craft your health and claim your well-being by employing Ayurvedic principles in your home, kitchen, and garden and on your humble meditation couch.

The Path of Ayurveda Lifestyle Wisdom

In many ways, lifestyle wisdom embodies an entire life journey taken up mindfully, daily. In this sense, Ayurveda lifestyle is a path to health. The Sanskrit word that describes this path to health is *swasthavritta*. The goals of swasthavritta are to maintain the health of the healthy, to avoid premature aging and untimely death, and to promote a healthy and totally happy life.

Some overarching themes from the science of Ayurveda, which impact us as we journey on the path to health, explain the connections between our state of health and the cosmos. I briefly address these themes below. Additionally, throughout this book, I introduce the three cornerstones of this journey, namely: sleep, sex, and food. These three areas are of greatest importance if we are to be truly healthy.

Unity of the Macrocosm and the Microcosm

Fundamental to Ayurveda is the understanding that the microcosm (in this case, the body), known as *pindanda*, is no different from the macrocosm (Nature, or the universe), known as *Brahmanda*. This means that you and your environment are essentially one. If you think about this, it's obvious. You and the universe are made of the same "stuff." What India's scriptures call the five physical elements (space, air, fire, water, and earth) comprise the human body and every other aspect of Nature.

The Macrocosm and Microcosm Are in a State of Constant Interaction

The interaction between an individual being and the world is represented by chronobiological rhythms—day and night, the turns of the seasons. There is a need to construct a lifestyle that acknowledges these rhythms. This lifestyle must allow the human body to adapt to the changes that are occurring in the environment. Western tradition has us following uniform prescriptions for every day of the year. Yet, to remain in alignment with a changing macrocosm, it is important that we change our eating and lifestyle practices to reflect the change of the seasons.

A Lifestyle Following Multiple Rhythms

Ayurveda health teachings (swasthavritta) include detailed hygiene routines (dinacharya) to be followed from the time we wake up until we go to bed as well as seasonal lifestyle precepts (ritucharya) that work in conjunction with the daily lifestyle according to the time of year.

The Three Pillars of Health

The three pillars of health, as mentioned previously, are sleep, sex, and food, and each of these is given extensive attention in the science of Ayurveda lifestyle. When all three are in balance, a human being is rightly nourished (not over or under), adequately rested (not more or less), and sexually active (in a balanced way). Lacking a critical balance in any of these three human needs, we can and will suffer from a myriad of disorders, ranging from headaches to infertility.

Throughout this book, I will discuss lifestyle practices to balance these three pillars along with other foundational Ayurvedic philosophies and health-promoting principles and traditions.

The Lifestyle Clock

In any period of twenty-four hours, there is a clock ticking, a clock that Ayurveda tells us to be mindful of because it maps energetic changes in the macrocosm with the change of time. Hence, we are asked to engage in life activities like sleeping, awakening, eating, and exercising in alignment with the macrocosmic energetic shifts. Without the knowledge of Ayurveda, we may still instinctively follow the clock anyway—since we are creatures of Nature, and thus, intuitively, we may do what is required of us, such as look for food around noon—but with Ayurveda's help, we can make sure that we are on mark. Ayurveda explains the reasons for the rhythm, and knowing the reasons helps us stay aligned with Nature's clock. That is why the chapters of this book are arranged according to time of day, beginning with waking up and ending with falling asleep.

At times, our busy lives seem to demand that we live in another rhythm in order to "get things done," and then we may miss the cues from our inner clock. Technology has made it possible for us to do anything at any time. We can cook food at any time of the day or night. We can darken our living quarters and sleep all day. We can stay up all night working on our computers. In these ways, our natural bio-cues can become tangled. If this has happened, then we can rewire our brain to follow Ayurveda's lifestyle clock. Following this clock externally allows our internal energies to sort themselves out and align with the rhythms of Nature.

Three Fundamental Forces in Universe

The reason this lifestyle clock is so important to us has to do with its relationship with the three fundamental forces described by Ayurveda called the doshas—pitta, kapha, and vata. I describe the doshas at some length in chapter 1, but let me mention them here in brief because our inner clock is influenced by them—they are in constant flux in the cosmos and impose a variability in the physiological processes of all living beings. In that sense, doshas drive our "life engine." The doshas are of three types and can be summarized based on their active (pitta), static (kapha), and variable (vata) nature.

Throughout life, from birth to death, it is the doshas that work nonstop to sustain the very process called "life" and what it takes to remain a living and functioning organism. The doshas bring about growth (pitta), sustenance (kapha), and ultimately dissolution (vata) or death of cells. They represent our ability to anabolize (kapha), catabolize (vata), and metabolize (pitta).

Kapha dosha is static in nature. The substratum of bottom-line solidity that we possess, the "is"ness of the body, or we can say the solid nature of the body, is represented by and maintained by kapha dosha. However, our solid body is not inert; rather, it is marked with chemical, metabolic, and thermal processes. This is the domain of pitta. Finally, the body with its solid and chemical nature is also alive with movement, vibration, motion, and rotation. Movement of both subtle and gross nature, from that of thoughts to that of the bowels, is the domain of vata dosha.

And what do the doshas have to do with our inner and outer clock? Everything!

Due to macrocosmic and microcosmic alignment, fluctuation of doshas in the cosmos impacts our inner clock. At particular times of the day, one of the three doshas will peak in the cosmos and thereby influence our individual state of physiology and psychology. Ayurveda advises a mindful protocol to work with this flux. Let us examine further.

Static energy: The static or dull state of energy known as kapha dosha peaks in the macrocosm typically from 6:00 a.m. to 10:00 a.m. and 6:00 p.m. to 10:00 p.m. Hence, at those times, the body and mind will reflect the corresponding kapha dullness, since macrocosm and microcosm are inherently aligned. Therefore, we may experience sleepiness, heaviness in limbs, and even desire to procrastinate important projects. Lifestyle wisdom dictates that we must consciously undertake activities of an opposite nature during these times, activities that are "active," to counteract physiological and psychological dullness, such as walking, working, or exercising, and not add to the dullness by sleeping, idling, or mindless eating that simply knocks us out.

Active energy: When the active and thermal energy state, known as pitta dosha, peaks—from 10:00 a.m. to 2:00 p.m. and 10:00 p.m. to 2:00 a.m.—it is best to engage in activities that counteract excess heat generation, rather than add to it. So Ayurveda advises choosing shade, mindful resting, deep breathing, gentle play, or even art therapy to calm a sharp mind state. In fact, one must eat a big enough meal to satisfy the increased appetite from cosmic thermal-energy increase. Conversely, subjecting the body to the direct rays of the sun, heavy exercise that generates heat, or a hot sauna may not be the best choice at this time of the day. However, the pitta in macrocosm can be put to good use to finish pending tasks, to write an essay or blog, or to accomplish anything else that requires the mind to be active.

Variable energy: Finally, when the variable energy known as vata dosha takes over in the macrocosm—from 2:00 a.m. to 6:00 a.m. and 2:00 p.m. to 6:00 p.m.—variability in all our physical and mental processes begins to manifest itself. Our energy, mental clarity, and even digestion become variable, and we may feel moody. In such a condition, I recommend you pause, regroup, and mostly wait it out (if possible) or only accomplish routine tasks. Practices that relax the being, such as meditation, yoga, and deep breathing, are also great at this time since they create a counterbalancing effect.

Thus, the same dosha influences us twice in a twenty-four-hour cycle. However, we are asked to respond differently each time. Table 1 summarizes this.

The Ayurveda daily lifestyle flow is based on keeping in mind these three fundamental energy states. Throughout this book, I discuss

TABLE 1 Daily Dosha Cycle

	Daytime	Nighttime
Static (Kapha)	6:00 a.m. to 10:00 a.m. Go against the flow: wake up; be active by choice.	6:00 p.m. to 10:00 p.m. Go with the flow: slow down more and more for better sleep.
Active (Pitta)	10:00 a.m. to 2:00 p.m. Stay active outwardly: work, eat, digest.	10:00 p.m. to 2:00 a.m. Stay active inwardly: do not work or eat; metabolize.
Variable (Vata)	2:00 p.m. to 6:00 p.m. Relax, regroup, take it easy; take a short nap if required to regain energy.	2:00 a.m. to 6:00 a.m. Sleep in first part and begin to wake up anytime 4:30 a.m. onward; a great time for yoga, meditation, and other spiritual practices.

the play of the doshas in each individual, the effect of the doshas on such topics as diet and exercise, and the need for each of us to bring the doshas into balance. The following list is an ideal daily routine according to the Ayurveda clock—in other words, based on the doshas. Each recommendation in this routine is based on the status of the fundamental energies at that time of the day. More information about many of these recommendations can be found in the chapters that follow.

Awakening: Wake up at or before 6:00 a.m. Wake-up time should be ideally an hour and a half before sunrise, as discussed in chapter 2, "Celebrating an Awakened Sky."

Elimination: Ayurveda provides a wealth of wisdom to ensure we take this aspect of our lifestyle seriously and benefit from its daily purification of body and mind, which is discussed

in chapter 3, "The Importance of Elimination." It is important to make this a habit; once it is, we can eliminate wastes and toxins at the right time, with ease, and without undue symptoms of "dis-ease."

Morning refreshing and spiritual practices: Splash your eyes, drink some water, bow to sun, perform the rituals revering the sun, and meditate—described in chapter 2.

Dental hygiene: Follow the three-step Ayurveda dental hygiene practice and the five-step plan for oral health as outlined in chapter 4, "The Art of Naturally Sparkling Smiles."

Self-massage with warm oil: Unless it is contraindicated, this practice is done before showering every day. See chapter 5, "The Delight of Oiling, Bathing, Sense Care, and Beauty Rituals," for detailed instructions.

Shower/bath: This follows oiling, always. For details and to construct your own bathing products, turn to chapter 5.

Five-sense self-care practices: Most of these practices are done after bathing or showering. See chapter 5.

Exercise: Any cardiovascular exercise must be done before eating. See chapter 7, "Sleep, Sex, and Exercise," for additional instructions on exercise.

Yoga and pranayama: Yoga poses and deep breathing can be accomplished either before an oil massage or after bathing and either with cardiovascular exercise or as your main form of exercise. They can also be done independently at any later part of the day as long as your stomach is somewhat empty. Refer to chapter 7 for details on exercise and yoga.

Meditation/worship: This is optional since formal worship rituals are a culturally prescribed practice and are not a universal recommendation. Either way, whether you have an altar or not, a few minutes of connecting with universal divine presence in silence or through chants is recommended. I share morning, bedtime, as well as mealtime *mantras* (sacred sounds, words, or phrases that are repeated during prayer or meditation) in appropriate sections.

Breakfast: The first meal of the day must be eaten before 8:00 a.m. You can, of course, eat it much earlier, as long as you are done with your morning practices. It all depends on what time you get up. The earlier you begin your morning routine, the sooner you will become hungry. For the best bio-regulating benefits, you must try to stick to the same routine—even on weekends! See chapter 6, "Crafting Sacred and Seasonal Meals," and appendix 4, "The Ayurvedic Diet Resource Guide," for recipes as well as seasonal recommendations. Always eat breakfast, or any other meal, according to the season and based on the strength of your digestive fire. The digestive fire is not necessarily dosha-based. If possible, eat all your meals facing north or northeast. You will find these suggestions and more in chapter 6.

Post-breakfast until lunchtime: Plan on doing your most productive and intellectually challenging work in these morning hours. This is pitta time, which helps the mind solve problems and sort issues most expediently.

Lunch: Lunch can be the biggest meal of the day since it is the time when sharp energy, or pitta dosha, peaks. This impacts the digestive fire, which also peaks at this time. Lunch should ideally be consumed between noon and 12:30 p.m. and should never be eaten after 2:00 p.m., which is when vata time begins, and the digestive fire can become a bit erratic and troublesome in digesting a full meal. If for any reason you have to miss lunch, then after 2:00 p.m. you can eat a light, warm snack or drink boiled, spiced milk. Chapter 6 provides the seasonal dos and don'ts and appendix 4 provides the recipes.

One hundred steps: If you can, after lunch sit in thunderbolt pose (*vajrasana*) and then walk one hundred steps. This little bit of physical exertion counteracts energy of dullness or kapha building up in the body. Whatever your doshic constitution may be, do not lie down on your bed or slouch in your chair to take an after-lunch nap. After a little bit of physical exertion, return to your work.

Five-minute pause at 2:00 p.m.: An early afternoon relaxation break, even just a five-minute pause, is important because the variable energy state, vata, is about to begin. This break will help center you in advance. Sipping warm water is good as heat counteracts vata (for energy- or dosha-balancing rules, see chapter 1, "The Science and Spirituality of Ayurveda"). Separately from the hot water (as we never mix the two), you can also enjoy a tablespoon of pure, raw, uncooked honey. This is especially good if you are losing energy. Then you can once again return to your work. After 2:00 p.m., however, try to keep the work you do light, certainly not physically intensive work. Once again, this is the time of vata, and it's not when you want to help a friend move to a new apartment.

Five-minute pause at 4:00 p.m.: If you skip the break at 2:00 p.m., it will be critical to take a snack break at 4:00 p.m. And you could take both breaks if you can fit them both into your work schedule. These five-minute self-care breaks go a long way toward supporting your well-being. This is a great time to enjoy a seasonal fruit by itself, to have a small portion of a vata-balancing cooked snack (either sweet or savory), or to drink a hot beverage. Do not, however, have the beverage with a snack and do not eat dairy or yogurt with the fruit. See chapter 6 for snack suggestions and information about the recommended size and seasonal appropriateness.

Exercise option: From 5:00 p.m. to 5:30 p.m., you can include an evening yoga and pranayama session. This allows you to center yourself for the evening ahead. Yoga also relieves you from fatigue that can build up during a working day. This should be a lighter session overall than the morning session as the energy at this time remains variable. If you have time constraints (you have to get dinner together or help the children with their homework or you have myriad other tasks pulling at you), then at a minimum, plan on a short walk or simply sit in a quiet area and do deep-breathing exercises with your eyes closed. Even five minutes of this will help reenergize you. See chapter 7 for ideas.

Dinner: Have your evening meal before 7:00 p.m. It should be the lightest meal of the day as static energy has begun, so your digestion may not be as sharp as it was in the daytime. This meal should, of course, be both seasonally attuned and easy to digest. See chapter 6 for meal ideas and rules. If you are skipping this meal, then at least sip hot water or, if your digestive fire permits, drink boiled spiced milk slowly and calmly.

Post-dinner until bedtime: If weather permits, after dinner, take a peaceful walk, by yourself or with family or friends. Then engage in pleasant activities you enjoy—read, practice self-care and self-love, pray, meditate, meet with friends and family. This is not a time to do much work on the computer, go through files, handle bills, perform heavy housekeeping, do chores, and so forth. Do only the easy, routine tasks that also allow you to enjoy pleasant company, entertainment, or spiritual study opportunities.

Pre-bedtime practices: To benefit from the static energy that ends at 10:00 p.m., you should prepare for and go to bed by 10:00 p.m. The kapha energy in macrocosm will help induce sleep in microcosm (that's you!) more efficiently. See chapter 7 for rules and recommendations regarding a good night's sleep. If you are active sexually, Ayurveda recommends that it is better to have sex at night before sleeping than in the morning right after awakening. Chapter 7 also contains recommendations on Ayurvedic sex practices.

Bedtime: Try to incorporate the good sleep practices of Ayurveda, given in chapter 7, into your routine. Even if you do not have sleep issues today, these practices will prevent problems from coming up in the future. Certain spiritual contemplations and nighttime mantras are also elucidated in chapter 7.

How to Use This Book

This book is designed to support your understanding and application of the precepts of Ayurveda lifestyle wisdom. I recommend that as you go through chapter 1, "The Science and Spirituality of Ayurveda," you make notes on whatever seems most pertinent to you. Then, in the chapters that follow, feel free to turn to any topic that most interests you, in whatever order suits you best. In this way, you will find all the necessary information you need to construct your own personalized lifestyle using Ayurveda lifestyle wisdom.

Later, you can return to the book at your leisure, and I hope often, to continue your journey of exploration. Ancient Chinese philosopher Lao Tzu has said, "A journey of a thousand miles begins with a single step." So, simply relax and take one step at a time, and even as you take this single step, you will come closer to your goal of vital health and abiding well-being.

Ayurveda lifestyle wisdom is applicable in sickness as well as in health. It protects the health of the healthy, and it restores lost health in the diseased. It does the latter indirectly, by connecting us back to the larger rhythms, the intelligence of Nature. After all, it is the distancing from Nature that is at the root of all disease.

Hence, no matter what stage of life you are in and what grave diagnosis hangs over your head, the good news is that you can begin to live an Ayurveda-inspired lifestyle today. You can check in with your doctor if you wish, as that is always a good idea, but these practices are not "medical," as such, and do not demand a change in your prescriptive regimen at all. Mostly, let common sense guide you as to what lifestyle changes you are ready to implement right away and which ones you wish to explore later, or never. It is never a compulsion.

If you are working with an Ayurveda practitioner already (for overcoming a specific disease), then I am sure he or she will be pleased you are reading this book and implementing its recommendations, which complement disease management (typically the domain of an experienced practitioner, not this book).

Each and every practice laid out in this book is sourced from the ancient and authoritative core texts of Ayurveda (known as Shastra), and hence, you can be confident that you are interfacing with authentic knowledge, made accessible for modern sensibilities. The lessons on lifestyle are not based on "maybes." You can learn from the ground up so that you can begin to use your own discrimination and experience to see that Ayurveda lifestyle wisdom is indeed reflecting a universal truth.

In the end, let me suggest that you practice patience. Ayurveda lifestyle is no quick fix, but if you sincerely follow the advice laid out in this book, within a few weeks you will begin to experience tangible benefits such as a perceptibly reduced stress level, improved sleep, better immunity, increased physical stamina, improved mood, greater mental clarity, enthusiasm, cheerfulness, and enhanced creativity.

You deserve health. When you follow Ayurvedic injunctions on right living, eating, thinking, sex, exercise, sleep, and leisure, you will be living a lifestyle that is resonant with Nature's intelligence. This lifestyle will protect your life and enhance your physical, psychological, social, moral, and spiritual health. You will manifest the health you deserve.

A Well-Lived Day

Sometimes I like to think of the world of Ayurveda as a great mystic forest filled with healing foods, medicinal rivers, and waterfalls that convey blessings. This forest dwells outside the periphery of a notorious urban landscape, which incessantly robs us of our health and well-being. Anyone who enters the forest of Ayurveda and merely sits in the shade of its vast and ancient trees is greeted by the ancient sages who teach the lesson that true health is the birthright of every human being. This lesson tells us that each of us is a self-healing entity who can utilize Nature's abundant tools to restore, renew, and recreate ourselves and that we can do this at any time of our choosing.

As you turn and start walking toward Ayurveda's enchanted forest, the world as you know it today—with its conflicting medical theories, alarming side effects, collapsing short-lived studies with millions still suffering from uncontrolled, ravaging diseases, and drugs that punish with untreatable and irreversible consequences—will be left behind like a bad dream.

There is a winding path through this enchanted forest of Ayurveda. Walking this path requires our inner wakefulness and our acceptance of personal responsibility for navigating our lives. Slumbering, self-deceptive, and passive states of mind are not helpful to those of us who wish to walk the Ayurvedic path.

Habits of self-neglect and self-betrayal may initially seem easy. Like weeds, they crop up and thrive through our inattention. Bound in self-defeating habits and addictions, dependencies, and negativities, many of us live quite artlessly. The lifestyle of Ayurveda is itself an art form, a means wherein we are encouraged to meditate on, to plan, and to weigh carefully our options—and, only then, to choose.

Once we enter the forest, the beauty of the exotic and majestic tree of mindfulness begins to naturally make us more attentive, to help us find and get rid of our own "weeds": habits of laziness, gossiping, oversleeping, slouching, missing meals, overeating, and general chronic mismanagement of time and space. These are the bad habits that undermine our health and create stress in our lives. With a little effort on our part, this tree of mindfulness enchants us into becoming mindful.

Ayurveda lifestyle wisdom, learned with patience and allowed to soak into your soul, acts as a weed destroyer. The knowledge contained in this wisdom has the power to recondition your consciousness and take you beyond your negative habits so that slowly and steadily you transcend the default modes that no longer serve you and gratefully learn new ways of self-care.

For thousands of years, my family has shown humanity a joy-filled path to abiding health of body, mind, and soul. And today, I share my knowledge, most humbly, with you. I invite you to make every day a health-protecting and health-reclaiming day, simply by the art with which it is lived. I remember my teacher Baba telling me that "*a well-lived day is medicine unto itself.*" Indeed, his wisdom teachings gain significance more than ever today, and I am excited for the amazing health and well-being that will manifest through this book.

CHAPTER I

The Science and Spirituality of Ayurveda

 When I was nine years old, my grandfather, Baba, told me, "Little Shunya, the universe is a book of knowledge, and even fishes and birds can read this book. So must you."

That day, I learned all about natural laws that are upheld unconditionally by all living creatures, at all times, and the creatures are in turn guarded and protected by these universal laws. Even the inanimate world collectively participates in a tacit pact of continuance within the field of universal intelligence. These invisible laws are not religious and are, in fact, impersonal yet omnipresent; they keep us healthy and allow us to become our healthiest, if we align with them. Since these laws are made available to us through Mother Nature, they are also called Nature's laws.

These inviolable laws are called *Rta* in the Vedas. Rta—which is pronounced "ruh-tah" but with a slight trill on the *r*—is the root word for *rhythm* in English. Apparently, since we humans have choices, we have the option to neglect these natural laws, or worse, completely forget about them. So we have to relearn them and make a conscious effort to reconnect with them.

"Let us call them 'pure laws,'" Baba said, "because when we follow pure laws, we return to our pure being, which is always healthy and laughing and playful."

"But I am healthy, I laugh, and I am always at play, so why do I need to guard these laws called Rta, or rhythm, Baba?" (I was learning English at school, and that night, I was very proud of our grown-up conversation.)

Baba said that we must relearn because as we grow older, we humans forget who we are and where we come from. The fishes don't forget who they are, so they need not go to fish hospitals to revive their life essence. The lotus growing in the pond behind our home never questions its identity. So it blooms with all its might and fiercely defeats the dark, downward pull and stench of the muddy, cloudy water below. It exclaims, "Look at me!" Even the rocks know how to be rocks. The rivers' inner knowing is the flow, and onward they flow, a course predetermined by Rta.

"But we humans, we get the worst disease of all—the disease of forgetting who we really are. We forget that we are beings who come from Nature and that we must respect Nature. We now need a map to return back to our natural state," Baba explained.

"Fortunately, what is truth can never be wiped out simply by ignoring it. It simply is. When we respect the outer rhythm, the inner rhythm gives us health. Your mind, body, and soul will become aligned, and you will no longer have to look beyond this to discover the ultimate truth of health, life, and happy existence. It is as if infinity will reveal itself to you from within. That beautiful moment is the state of perfect health. And it is not a magical or mystical encounter. It is just you and me remembering our true nature and thereafter living with self-confidence in our own ability and right to heal by intention, sacred thought, and Nature's pure ingredients—sunshine, air, earth, and foods that are soul satisfying and naturally sourced according to the Rta of seasonal intelligence," said Baba.

Baba explained that there has to be constant interaction between inner life and the outer life of Nature. Hence, living a daily life that can uphold Rta is important.

"Does the bird in the nest, the beetle on the rock, and the lofty banyan tree that I love to climb and swing from also follow Rta? Do they, too, read Nature's book called Rta?" I asked.

"Yes, Shunya, my child," said Baba. "The fundamental spiritual truth, the one common reality that underlies all diversity, due to which the sun shines, the wind blows, and our Earth is upheld in its orbit, which is applicable to all creatures at all times, and at the same time dwells in each creature's heart as the innermost health and self-love secret—this Truth, with a capital *T*, itself translates into this universe as the divine cosmic law Rta."

In my child's imagination, a huge book on Rta, perhaps four times bigger than our ancestral home in India, came to my mind. I imagined climbing it (like the monkey my father said I was) and reading each word on cosmic rhythms with glee. It was the most comforting image that I remember in my childhood (while my friends dreamt of dolls, I dreamt of a book that would never end, and amid whose pages I would have countless adventures). With this imagery, somehow I knew that if I ever needed to, I would go to this book and figure out what to do next.

A few months later, when my mother closed her eyes one night, never to open them again, I asked Baba if this was in the book too. He said, yes, all mothers stay in one body only so long. Sooner or later, they have to become part of Mother Nature herself, from where they came to us to begin with, so they can look after us even more. That made tremendous sense.

And I found out that the book, though it touches infinity, is not two stories high after all; I could keep it nicely tucked in my bookshelf. By now, the book had a name—it is the classical Ayurvedic text, Charaka Samhita, composed by enlightened Sage Charaka from the third and second centuries BCE. When I became a mother myself, I kept this one text close to me. I read from it and went through its pages expounding the wisdom of life, from beginning to end, many times, again and again. I knew that from this sacred text, I was receiving the same loving wisdom my physical mother would have offered as nourishment for me if she were with me.

In my pregnancy, as I flipped through the Charaka Samhita, Baba's wise eyes and deep voice leapt from the pages, teaching me loving lessons of wisdom.

When my son, Dhruv, was a toddler, he sketched lines through the book with his crayons. I did not stop him. I knew that through the pages of this book, Mother Nature was blessing him. And she did. My son is a blessing to me. When he is ready to receive, I will give him this same text, with his lines awaiting him.

Now I, Shunya, have become an aging teacher to many young, eager students, just like my Baba was to me. From this very text, I share the wisdom of the cosmic rhythms and the merit of respecting them. I teach all who come seeking relief from the disease of forgetfulness. In each instance, the book of Nature imparts exact knowledge, and this allows me to remain in all interactions worldly yet sublime, spontaneous yet balanced, and vulnerable yet in my power. What I share is Ayurveda's natural blessing for all.

The Concept of Rta

Does a single planet go off its orbit and wander in the galaxy? Does our own Earth not spin on her axis always at the same steady pace? Does Nature not follow her own luxuriously sensual rhythm and dutifully gift us a fragrant and flower-laden spring after every cold and barren winter? Birds and other animals and even plants follow a divine rhythm, knowing when to eat, mate, and play; when to migrate or hibernate; and when to let go of a precious skin they once were attached to but have outgrown.

All beings and creatures in Nature know intuitively when to flower into their being and when to surrender and dissolve. There is a time for the bud to burst forth and then to blossom, to be at the zenith of her sexual self—potent and charged as a magnificent flower—and to invite the dance of birds and bees to herself.

Then, without a qualm, the flower knows when the time comes to drop one petal after another till this magnificent creation once again rejoins the soil. And from this soil grows yet one more bud.

A plant doesn't have to do anything extraordinary to go through these stages. This dance is choreographed by Nature. The plant isn't afraid of so-called death because in this rhythm, death is simply a transition from one form to another. Resurgence is guaranteed by Nature herself.

Deeply rhythmic creatures ourselves, we are reminded daily of this important fact as we watch the rhythm of the setting sun and the rising sun, and in that one instant of sunset or sunrise, we become one with the truth of Nature. And then our busy minds run off to this and that, yet again forgetting our truth, even as every moment in consciousness pulsates with the rhythm of slipping into the next moment in consciousness. *What will that moment be like when I will awaken to my truth of health?* Ask this of yourself.

 I remembered Baba's words to me one night as we watched the night sky decorated with a billion shining stars, "Shunya, may you remain forever steadfast in your orbit, like Earth is on hers, and the planets are on theirs. They follow Rta. You should uphold it too, through your living it in daily life."

I was concerned that night, and perhaps my face showed it. So Baba reassured me that I had to do nothing different or special to keep his word but simply continue living the lifestyle we were living then, even when I was old like him, perhaps even on my last day on Earth.

I could not imagine that far out, but I liked that suggestion, so I said yes. Besides, the life we lived wasn't hard on us. Who would want to give up waking to the delicious aroma of foods cooked fresh with digestive and delicious spices? Why would I stop bathing with hand-crafted herbal hygiene products? And why stop loving my entire body with warm, soothing oils? This and so much more was my inheritance. Yes, I said, of course, yes.

The universally applicable laws of Rta are not a list of rigid rules, nor an elaborate statement of dos and don'ts. Nature reassures us by her regularity and predictability of events and knowledge. Cosmic mathematics, a natural, inviolable framework (such as the delicately balanced ecological chain, which is the interdependence of all living beings, plants, animals, and humans); metamorphosis and transformation through fire and other principles (inner and outer); and the forces of Nature, such as electricity and thunderclouds—all of these are a part of Rta.

Social, moral, and psychological order and harmony in the universe are also ordained through Rta. Why a mother loves her child is a fact from the book of Rta, and why an ant hoards food before rains arrive is yet another truth of Rta. How the human body and mind dance to the strings of sun, moon, and wind—this too is Rta.

Explaining all of this to me, my Baba said, "Shunya, let us resolve to preserve Rta on Earth." And I said, "Yes." ✒

I invite you to experiment with Nature's rhythms and understand how your being is truly a poetry of rhythms. Your breath has its unique rhythm. Any break that occurs in that rhythm due to stress or inhaling pollutants or just not being mindful in your day-to-day life leads to distress and to serious consequences for both body and mind. Nature's truth is simply asking you to follow your natural rhythm. This is why simple deep breathing (pranayama) and becoming aware of your natural, relaxed in-breath and out-breath can bring you into balance and enhance your immunity. After all, it brings you back into your rhythm!

Thus, Ayurveda teaches us to respect the intelligence of the hidden laws of this rhythm, Rta. From the womb of Rta, Ayurveda's health-giving lifestyle is born. Availing ourselves of the wisdom of Ayurveda, human beings can, from the deepest recesses of our own beings, begin to heal ourselves. Baba used to say, *"When the knowledge of Ayurveda is internalized, one does not love or reject life's rhythm but becomes the rhythm itself. One is no longer on two sides of the truth. One becomes the truth."*

There is a master pattern and a perfect form through which universal intelligence operates. Ayurveda lifestyle wisdom works in cooperation with this intelligence, Rta, and employs it at every level in delivering health and well-being.

Respecting Natural Rhythms in Ayurveda

The sages of Ayurveda recognized that Nature is the source of constant change. Nature is the bedrock for the process of change, the keeper of the ingredients of change, and indeed, the very resolution or transformation that is achieved as a result of these changes. If we want to cultivate health, we cannot afford to remain oblivious to the changes in Nature.

The rhythmic lifestyle of Ayurveda follows Nature, and if you decide to live according to this lifestyle, you too will begin to feel supported by Nature—from within yourself. You can discover the deep nurturance that is always available in Nature and gradually become one with the great natural rhythm. Be assured, Ayurvedic principles are Nature's own principles. Ayurveda is a medical science that is always in compliance with the laws of Nature.

Ayurvedic wisdom teaches us to live in harmony with Mother Nature, called *Prakriti* in Sanskrit. While the word *prakriti* popularly denotes mind-body constitution types in Ayurveda, it is also used to denote Mother Nature. Figuratively speaking, Prakriti is the mother of the material universe and is one of the key concepts in Ayurveda. Prakriti is the subtlest matter, stuff from which the manifest gross universe is created. Prakriti, and Prakriti alone, is the primal cause of creation and everything that is seen, heard, felt, and smelled in this world. Therefore, the material world and our material bodies exist because of Prakriti.

Through an encompassing vision of Mother Nature (Prakriti), Ayurveda invites us to meditate and reflect on the interconnectedness of macrocosm (environment) and microcosm (individual being) at every level of existence, from an ant to a human being. Ayurveda aids our recognition of the fact that our universe and its timeless components—time, space, seasons, sun, moon, crops, herbs, and the creatures that populate it—have perpetual rhythmic influences emerging from a common source, Prakriti. These rhythms, which affect us at different times in different ways, play a significant role in both restricting and facilitating our well-being.

This is why, in Ayurveda, we work with natural changes. We understand Nature's ebb and flow, and we try to understand what Mother Nature (Prakriti) is asking of us through her rhythmic changes. We learn to dance to Nature's rhythm, and we take powerful lessons from her book of wisdom and incorporate these into our lives.

Health is certainly not as complicated and contrived an effort as it is made out to be, provided you consciously decide to stay as close as you can to Mother Nature. In other words, Ayurveda asks you to align with the rhythm of your natural bio-existence. It is true that certain factors over which you have no control affect your health—your genetic inheritance, for instance—yet, there are other, equally powerful principles that come into play with the natural laws of Rta. Having knowledge of Nature and how to live close to Nature is more important to your health than popping a pill.

Through the lens of Ayurveda, the role time plays in health is unmistakable. Time, expressed through Nature's rhythms, is the greatest healer. Ayurveda's approach to treatment emphasizes the factor of time (*kaala*). Your role is only to assist Nature by respecting her rhythms and not interrupting them. Indeed, being in rhythm with Nature is the best medicine!

Thus, Ayurveda establishes its foundational healing principles in the intelligence of Nature's rhythms. These rhythms are of three kinds: diurnal, lunar, and solar.

Diurnal Rhythm

Ayurveda invites conscious seekers of health to commune with Mother Nature in peace and mimic her ways. This is why Ayurveda sages teach us an inspired and enlightening daily routine called dinacharya, which teaches humans to follow the rhythm of the sun and rise when it rises, and to eat and be intense at work or play when it is in full form at midday. As the sun slowly travels across the sky and sets voluntarily with the cooperation of Earth swirling in her own magical ballad, we should follow Baba's words of advice: "*Now rest your being and surrender; accept what is and what is yet to be; and with family and love in your heart, make peace with the day. Prepare for slumber.*"

But what did we do? We invented the lightbulb and then the Internet. The "light" may go off in the macrouniverse, but in the microuniverse of the modern human being, the lights are on, and the night is still young. Nature may slumber—who cares!—but we are boldly awake.

For such a person, anxiety, insomnia, unprocessed food and emotions, and a restless state of mind, as well as chronic diseases come to dwell in the body and mind. If only we had rested and in restfulness witnessed the truth of our health. In rest, we would have rejuvenated and revived ourselves to come back out at sunrise for adventure, exploration, and play. But we proclaim our modern lives to be against the divine rhythm, and we pump into our blood more antidepressants, more sleep aids, more health aids—making the pharmaceutical industry rich while we impoverish our own natural potential for self-healing, self-actualization, and self-realization. Alas, we forgot the rhythm that teaches us how to be at peace with what is.

Thus, Ayurveda's lifestyle describes in detail the timing for activities and foods in relation to the rhythm of day and night. This flow is designed to keep the rhythms of day and night in mind and to accept the effect of natural light—and its lack—on living systems. This entire book elaborates dinacharya, daily routines, in detail, chapter after chapter. If you experiment with these simple suggestions, you will quickly notice how your health improves without extra expense, side effects, or dependency on drugs.

Lunar Rhythm

There is a nightly regimen (*ratricharya*) recommended by Ayurveda that connects our being to the moon or the lunar rhythm. As the moon rises in the sky, we are advised to become more introverted and slow down our activities more and more (rather than getting more and more active, as some of us tend to do, especially since the invention of the Internet).

If we were to pause long enough from our preoccupations at nighttime and simply gaze at the moon from a window or balcony, we would discover that moon rays have a special calming and relaxing effect on our minds. In summer, perhaps we could even choose to sleep directly under the moonlight (and starlight).

To support the moon rhythm even further—that is, inviting an inward flow of consciousness and bodily energies—Ayurveda recommends self-massage with warm, soothing oils before bed, the application of calming essential oils, and of course, meditation and prayer, which act as moon-blessed treasures on the way to the heaven of sleep. In sleep, the body goes back in time and heals itself. In sleep, every cell can rest. In sleep, the mind lets go of the troubles and prepares for the next day.

Ayurveda sages suggest we welcome sleep, prepare the chamber of sleep mindfully, and enter into divine slumber when Nature and her creatures are enveloped by the great goddess of sleep (known by her various Sanskrit names as Mahamaya, Mahamoha, and Mahanidra). Here is a resolution for sleep: "Wakefulness, it lies like a dormant seed in my sleep, but tonight, I will sleep."

Thus, nighttime is not dismissed as simply that part of the day in which we must somehow or other sleep. The purpose is not simply to recover enough energy that we can go into "the important time," daytime, when we can fulfill our ambitions! Many people consider sleep to be an unavoidable biological obligation they must fulfill. They develop a dread of nighttime and think of their sleep hours as time wasted. From an Ayurvedic perspective, the night is perhaps the most important part of the twenty-four-hour cycle—the part when we rejuvenate and refresh ourselves by connecting with the moon and embracing the lunar rhythm of mindful restfulness.

Solar Rhythm

The sages explain how the solar rhythm presents itself through the cyclical change of seasons and suggest how we humans can live in synchronization with the solar rhythm by understanding the concept of seasonal lifestyle, or ritucharya.

In summer, when our internal heat matches the external heat, Ayurveda recommends eating cooling, moistening, tempering, and calming foods. In summer, walks in the moonlight, playing with fragrant white flowers, and watching our own tempers are good ideas. Summer demands from us that we eat certain foods that cool us. (These are shared in chapter 6.)

In winter, the cold without and the cold within benefit from hot, spiced, and warming foods—soups and stews—exposure to sun, and lots of sexual and creative activity. Whatever kindles the inner fire is a good idea.

In fall, the wind blows, and the inner universe becomes shaky. It is important at this time to stabilize our routine of eating, sleeping, and eliminating. Becoming steady in our ideas and convictions may help us to deal with this season of change.

Spring, on the other hand, requires letting go—allowing the melting to occur—and, to balance this melting, the foods for spring are pungent, astringent, and bitter. Romance and renewal are one. Allow the blossoming of your true nature, and thrive.

Ayurveda sages had the insight to guide us to a seasonally attuned lifestyle. They understood that just as seasons affect the plants and trees, we are affected by seasonal changes.

The concept of having the same diet or the same level of exercise throughout the year doesn't seem rational in light of this flux of seasonal attributes. Ayurveda recommends specific protocols for spring, summer, rainy season, fall, early winter, and late winter. Chapter 6 provides detailed guidance on food groups, tastes, and activities that, when practiced daily, prevent seasonal infections and protect from diseases such as heatstroke in summer or allergies in spring.

FROM POWERLESSNESS TO POWER: ANANTA RIPA AJMERA'S STORY

What I most appreciate about the Ayurveda system of health and healing is that it brings out the best in each of us. And when our best is established, how does disease stand a chance?

A conscious, health-evoking lifestyle is something that we get to carve out for ourselves, body and mind, meal by meal and thought by thought. Our life's script is in our own hands. There is no need for us to remain paralyzed by the erroneous concepts of powerlessness and helplessness that afflict so many people. One shining example of this is Ripa Ajmera, who lived most of her life with poor health and turned her health around by following Ayurveda lifestyle wisdom. Today, she is not only fully healed but is able to show others how to reclaim their health with Ayurveda. Ripa is an example of those who have taken their life script into their own hands.

In terms of the externals, Ripa Ajmera's life always seemed impressive. She has beauty, a degree from a prestigious college, and lots of friends and potential dates. On top of this, she was born into a lifestyle of expensive vacations, fine jewelry, and all the clothes and shoes she could want. What more could a girl need, right?

Internally, however, Ripa was devastated by an eating disorder that she had struggled with since age twelve, and her sleep was punctuated by violent nightmares that were flashbacks of terrifying experiences in her childhood. When Ripa was in her mid-twenties, her hair was falling out, and her face had constant blemishes. Along with that, she was also afraid to eat. She had trouble digesting food, intermittent but inexplicable stomach pains, and a great deal of pain in her joints. Ripa felt powerless; she felt she was a prisoner of her own body.

Ripa heard a lecture on Ayurveda I gave at Stanford University and immediately resonated with my suggestion that those who wish to serve others need to begin by practicing loving-kindness to themselves. This "loving-kindness" was following Ayurveda's lifestyle practices, which make an individual whole and healthy. Unless we ourselves are whole, as I said in the lecture, there is no way we can impart wholeness to this world.

After the lecture, Ripa talked to me at length about her ideals for social service. But with my own years of experience in healing souls with physical and emotional trauma, I knew intuitively that this young woman's ideal of giving back was actually based on her not having received enough in the first place.

When she asked, I told her, "Yes, you can apply to be my student," but I admonished her that before she could offer the gifts of Ayurveda to others, she would have to learn how to give them to herself. She looked at me unblinkingly, as if accepting my challenge. Ripa joined the awakening health self-care course that my team and I teach for beginners, and she later transferred to a one-year self-healing immersion program. Ripa's health had begun to turn around within the first few weeks.

By the end of six months, Ripa almost forgot she'd ever had stomach or menstrual cramps, and she had lost her dependency of several years on ibuprofen. Her skin cleared up, and she radiated good health. And today, five-and-a-half years after she first began her practice of Ayurvedic principles, Ripa can't even remember the last time she visited a doctor.

Because I feel a person's first steps with Ayurveda are so important—it's when you have the opportunity to see and feel most clearly the transformative effects of this practice—I'm going to share some specifics about what Ripa did in the beginning to bring these principles into her life. Understand that she had been *trying* to take care of herself. For breakfast, for instance, she wasn't eating Pop-Tarts; she ate a bowl of commercial cereal with cold milk and, on many mornings, sliced fruit. She thought of it as a healthy breakfast, but this is not Ayurveda's view.

Milk is never easy to digest, but when it's served cold, it is extremely difficult for the body to deal with. Combine cold milk with raw fruit, and you're asking your digestive system to

process a poison. I discuss why certain foods are incompatible in chapter 6; here, it's enough to say that Ripa was demanding enormous energy from her body every morning just to digest what she thought of as a healthy start to the day.

So, as a first step, Ripa changed what she ate for breakfast. She began drinking cooked, spiced milk and hot cereal. Within a few weeks of studying Ayurveda, she realized that she often ate incompatible foods, food combinations that generate toxins and disturb the digestive process. Almost as soon as Ripa stopped consuming these antagonistic foods, her stomach pain disappeared.

Another of Ripa's problems, acne, was also connected to her impaired digestive process, which created toxins that disturbed her skin. She had always obsessed about the pores of her skin and battled the topical bacteria—the mainstream view of treating acne—but to no avail. Following the rules of Ayurveda, Ripa improved her digestion by eating compatible foods, eating according to the seasons (see chapter 6), and living in a way that ensured prompt elimination (see chapter 3), and—presto!—her skin cleared up. Now, her blemish-free skin glows. She gets compliments on it all the time.

Ripa's body also responded immediately to daily rituals of relaxing warm oil massage (see chapter 5) and a more judicious implementation of exercise. She had been attending yoga classes in which the teachers played loud music and presented a multitude of postures per class, having students perform all sorts of acrobatic feats. "Right after class, I would feel amazing," Ripa said, "but after a while, I noticed that I never had any energy. I had to stop all exercise for about a year and a half to recover my strength. Then, it was so freeing to relearn yoga from Acharya Shunya—to learn that practicing only one *asana* (yoga posture), with full focus, devotion, and intention, could give me the experience of spiritual oneness and inner power I had been seeking all along." As a result of the gentle massage and gentle exercise, all of Ripa's aches and pain subsided before the end of her first year of Ayurveda practice. As she indicated, Ripa fell in love with the slow and spiritualized yoga teachings I provided. These perspectives on yoga are included in chapter 7.

The root cause for many of Ripa's ills was, of course, in her mind, and it took a little longer to address. I can't document exactly when her mind made a complete U-turn, but it did, and it started at the very beginning. In her very first class with me, Ripa told me later, she experienced a surge of unexpected hope, an intuitive feeling that she was finally safe. This was true; she was safe. She had found a knowledge that is timeless. Ayurveda's optimistic, life-sustaining wisdom would never allow Ripa's mind to remain lost in self-defeating patterns. The early morning practices and the spiritual mantras and contemplations she learned and practiced daily connected Ripa's mind with something beyond itself—beyond time, space, and all such limitations.

My students have the privilege of taking on a new name, inspired by the fire of Vedic wisdom, and Ripa asked me for one in 2014, feeling that she had truly become transformed. I named her Ananta, which means "the limitless one." Her formal name is now Ananta Ripa Ajmera.

Ananta Ripa no longer feels alone or at the mercy of a cruel world. Patterns of anorexia and anxiety have fallen away to make room for ideas and ways that are illuminated by the wisdom of Ayurveda. Now, she receives wisdom and guidance from her own healthy mind, which is connected to her spiritual Self.

A gurukulam—a traditional, guru-led school and learning community—was the dominant model of education for several thousand years in India, but in recent history, it has somewhat fallen out of use. The gurukulam education—whose revival in the twenty-first century I have pioneered with the establishment of my own gurukulam in California—is different from all other classroom education in Ayurveda. For starters, the highest and purest intellectual knowledge from source texts is made experientially accessible in ways that directly impact the physical, emotional, psychological, and social well-being of the student. The student is not asked to memorize but to internalize the wisdom and live the practices. The student is not asked to take written tests and regurgitate rote learning, but is encouraged instead to demonstrate the truth of wisdom via the blessings of a spiritualized education process—namely, restored physical health and immunity; improved self-esteem, self-control, and ethically evolved, socially responsible beliefs and ideas; and finally, a recognizable radiant soul connection.

An ancient Atharva Veda verse puts it this way: "Make room for your own elevation. Release your imprisoned Self from the fetters of body and mind. Freed, traverse the new pathways of your own choice and making."[1]

Naturally, I take personal interest in the lives of my sincere students, and after they touch their own infinite potential, I groom them to become humanitarian wellness leaders.

Ripa's talk of serving the world has now become her reality. In making her leap from needing help with her life process to becoming whole and then to giving help to others, Ripa has thanked Ayurveda every step of the way. Under my guidance, Ripa completed a successful pilot program at the Alameda County Probation Department. This led to her becoming certified to train prison staff and police officers across the state of California in Ayurveda lifestyle practices and yoga. She also serves as an associate faculty member at my school and leads the school's yoga classes. She teaches Ayurveda at Stanford University School of Medicine's Health Improvement Program with another student. Ripa is also creating pilot programs to empower corporate and healthcare employees and exploring opportunities with state-level public health departments to spread knowledge of the living practice of Ayurveda.

The anxious, depressed, and painfully thin young woman has flowered into a graceful, well-nourished, powerful leader, living the life of spirituality and service she always dreamt of, from a place of authenticity.

Isn't this beautiful? This young woman's story illustrates my contention that the central message of Ayurveda is always positive. Optimistic, truth-seeking, exuberant, and life-celebrating Ayurveda lifestyle wisdom revitalizes and reconnects us with our own spirit source. Thanks to the sages' brilliant insights that ensure we heal the body and emotions in one sweep, health does not remain a farcical product of technology with deadly side effects in Ayurveda, but becomes a real, achievable, and realistic option, courtesy of the activation of our inner self-healing power via alignment with Nature.

After adopting even a few aspects of the Ayurveda way of life, individuals like Ananta Ripa Ajmera begin to feel hopeful, even excited. They begin to feel in control; they see that what they eat and how they live can heal their bodies in a way the prescription drugs never could. That is why, over these years, I have counseled the sickest of the sick to put aside their disease

consciousness when they come to study or heal with me, and to simply immerse themselves in implementing Ayurveda's lifestyle wisdom, one practice at a time. That is usually enough to turn the tide of "dis-ease" toward health. Tiny changes in lifestyle and foods begin to yield positive and unexpected health results. Indeed, Ayurveda imparted to Ananta what endless doctors and therapists had failed to impart.

Unity of Macrocosm and Microcosm through Rta

A fundamental tenet of the Ayurvedic system of medicine is the principle that the macrocosm (the universe) and microcosm (the individual being) are similar. We human beings are made of the same "stuff" and regulated by the same rhythms as the rest of the universe. The sun, moon, and wind that influence our outer universe also influence our individual bodies through the corresponding principles called the doshas. Within the sphere of the body, the sun is represented by pitta dosha, the moon by kapha dosha, and the wind by vata dosha.

Just like disturbances in Nature such as storms, cyclones, hurricanes, tidal waves, floods, and droughts dictate the quality of life on our planet, diseases come to our bodies when there are disturbances in the three doshas because doshas represent the personal Rta, or the regulating intelligence in our bodies.

Thus, it is of paramount importance for us to keep the doshas in balance. Balancing the doshas is akin to keeping our environment in balance. While we cannot do much to influence the effect of sun and wind on the planet, we can, in fact, do a great deal to balance these influences within ourselves by balancing their counterparts in our bodies—vata (wind), pitta (sun), and kapha (moon). The best part is that you don't even need to identify your dominant dosha. By following the universally applicable lifestyle that is explained in this book, your doshas will come into balance and will stay balanced, inevitably.

This entire book is, in essence, teaching the wisdom of living so artfully that whether you remember my descriptions of the doshas, or not, will not matter. Simply by living your day according to the practices prescribed and by eating the foods prepared with recipes provided, your doshas will become balanced. It will happen without your giving it any thought at all.

I have found, however, that some students have an academic curiosity, and for them I describe the doshas and their cycles in the following sections. If this interests you, I suggest that you pay special attention to the signs and symptoms of dosha imbalance so that you can watch out for these in your own system. You may also be interested to learn about Ayurveda's understanding of why these imbalances occur and how these disturbances can be prevented or corrected through simple lifestyle measures. You can also skip this section for now and refer back to it later.

The Three Doshas

The five great elements—or states of matter, as they are known in the Indian philosophical traditions—are space, air, fire, water, and earth. These are the building blocks for all of life and for inert objects as well. Everything in the universe is created from these five elements in a particular ratio. Just as matter and energy are interconnected on the continuum of existence, these five great elements (*mahabhutas*) can be

thought of as both energy and as subtle forms of matter (as opposed to their gross forms that we are most familiar with, such as the actual substance of water).

According to cosmic law, the five elements combine within a living body, and from them arise the primary life forces that perform various functions in the body for its upkeep and health. Ayurveda names these life forces the doshas, and they assist in the operations of Rta. When the doshas are in balance, Rta is upheld, and we enjoy health. When the doshas are imbalanced, Rta breaks down, and we experience ill health.

As already mentioned, the three doshas are vata, pitta, and kapha. One of the classic ways to understand the doshas is to view them as expressions of the basic elements in physical creation. Following is the nature of each of the doshas:

- Air and space elements combine to form the force of vata.

- Fire and water elements combine to form the force of pitta.

- Water and earth elements combine to form the force of kapha.

The Doshas in Health and Disease

The doshas are invisible, subtle matter states, like energy. These three energies, acting together, regulate and orchestrate the entire physiology of the living body. The doshas regulate and sustain all of our biological functions and impact our psychology as well. In a general sense, vata represents motion, pitta represents transformation, and kapha represents arrest.

TABLE 2 Doshas' Physical Qualities

Vata	Pitta	Kapha
Dry	Fluid	Heavy
Light	Light	Cold
Cold	Hot	Soft (yielding)
Rough	Slightly oily	Stable, sturdy, firm
Clear	Penetrating	Slimy or sticky
Subtle	Sharp	Smooth
Mobile	Yellowish	Dense, formed, or compact
Invisible	Foul smelling	Slow, inactive, or dull
Formless	Sour and pungent	Whitish

The identification of these three doshas demonstrates the genius of the ancient Vedic seers of India. With their divinely tuned vision, these enlightened beings saw the interconnected nature of this universe and identified the role of the synchronous forces they called the doshas. The understanding of these sages was simple and profound. The outer becomes the inner. The inner dances to the tune of the outer.

To better understand how the three doshas operate within us, consider the summary of their physical attributes in table 2, and then read further for the explanation of their functions.

Vata: When vata functions normally, we experience enthusiasm. Vata regulates inspiration, expiration, and all movement, including our thoughts, the processing of physical tissue, and the elimination of excrement.

Pitta: When pitta functions normally, we are cheerful. Pitta regulates vision, digestion, heat, hunger, thirst, and softness in the body, governing both physical luster and intellect.

Kapha: When kapha functions normally, we are content. Kapha regulates physical structure, strength, forbearance, and restraint through its tendencies to be smooth, firm, and binding.

Stabilizing the Unstable

The doshas respond easily to changes in our biorhythms, food, and lifestyle. When the doshas respond by becoming imbalanced, we notice the onset of uncomfortable symptoms and, over time, disease.

This is the reason Ayurveda suggests studying the nature of doshas and understanding what triggers their imbalance. In this way, we can develop a natural lifestyle that keeps the doshas from becoming imbalanced. And if, due to the errors of our ways—either because we have forgotten or because we knew no better—an imbalance has already occurred, then an Ayurveda-inspired lifestyle can reverse dosha imbalance by counteracting the precipitating causes. When doshas are imbalanced, they undergo several changes.

STAGE ONE
Increase or Accumulation (*Sanchaya*)

The first-level change indicates a general, nonspecific "increase" of doshas and consequent accumulation in specific sites within the body. This buildup is not only due to food and lifestyle choices we make, but also to natural causes outside our control, such as time of the day, seasonal changes, and so forth. Excess vata accumulates inside the large intestine, pitta accumulates in the lower stomach and small intestine, and kapha accumulates inside the chest and upper stomach.

STAGE TWO
Excitation or Aggravation (*Prakopa*)

If the accumulating doshas are not counteracted by food and lifestyle, they keep accumulating and build up to such a critical level that they begin creating adverse symptoms. This stage is called the stage of "excited" or "aggravated" doshas. Once again, doshas get aggravated not only due to excess consumption of dosha-aggravating foods or lifestyle, but this can also happen due to fluctuating natural rhythms, such as change of season and so forth.

STAGE THREE
Pacification or Alleviation (*Prashama*)

The previously built-up dosha becomes "spontaneously pacified" due to changes occurring in the macrocosm (seasons, time of day, and so on), or it can be "artificially pacified" when we employ the science of Ayurveda, mindfully eating a specific dosha-balancing diet for a preplanned duration or by following specific dosha-balancing lifestyle practices. This arrests and even restores the healthy (nonsymptomatic) level of the doshas.

STAGE FOUR
Spread or Dispersion (*Prasara*)

A fourth level includes spread or dispersion of the doshas from their native site to other sites or organs in the body, causing yet more symptomatic complexity and creating conditions ripe for future disease. Fortunately, by implementing Ayurveda lifestyle wisdom, there are things we can do during the first three stages to entirely prevent stage four from occurring. This is also how three more, increasingly pathological, stages of dosha variation are prevented (these advanced stages are not described here because they are beyond the scope of this book), and disease is thereby entirely prevented.

What Can You Do?

The best thing you can do to maintain your health is to become aware of the dosha changes and gain appropriate knowledge to offset accumulating doshas. This book will provide the required information in detail.

In the first stage of buildup or accumulation of doshas, since the body is an intelligent

TABLE 3   The Increase and Decrease Principle

	Choice 1	Choice 2
Action You are cold.	You drink chilled water.	You drink hot water.
Effect You are shivering.	**Like increases like** Shivering increases. (Try it!)	**Unlike will decrease** Shivering decreases. (Try it!)

self-healing entity, desire arises to consume food and drinks of a nature opposite to that of the accumulating dosha (to offset the buildup).

This is Rta, or Nature's intelligence, inside our bodies and minds in action: Mother Nature's way of nipping in the bud many potential diseases. Many of us, however, fail to recognize these natural cravings as messages from the self-correcting doshas and continue instead to live and eat by our habits. So here is what we can watch out for:

- When vata increases or accumulates, a dislike for rough, dry, and cold foods and drinks will arise, and there will be a corresponding craving for warm, cooked, soft, moist, and oily foods.

- When pitta dosha increases or accumulates, we develop an aversion to fried and spicy foods and to prolonged sunlight and instead crave cooling foods, cold drinks, and a shady environment.

- When kapha begins to increase or accumulate, we dislike dairy and fatty, oily, and rich foods and crave light fare that is

easy to digest, along with hot drinks and stimulating spices.

If doshas are not overcome in the first stage, by following the cravings, the second stage of dosha aggravation (with yet more symptoms) may manifest. But once again, few of us recognize these symptoms as dosha aggravation. Once these symptoms have begun, Ayurveda recommends beginning immediately to make the changes that will restore balance to the doshas. Here are some guidelines so you can begin to recognize the dosha symptoms:

- Vata aggravation may cause gas, distention of the abdomen, and a feeling of fullness inside the gastrointestinal tract. A desire to seek warmth through food or drinks may also be present.

- In the case of pitta, the yellowness of urine and stool may slightly increase along with an increase in body heat, with even some minor anger and irritability.

- When kapha is aggravated, the stomach and chest may feel heavy or moist, as if filled

TABLE 4   The Vata Cycle

Accumulation	Dryness (be it cold or hot) excites vata dosha's qualities of dryness, roughness, lightness, mobility, and all other windlike attributes. Hence, a dry atmospheric heat and the dryness of raw foods, dried fruits, certain lentils, beans, and even certain drier oils (olive, mustard) can cause the accumulation of vata.
Aggravation	Coldness provokes all vata qualities and the conditions associated with vata: pain, constipation, sleeplessness, and so forth. So whenever our bodies become cold, arthritis or other odd aches and pains may begin to act up, our stools may become harder, our breathing may become labored, and our minds may become restless.
Pacification	Heat counteracts cold, and oiliness counteracts dryness. Thus, application of heat and oiliness as in the use of a warm sesame oil massage pacifies an aggravated vata dosha.

TABLE 5   The Pitta Cycle

Accumulation	Qualities such as sharpness, lightness, and oiliness cause pitta to accumulate over time. Alcohol is sharp and light; sesame is sharp and oily; and sautéed, spicy foods are sometimes sharp, light, and oily.
Aggravation	Heat aggravates an already accumulated pitta. Heat sets off pitta and makes it flare up like fire. So the heat of the sun; the heat of fiery foods like garlic, peppers, alcohol, and fermented foods; the heat of sex; the heat of exercise; and mental heat such as anger and jealousy can spark pitta.
Pacification	Cold pacifies heat; dullness or slowness offsets sharpness; and heaviness offsets lightness. So dairy, which is cooling, heavy, and slow to digest is recommended in pitta disorders. The coolness of moon rays, of flowers, of expressing qualities like compassion, and of cool colors like blue and green can pacify an aggravated pitta dosha.

TABLE 6   The Kapha Cycle

Accumulation	Qualities of moistness, heaviness, and dullness increase kapha, as like increases like, and these are also the qualities of kapha dosha. Hence, eating cheesecake would increase kapha and so would a cold, rainy day.
Aggravation	Both excessive cold and hot can aggravate kapha. Think of water and the way extreme heat can make it a vapor and cold can cause it to harden into ice. Either extreme changes the form of water. This is why in the spring sun kapha melts and comes out as liquid phlegm (allergies), and in the cold of winter kapha again gets stirred up as a congested mass.
Pacification	Generally speaking, dryness counteracts kapha's intrinsic moistness; lightness counteracts kapha's heaviness; and a dry heat counteracts kapha's damp cold. The sharpness of ginger counteracts kapha's dullness, and mobility through exercise counteracts kapha's slow-moving tendency. Exercising (mobility), eating a small quantity of easily digested food (light) with spices (hot and sharp), and then long periods of fasting between meals is recommended to balance kapha.

with fluid, and some overall heaviness and lassitude may be present.

Fortunately, simply returning to the roots of living according to Nature through an Ayurveda lifestyle will correct dosha imbalance. Is this not wonderful? We simply have to live according to Ayurvedic principals, and balance is restored and disease averted.

Since the doshas respond to specific foods, thoughts, and lifestyle choices, it is possible to eat different foods, think different thoughts, and make different lifestyle choices in order to pacify the doshas and thereby regain balance. A fundamental Ayurvedic principle is at work here: like increases like; opposites decrease each other

(samanya vishesha siddhanta).[2] According to this doctrine, combining the similar brings about an increase in a given dosha, whereas combining the dissimilar brings about a decrease in a dosha.

Applying this principle, it is clear that those foods and activities that are similar to a dosha in quality or function will increase the dosha, whereas dissimilar foods and activities will decrease the dosha. Let's look at this in table 3.

At this level, of course, it's common sense. The doshas, however, are more complex than the simple example in table 3. This principle has been put to great use in Ayurveda, and you will come across many practical applications throughout this book. The principle is further elucidated in tables 4–6.

TABLE 7   Natural Factors Associated with Dosha Aggravation

FACTOR	VATA	PITTA	KAPHA
Age	Peaks at end of middle age or start of old age	Peaks after puberty to end of middle age	Peaks between birth to puberty
Time	2:00 a.m. to 6:00 a.m. 2:00 p.m. to 6:00 p.m.	10:00 a.m. to 2:00 p.m. 10:00 p.m. to 2:00 a.m.	6:00 a.m. to 10:00 a.m. 6:00 p.m. to 10:00 p.m.
Seasons	Accumulates in summer Aggravates in rains/ late summer Pacifies in autumn	Accumulates in rains/ late summer Aggravates in autumn Pacifies in early winter	Accumulates in late winter Aggravates in spring Pacifies in summer
Digestion	Accumulates at middle of digestion Aggravates at end of digestion Pacifies at beginning of digestion	Accumulates at beginning of digestion Aggravates at middle of digestion Pacifies at end of digestion	Accumulates at end of digestion Aggravates at beginning of digestion Pacifies at middle of digestion

The following lists describe the symptoms you may experience if any one, two, or all three doshas are in a state of aggravation. Again, aggravation may be chronic or simply what you are experiencing due to seasonal and other transient factors. Feel free to note anything in the lists that applies to you right now. You can always come back to these lists in the future to explore what is going on with your doshas. It will be eye-opening.

Symptoms of Aggravated Vata Dosha

- Unexplained emaciation or thinness
- Astringent or bitter taste in mouth
- Dry, rough skin
- Insomnia or sleep disturbances
- Weakness or unexplained fatigue
- Tremors, cramps, and muscle spasms
- Constipation and flatulence
- Mood swings
- Increased pains and aches
- Increased experience of cold
- Increased desire for hot climate
- Increased desire for hot foods and drinks

TABLE 8   Lifestyle Factors Associated with Vata Dosha Aggravation

Factors That Aggravate Vata Dosha	Description
Tastes	Excessive eating of foods dominant in bitter, pungent, and astringent tastes
Cold foods	Drinking cold or chilled water, eating cold or frozen foods and drinks
Dry foods	Eating dried pulses, dry chips, and raw salads
Avoiding fat	Eating a zero-fat or low-fat diet, avoiding dairy (vegan diet)
Mealtime	Fasting, skipping meals, irregular eating schedule, wasting diseases (such as anorexia), excessive dieting
Natural urges	Suppression or premature prompting of natural urges such as the urge to sneeze, urinate, pass stool, and so forth
Activity level	Improper running, jumping from high places, carrying heavy loads, overworking till exhaustion
Physical trauma	Fractures, joint dislocations, and other physical traumas, impacts, and injuries to the body
Commuting	Driving long hours without stopping, excessive riding, walking long distances (hiking), or making long journeys on rough roads more than occasionally
Sex	Indulging in sexual intercourse repeatedly and not taking long enough breaks or stopping to recover
Sleep	Staying awake during the night (especially after 10:00 p.m.)
Senses	Nonstop TV watching, playing video games, talking on the phone, staring at computer screen, or typing
Emotions	Indulging in chronic fear, grief, anxiety, work-related tension, and heightened day-to-day stress

TABLE 9   Lifestyle Factors Associated with Pitta Dosha Aggravation

Factors That Aggravate Pitta Dosha	Description
Tastes	Excessive eating of foods that are predominantly pungent, sour, and salty
Sharpness	Eating foods that cause burning in the stomach during digestion (such as vinegar and sharp fermented foods)
Hotness	Eating foods that are fire-dominant in their own elemental natures, including yogurt, fish, mustard, alcohol, sesame, sour fruits, buttermilk, peppers, and horseradish
Temperature	Consuming food that is so hot to the touch that it might burn the tongue
Mealtime	Fasting or skipping meals or neglecting to satiate your hunger or thirst
External heat	Prolonged exposure to sunlight or other heat-increasing agents such as hot showers, sauna, heated pools, and hot tubs
Sex	Excessively indulging in sexual intercourse or having sex while suffering from indigestion
Emotions	Indulging in intense emotional states of anger, sorrow, or fear

Symptoms of Aggravated Pitta Dosha

- Feeling hot even if weather is not hot
- Yellow discoloration of skin, eyes, or urine
- Difficulty sleeping
- Burning sensation on the skin
- Increasing anger and irritability
- Increased sweat
- Increased boils, acne, rashes, or other skin eruptions
- Pungent and sour taste on tongue
- Increased desire for cold food and drinks

Symptoms of Aggravated Kapha Dosha

- Feeling cold even if weather is not cold
- Increased drowsiness
- Increased saliva and phlegm secretion
- Joints that feel heavy
- Overall increase in heaviness
- Experience of dullness in body and mind
- Increased flabbiness and loose joints
- Increased hardness of tissues
- Cough, cold, or lung congestion with phlegm and labored breathing
- Weak digestive power
- Sweet and salty taste in mouth

TABLE 10   Lifestyle Factors Associated with Kapha Dosha Aggravation

Factors That Aggravate Kapha Dosha	Description
Tastes	Excessively eating foods that are predominantly sweet, sour, and salty
Coldness	Eating foods that are cold in temperature (cold meats, ice cream, chilled drinks)
Liquidity	Consuming foods that are more liquid than solid (soups and stews) or excess drinking of water and other fluids throughout the day
Heaviness	Excessively eating heavy foods, such as black gram lentils, dairy, sweets, fish, and shellfish
Hardness	Regularly eating foods that are hard to digest, such as poultry and meats
Oiliness	Eating foods that are very fatty, such as fried foods
Sliminess	Consuming foods that have a slimy quality, such as okra
Sourness	Excessively eating foods that are fermented (vinegar or yogurt)
Mealtime	Overeating, eating frequently, or snacking between meals
Activity	Remaining sedentary; getting little exercise
Sleep	Getting too much sleep or sleeping at all during the daytime
Attitude	Insufficient or inadequate mental activity; being lazy
Metabolism	Chronic or occasional nonefficient or dull state of metabolism

Natural Causes of Dosha Aggravation

There is a natural fluctuation of doshas due to the time of the day, the season, the stage of digestion, and also a person's age. This fluctuation follows a set pattern throughout the day and from birth to death. It is natural in the cosmos for the doshas to build up, peak, and then subside. We cannot intervene in this natural rhythmic rise and fall, but we can understand and work with it. Table 7 provides a brief overview of the dosha fluctuation patterns based on your age, time of the day, current season, and stage of digestion. A review of this table will help you better understand why you are experiencing a particular symptom or cluster of symptoms.

Lifestyle-Related Dosha-Increasing Causes

Now we come to dosha-increasing factors that are within our control. Note those items you indulge to excess—and note as well that you probably are aggravating all three doshas. (Most people do.) You do not want to focus on just one dosha here—the goal is to keep all three in balance. And just in case you are wondering, in Ayurveda, we never work on increasing a depressed dosha. We simply work on pacifying aggravated dosha. This takes care of the triangulated balance with the other two doshas. Tables 8–10 highlight the specific factors that lie at the root of dosha aggravation. By studying these tables, you can gain insight into your lifestyle choices that may be contributing toward a specific dosha aggravation. For example, you may understand from the table that it is your penchant for chilled water and foods year-round that is causing you excess gas and bloating (vata symptoms). These lists can be quite educational in terms of the effect of our choices. Browse now or come back to these lists at your leisure.

Restoration of Doshas with Lifestyle

This entire book teaches you how to live so that your doshas do not become imbalanced or, if they have, so that they return to balance. So even if you see several causes of dosha aggravation in tables 8, 9, or 10, by adopting the practices described in this book, you will regain balance within a few months. The following lists provide some of the simple practices you can begin to embrace to achieve total balance and abiding health.

Vata-Balancing Choices

- Eat more sweet, sour, and salty foods.

- Add adequate fat in your diet—cook in fat or add oil on top.

- Eat the heavier, more substantial foods that ground vata dosha.

- Eat foods when they are still hot or warm, and drink only warm water.

- Indulge in warming comforts, such as hot tubs and hot showers.

- Practice daily self-massage with warmed oils.

Pitta-Balancing Choices

- Add more astringent, bitter, and sweet tastes to your meals.

- Ensure foods don't burn your tongue or belly on eating (nonheating potency).

- Choose foods that take more time to digest (such as whole grains).

- Add ghee, or clarified butter, to cooking.

- Look for cooling comforts like walking under the cooling moonlight, cooling sherbets, and cooling scents.

- Moderate sexual activity and exercise regimen to prevent overheating.

Kapha-Balancing Choices

- Eat more bitter, pungent, and astringent tastes in your diet.

- Choose drier rather than moist foods (raisins versus grapes, for example).

- Plan regular detox and fasting protocols.

- Drink hot water and eschew chilled water at any cost.

- Exercise. (The more you exercise, the better you will feel!)

- Reduce your sleeping and sedentary time.

As you can see, Ayurveda has you covered. Ayurveda conceives of health at a grand scale—health in which even the sun, moon, and wind are entreated to stay on their respective courses. (If they didn't, then cosmic chaos of unimaginable magnitude would follow!) Likewise, the inner doshas—vata, pitta, and kapha—have their respective rhythms, and these are upheld by a conscious lifestyle.

The Spirituality of Ayurveda Lifestyle Wisdom

The science behind Ayurveda, as discussed above, forms the key concepts and principles of this ancient system of health and healing, but one of the important things that makes Ayurveda unique is its spirituality aspect. Ayurveda contends that every human being is, at heart, a nonphysical Self that is having a physical experience through the outer material wrappings of body and mind. Any and all healing is the expression of our own source, this Self called the Atman. The ultimate spiritual reality is described in Sanskrit as satyam, truth. *Truth* is a confusing word because what I see as truth may not be what you see as truth, and we may both have a different idea of truth than another person has. Throughout history, religious wars have been fought over various versions of the so-called truth.

The ancient Vedic texts, however, clarify that we're not talking about ordinary truth here. We are talking about the impersonal and fundamental truth of consciousness, truth that is the Ultimate Reality. This truth is that which transcends realities of a relative order (including the gods of humans) and yet is, at the same time, imminent and ever-present in the phenomenal universe.

A single seed contains in its womb the potential for an entire forest. Yet, when a single seed is split open, all it contains inside itself is emptiness known as *shunya*. This emptiness is consciousness, the unseen reality that cannot be heard, seen, smelled, touched, or tasted—it cannot be measured by any scientific instrument, nor restricted to any religious point of view. Yet, at the same time, it holds the potential of a tangible universe. An entire forest can grow from this one potent emptiness within the seed. Truth is pure consciousness. It is, according to the ancient Veda, formless and absolute existence, consciousness, and joy.

It is this reality, this truth, that sustains each one of us as the indwelling Self. Since the body and mind that encase this Self are iterations of food, both subtle and gross, these encasements undergo endless change. The Self, however, which is what we are inherently, has an independent existence and is of a higher order of reality than the body and the mind. You, the Self, are not limited to the overwhelmed mind and the decaying body that you may identify yourself to be. And this is why health is never really far away.

When, due to spiritualized lifestyle practices, we begin to think *wellness*, we also begin to experience wellness. When we think *expansion*, we create expansion. When we think *joy*, we become joy. Baba told me, "*Free from evil, old age and death, grief, hunger, and thirst, your soul's desire is for experiencing its own glorious truth, so understand the intention of your Pure Being—forever seek it, your Self. One who finds and understands that Self attains every world, every desire.*"

And this is where what I teach in reference to Ayurveda lifestyle may differ from most other teachers of Ayurveda in this modern world. I am telling you that, yes, do learn through the pages of this book how to take care of your body. I will teach you all about health. But our work together is not based on the premise that you need this book right now because there is an inherent gap between you and your healthy Self.

I am saying that your true nature, your Self, is already flawlessly healthy. So you are invited to quit thinking thoughts such as *I want health.* Think instead, *I am health. And this Ayurveda lifestyle will simply aid me (the mind-body–based me) to live in closer proximity to this inner perfection, my true Self.* Hence, you will be celebrating your own healthy Self, through the inexplicably growing health of body and mind in daily life.

To me, good health means saying hello to your own inner, perfect nature. And knowing this perfect nature of yours, you can take rest in it. You can at the same time implement whatever

changes you may feel will help your body and mind, but you can do this with a sense of joy and an expectation of positive outcome—not from a place of worry, obsession, or lack. So you shift your perspective from a place of suffering to a place of inherent freedom. And you then operate from that inner space of freedom.

But until you have that perspective shift, in my experience, you're really operating under stress and pain generated from ignorance of Self. It may be very low-level chronic stress, but we are so accustomed to chasing everything that we even begin chasing health!

The stress from the pain of separation from your true nature, your higher Self, is a private, painful sorrow. And in my opinion, that is the essence of spiritual suffering. People can say to us, "You're not good enough." This happens all the time, sure, but when we begin saying to ourselves, "I am not good enough; I do not deserve health," or "I suffer from disease because that is what I deserve," then this is the sign that spiritual disease has set in. We have abandoned ourselves and forgotten that our true Self is always healthy, worthy, and pure love. Shame represents, after all, the original disease, the spiritual disease of Self-betrayal and forgetfulness of our true Self. Shame is a seriously painful experience; it saps away our joy and well-being.

Hence, I wish to address this spiritual forgetfulness, too, of your true nature, even as you go about learning practical, tangible, hands-on ways to increase health.

What I want you to remember is this: You are that eternal source of health. Your true nature is boundless, inexhaustible health. You may have made choices that were not always the best, and these choices may have brought you to a place of imbalance or even disease. But you are not a mistake. You are perfect.

You can say this, right now: "My true nature offers me limitless opportunities for self-renewal. Simply by living consciously through the art of an inspired lifestyle, I will experience my inherent perfection."

This is why the Ayurveda sages teach us to first discover and then honor our *svadharma*. The concept of dharma, or righteous living, is inherent to the Indian philosophies, and svadharma is that lifestyle that supports the immortal Self. This Self is not the body that comes with a limited warranty, nor is it the mind that constantly changes with new information and is often affected by mood swings. The immortal Atman that lies beyond body and mind is a reflection of the highest truth; it is a universal, infinite, eternally awake, and living presence.

It might be helpful to see how this teaching changed the life of one of my students, a young mother named Kristin Mattias.

WHAT DOES SVADHARMA LOOK LIKE?

Kristin, in the process of her studies of Ayurveda, moved from a job as a patient-relations coordinator for a liver-transplant team at a local hospital to become the food manager at her daughter's Waldorf-inspired school. That job change was quite significant, but it wasn't the most important of the changes that Kristin experienced. After making a few dietary changes for herself and her young daughter, Kristin was intrigued by the spiritual philosophy of the Vedas—most particularly the idea of moksha, which means "freedom from the suffering of mind, body, and world and being in union with your highest Self."

I told Kristin, "Moksha is your birthright. You were born free. You just forgot. Moksha, however, is accessible right here and now, in every moment. You experience a moksha moment when you see through your ignorant identification with powerlessness, when in fact, the supremely indestructible, supremely powerful, and eternally healthy Self is your true nature. The conscious dropping (*kshaya*) of your worldly, limited beliefs around your body, disease, and relationships and the acceptance of your inherent, invisible, limitless, inexhaustible, infinite nature is moksha."

As Kristin started to think about this startling idea of moksha and how she might integrate this concept of spiritual freedom into her life, she saw that she had been focusing on her shortcomings and not thinking of herself as the free, whole person that she knew she was.

"I was so overwhelmed with all of the responsibilities and decisions that a new mother has to make. Do I co-sleep? Do I vaccinate? Is she getting enough breast milk? When do I introduce solid foods? Which medicine do I give—and not give!—when she is sick? The questions went on and on. The responsibilities felt like a burden—and there I was, focusing on all the things I *wasn't* doing rather than looking at the love and nurturing I could give my child. I was clouded by self-doubt and self-criticism, and I had forgotten my divine, whole, and complete innermost Self!"

Remembering the spiritual Self, Kristin came back to her belief in herself—as a person and as a mother. She let herself take personal time—for walks, meditation, and writing in her journal about her connection to her higher Self, to God, and to Nature. "This made a huge difference," Kristin said. "In this personal time, I was able to drop the negative talk, the overthinking, the judgments. I was able to focus more on my inner light and on my child."

Kristin, who is a superb mother, has three children now and continues to reach for her higher Self over the worries and concerns that are of a lower order. Kristin has a mantra today: "I am inherently free, and therefore, capable of rising above the chaos of the world." She calls these flash realizations "moksha moments" because, as she puts it, "In that instant, I recognize my inherent freedom, and claim it!"

In the world of forgetfulness, a turn inward, toward the Self, is a turn taken in the right direction—a turn toward home. The path home is the path of svadharma, and home is, of course, the expansive, infinite, eternally loving embrace of our true Self.

When the cosmos is represented inside you as your own universal Self, surely the cosmos must be expressing and celebrating something unique through you. Whether you have discovered this or not, there is a special life purpose just for you.

Hence, through the pages of this book, even as I expound on Ayurveda lifestyle, I am also asking you to live your dreams and to live your most honest version of your Self. I am asking you to seek what is unique within you and then shine the light on that, without shame, fear, or disappointment. This version of you will activate total health, swastha. It is a reclaiming of health from deep within.

What Constitutes Health in Ayurveda?

The Sanskrit term for health is *swastha*, which means "to be established in one's own essential nature or natural state." According to Ayurvedic sage Sushruta, true health manifests through a state of balance in all the dimensions of human existence—body, mind, and soul. His all-in-one definition leaves no aspect of our existence outside its parameter:

Samadoshah samaagnash cha samadhaatu malakriyaha

prasannaatmendriya manaha svastha ityabhidhiiyate.[3]

The translation is this: "A person who has the equilibrium of dosha, *agni* (digestive fire), *dhatu* (tissues), *mala* (impurities), and other activities of the body; who has happiness of Atman (soul), *indriya* (senses), and *manas* (mind) is called *swastha* (healthy)."

First, this definition of health covers physiology in the equilibrium of bio-energies and tissues as well as digestion and the process of elimination. The term *equilibrium* implies that balance in these functions is the optimum state as opposed to a mode that is either hypoactive, hyperactive, or in any way erratic.

The senses, which involve both the physical and the mental, must operate optimally for health—the sage uses the term *happiness*, which implies to me that the senses are used with ease and in the long term as opposed to being over- or underused or put to self-destructive use.

The mind of a healthy individual must also be in a balanced state, which means operating with its native intelligence mode and able to exercise discernment in choosing between beneficial and nonbeneficial options that will promote happiness or unhappiness, respectively.

And health in all of these areas—mind, senses, and body—is not enough for true health, which according to Ayurveda, must also involve a state of *prasanna*, signifying "health of the soul." This final level of good health means that the individual soul feels connected with a higher soul—which we would call God or a source of superintelligence—and also experiences life to be happy, beneficial, purposeful, and meaningful. The health of an embodied soul is directly related to the moral, ethical, social, and interpersonal well-being a person experiences.

So it is easy to see that Ayurveda's holistic approach to health, tying together the physiological, psychological, spiritual, and social dimensions of health, is in stark contrast to that of mainstream Western medicine, where a person is seen as a patient, and a patient is often no more than an ailing lung or peaking lipid profile. In my observation, Western medicine classifies the human being into body and brain, dismissing the issue of consciousness altogether, while Ayurveda considers, and treats, the whole human being: body, mind, and spirit. Ayurveda will not neglect one dimension while focusing on another; all are seen as equally significant.

The various Ayurveda lifestyle practices impact more than just one dimesion. Putting fresh flowers in your house, for instance, may please your senses and mind, and as well, they could affect your relationship with others who live there. Following Ayurveda recipes and food recommendations could impact your physiology as well as your psyche. Meditation may not only lower your blood pressure but also calm your mind and connect you to a sense of a spiritual power beyond your mind.

So think of this path as more than just a way to address a specific ailment with its annoying symptoms. Implementing Ayurveda lifestyle wisdom into your life is a way to craft wellness for yourself, a way to heal the whole person.

 As a little girl, I knew a lot of important-sounding Sanskrit words from listening to Baba's daily discourses to his students, but even though I had heard the word *swastha* used a lot in my home, I didn't really know what it meant. I asked Baba.

"It means health," he said, "but this is not just a matter of a healthy body. It refers to total health. It is a special, wonderful state of the body and mind and, of course, your heart that allows you, little Shunya, to play and climb trees and fall down and get back up again quickly."

Baba said that this condition of total health helps the body fight off invisible invaders called *krimi* (germs) and *krumi* (parasites), so they can't make us fall sick. Swastha protects us when seasons change, so we won't cough or have to wipe our nose every spring or have to deal with boils from eating hot mangos in summer. When we are swastha, we simply sail through changes in the seasons because all the five elements are in harmony within us.

"Yes, Shunya," he told me, "when you are swastha, you feel balanced. I will not need to tell you what that feels like. This is a feeling you know. When you are swastha, you feel enthusiastic; when you are swastha, you feel generous; when you are swastha, you feel grateful to be alive; when you are swastha, you know you are one with God and all of Nature, which is God's body."

With a magical smile, Baba added, "When you are swastha, little Shunya, you feel happy, and you spread this happiness everywhere around you." Then Baba turned to his students and made a statement that, decades later, I still repeat to my own students: "*sukha sangyakam aarogyam*—remember, happiness is nothing else but health."

In an evening discourse, Baba once explained that the state of swastha, true health, means being established in your own highest Self, and since the Self is nothing else but bliss, naturally you are happy. I was in the lecture hall that day, sitting in the back and leaning on my mother, my face hidden in the folds of her cotton clothing, which held her scent. In that safe place, I listened to Baba's every word, and I smiled. Baba spoke quietly, yet in my heart, I was growing more excited.

True health meant connecting with my own divine Self, which meant happiness for me and for everyone else as well! This was becoming thrilling!

What my soul understood that day was huge, but because my mind was that of an eight-year-old, I could begin to explain it to others only decades later. My soul's wisdom had preceded my mind-based vocabulary.

Later that night, just before bedtime, Baba beckoned me to join him. I would immediately climb into my grandfather's peaceful lap and put my ear to his heart, ready for a private teacher-student dialogue (*satsangha*). Doing that stirred so many ancient and wonderful memories in my little being.

He held my head and, looking steadily into my eyes, said, "Shunya, remember swastha is your true state. You are a divine being. You have a right to be healthy and, therefore, happy. Simply evoke swastha from within you. Simply have patience when challenged in body or mind, and do not quit or swerve from your path of self-care and self-love and self-worth until your swastha nature once again shines through you. And it will. Truth can never be contained for long. Clouds can hide the sun only so long. Your true nature simply is, and it is never far from you. Disease is only a symptom of imbalance. Balancing practices will once again evoke your inner swastha."

After those words, Baba fell quiet, and I remember simply lying on his heart, complete in the knowledge of swastha, and breathing together, one breath, master and disciple, until I fell asleep, and my mother or father carried me to my bed. ✎

Baba was referring to an interesting concept advanced by Ayurvedic medicine: we all are self-healing entities.[4] If we are in an imbalance, we can correct this misalignment by making lifestyle adjustments. It is these adjustments that will activate our inherent self-healing mechanism.

This is why Ayurvedic remedies, including lifestyle adjustments to prevent disease and optimize health, mainly work toward creating an optimum environment—both within and around a body—to set the stage so that the body's supremely intelligent, natural healing process can take over and restore the body to balanced health.

CHAPTER 2

Celebrating an Awakened Sky

The science of Ayurveda recommends waking up while it is still dark outside. A serene beauty and stillness envelop the Earth at this time. Though it is still dark out, the early morning darkness seems to be softer than nighttime, almost as if it's infused with a divine light. And rising this early benefits your body, mind, and spiritual practice.

 When I was a child, my eyes would open to the expectation of light, even before greeting the light itself. That is a special feeling. Witnessing the phenomenon of light banishing darkness every morning would chase away many mind-based falsehoods or concerns. Refreshed and reassured, I would embrace the day.

In Sanskrit, the language of the Ayurvedic sages, this time in the early morning is called *brahma muhurta*, "the time of God Consciousness," the time of perceiving the highest truth of universal consciousness. Naturally, it is an ideal time to meditate, contemplate, and acquire spiritual knowledge.

The Vedic sages calculated that this special time begins exactly one and a half hours before sunrise and lasts until the sun comes over the horizon. From this understanding, we can easily calculate when we should wake up, based on our location on Earth. In any case, we should try to wake up at some point before or at 6:00 a.m. and not later. There are scientific reasons for this, which I will go into later, in depth.

I'm happy that because my family's daily routine revolved around Ayurveda, I never had a choice to sleep in. All of my family members arose at brahma muhurta—and not just the humans, either. Even our family cow, Nandini, was always awake bright and early.

A big part of my life as a child was my trip to the river in the early morning with my grandfather. Like everyone there, our lives revolved around River Sarayu, whose history extends back to the *Rig-Veda* in ancient times. This beautiful blue river emerges from the glaciers of Mount Everest, the world's tallest mountain, and runs across valleys and gorges through tiny mountain hamlets and settlements to reach the city of Ayodhya in the plains of northern India.

Every day, Baba would wake me at the beginning of the brahma muhurta with a reminder that River Sarayu awaited us on her way to merging into the holy Ganges River (Ganga Maa, as we called her).

As a little girl, I would wonder to myself, "Why does the river await us? Does the river know us?"

When I asked Baba these questions, he replied with a gentle smile, his eyes sparkling, "Of course, because we are essentially one." ✒

The Beauty and Magic of Dawn

As individual beings, we share an inherent relationship with our environment. So when light begins to spread across the sky, our minds, too, begin to experience hope and courage.

When we gaze at the sky at this time, we know, deep in our hearts, that the sun will be here soon, and the dark night will be consumed by the spreading light, taking with it the fears, doubts, and ignorance that enveloped us as we slept. When we witness the transformation from dark to light, from night to dawn, there is a stirring of hope and a spiritual presence in our subconscious being, which begins to reveal itself, banishing ignorance and infusing our consciousness with divine illumination and intuitive knowledge.

For me, the early mornings are magical. At this time, the darkness of the night is slowly dissipating, and the light of the sun, even before it has tangibly announced its bold presence in the sky, is making its subtle but commanding presence felt. I cannot yet see the light, but I can sense the light in my heart, wherein dwells that one consciousness that connects us with the sun, moon, and Earth and all that we know and also all that we cannot fathom with our ordinary senses. It is during this time of outer stillness and inner silence that you can most easily connect to *Brahman*, the universal truth, and the one reality that is immutable and absolute.

 One beautiful morning when I was about six, Baba said to me, "Come, little Shunya, let us resolve every day to be awake for the breaking dawn, and let us rejoice in all its breathtaking, electric magnificence." Baba would often talk to me on our way back home from the river, and on that day, he explained how the early morning sun distributes blessings, including the gifts of health, wisdom, and peace for all of Earth's creatures, big and small. I liked this idea of gifts; it reminded me of receiving presents on my birthday and on Diwali (the Hindu festival of spiritual lights). My grandfather must have known this because he added, "But these gifts are different. These gifts are invisible, and you open them for the rest of your life."

That was enough for me.

Over the years, I would try my best to internalize Baba's words because he never repeated himself. Even when I was too young to understand his words, his eyes would share an invitation to be happy by simply rising before dawn. Four decades later, as I write these words about the benefits of waking up early, I remember Baba's eyes being lit by the first rays of the sun. ✒

The Significance of Brahma Muhurta

As night proceeds to dawn, all the creatures of Nature, big and small, are slowly awakening, following Nature's book of rules. Even the grass, plants, flowers, and trees are looking reenergized and awake to a discerning eye. Everything else is also stirring from sleep and pulsating with movement. It is our time to stir, too, as we are not separate from Nature.

Ayurvedic tradition tells us that those who awaken in brahma muhurta receive abundant health in body, mind, and soul. The physical benefits, alone, are quite profound: increased energy, eradication of depression, and improved digestion.

According to one classical Ayurveda text, the Ashtanga Hridayam, a healthy person should wake up at brahma muhurta to protect his or her very life. In this scripture, it is said that waking up early is tied to increased lifespan and longevity.[1]

In both the introduction and chapter 1, I mentioned how each part of the day is governed by a particular dosha, and now I will go into this daily timing of energies in greater detail.

Recall that in the early hours of the day, between 2:00 a.m. and 6:00 a.m., vata dosha is dominant and most active. Vata represents movement or variability, as opposed to kapha dosha, which represents dullness or inertia.

Kapha dosha dominates between 6:00 a.m. and 10:00 a.m. Finally, pitta dosha, which represents transformation and sharpness, is most active from 10:00 a.m. to 2:00 p.m.—at which point the cycle begins all over again. From 2:00 p.m. to 6:00 p.m., vata dosha is once again active, and from 6:00 p.m. to 10:00 p.m., kapha dosha takes over. And finally, once again, pitta dosha becomes dominant from 10:00 p.m. to 2:00 a.m. This cycle continues nonstop, ad infinitum.

It is useful to see how the world and natural phenomena around us reflect vata dosha's theme of movement in the macrocosm. Literally everything begins stirring at this time. Thus, by choosing to wake up at a vata time, prior to 6:00 a.m., we are adjusting our own lifestyles according to the overriding energy of the day. By doing this, we maximize our own health and energy.

Let's say that, instead of waking up early, we sleep through this active vata time. It's enjoyable to pull up the covers and stay in our warm beds sleeping, is it not? Initially, yes, it is. But Ayurveda says that this extra sleep can lead to challenges in body and mind in the future.

If we sleep late on a regular basis, acting counter to the energy of movement all around us in the cosmos, an inertia settles into our beings. We have reduced energy overall, and this leads to digestive problems and even a lack of motivation.

Right here lie the roots of imbalance: in our action, or inaction. As we are not separate from Nature, brahma muhurta is our time to stir, too. All must move at the right time for good health—arrested or delayed movement can be a problem. Nowhere is this more apparent than in the colon, which is the seat of vata dosha.

Get out of bed before 6:00 a.m. no matter what! This is what I have recommended to the hundreds of people who have sought my advice on chronic constipation. Before I prescribe herbs that assist elimination or even suggest changing the diet to add the oily quality (*snigdha*) that aids elimination, I first ask a client a number of questions, the first of which is what time they wake up. Some people are puzzled by this line of questioning. Why am I asking what times they go to sleep and wake up? Why am I not asking the obvious questions?

But those who have followed my advice to rise early have reaped the benefits. When we arise in the vata time of the day, our bowels will function naturally, eliminating waste and pent up gas. This clears the digestive tract, gets gas out of the stomach, and makes room for agni, or digestive fire, assisted by vata dosha, to flare up appropriately. Pay close attention to the words I'm using—you'll notice that "flare up" is also a kind of movement. This gastric movement then ensures timely hunger, timely digestion, and—hallelujah!—timely elimination the next time around.

The entire body clock begins to reset itself, just because we got up at the right time.

a way that we go to bed by 10:00 p.m. or earlier. According to Ayurveda, this is an ideal schedule for going to sleep and arising. How you can get into bed at 10:00 p.m. and then fall asleep quickly, with no tossing and turning, is a topic we'll discuss at length in chapter 7.

It is commonly understood that getting eight hours of sleep at night is ideal for health and daily functioning. Going to bed by 10:00 p.m. and then waking up at 6:00 a.m. or earlier, you may not sleep for the recommended eight hours. By waking up at brahma muhurta, however, you have opened your being to the gifts of cosmic energy and alignment with vata dosha, so you may not need the full eight hours of sleep after all.

Routinely, I go to bed no later than 10:00 p.m. and wake up no later than 5:00 a.m. So, for decades now, I've been getting only seven hours of sleep each night. Yet I have more physical energy and mental endurance than most people half my age. My students can attest that in the last ten years their teacher has not missed a single class due to ill health or fatigue. And I always accomplish what I set out for myself during the day with ease and energy left for spiritual practices before bedtime. I suggest that with an Ayurveda-inspired lifestyle, the quality of your sleep may count more than the quantity of your sleep.

If you begin to incorporate Ayurveda lifestyle practices into your routine, then you will find yourself going to sleep earlier and that the quality of your sleep has improved. Then, getting up in time to meet the rising sun will become your routine. Try it, and then you won't have to merely take my word for it.

The Proper Time for Sleeping and Waking

Since it is ideal to wake at or before 6:00 a.m., it is also important to plan our entire day in such

Exception to the Rule of Waking Up

There is an exception to this rule of waking up before sunrise. If one night you need to stay up especially late—an airport pickup, say—you should not wake up at your usual hour. Let's say you don't get to bed until midnight. Then your whole system is running two hours behind. In such a case, Ayurveda prescribes that you sleep one hour later than usual and wake up at 7:00 a.m. Rather than making up the full two hours of lost sleep, you instead make up only half of the time lost.

You could, on the other hand, suggest that your friend take a train, call a taxi, or find a different friend! But life and a friend stuck at the airport are not in our control. And we don't want to leave our friends hanging! So Ayurveda takes special circumstances into account and allows us to make up our sleep. But for one night—not night after night after night.

Every day is a twenty-four-hour wheel, and the choices we make for every part of this wheel impact our resulting state of health. Waking up regularly at brahma muhurta is not about simply setting the alarm for an hour or so earlier than you would otherwise. Our lifestyle choices throughout the twenty-four hours preceding brahma muhurta impact what happens on the wheel of life at this particular point. The food we eat, the sorts of activities we engage in, the time we go to sleep—all of our choices from the previous day, month, and year stack up on us. We are spinning constantly on the wheel of time from one sunrise to the next.

Thanks to a fixed bedtime and wake-up routine, every morning, my mind begins its habitual humming and wakes to the breaking dawn in its breathtaking, electric magnificence. Before the first rays of light materialize, my slumbering body stirs naturally, like the birds and flowers in my garden.

We Are Part of Nature

We humans have strayed a long way from Nature. After all, we have choices. Our windows, draped with heavy curtains or blinds, and our sound-insulated homes, barricaded from our life source, the sun, keep us well cocooned in our own world. We barely remember anymore that we are a part of Nature.

But Nature, being a mother, does not give up on us. With every sunrise, she sends us many reminders to not only wake up, but truly awaken to the truth of our connection with Nature. The golden radiance that spreads across the vast skies and lights up the horizon is meant to touch us as well and enlighten our consciousness. The divine radiance is meant to come in through our eyes, warm our lonely hearts, and illumine our isolated minds. How can the sunlight do this if we choose to keep our eyes shut?

Then, Mother Nature asks the birds to tell us all about the resplendent morning and its majestic beauty. The birds chirp away and sing profound songs about the merits of waking up early, but we can't hear them through our spongy, multicolored latex earplugs, the hum of computers, water heaters, or electronic devices that send simulated sounds of Nature to block out the true sounds of Nature coming alive with the rising sun.

Babies tend not to follow grown-up rules. They wake up spontaneously in the early morning, during the time of vata, to coo, cry, play, and even poop effortlessly with delight. We adults put a silicon nipple into their little mouths and hope that their diapers can wait a bit. "Sleep a little more," we tell our babies, "Mommy and Daddy are tired." Our pets are stirring early, as well; they yearn to join creatures of the natural world outside our four walls. But the alpha human continues to snore, so what choice do we give our animals but to curl up and sleep some more with us!

I've spoken a lot about the benefits of rising before 6:00 a.m., but nothing yet of the disadvantages that come to those who do not. Since kapha time starts at 6:00 a.m., sleeping past 6:00 a.m. will rapidly increase kapha (inertia). In other words, an inert sleep will increase an individual's overall inertia.

The longer we stay confined in our kapha sleep, the heavier we feel, the sleepier we become. When we finally do awaken, we don't feel refreshed in the way we would had we awakened during vata time. On the contrary, we feel groggy, dull, and even sleepier. Sometimes this heaviness lasts for several hours after waking up, and we begin to label this experience as fatigue. Actually, this is nothing more than kapha dosha, with its qualities of heaviness, dullness, and slowness, which has enveloped us and settled into every pore and channel of our beings.

When kapha increases in the macrocosm, our bodies, which are the microcosm, will mirror it. Hence, processes that were previously under the quick command of movement, such as regular functioning of the bowels, will now slow down considerably or, in some cases, come to a standstill. You get the picture.

In this way, through Ayurveda lifestyle wisdom, we can choose the activities of our day consciously. When vata, which is variable and active, peaks in the macrocosm (from 2:00 a.m. to 6:00 a.m. and from 2:00 p.m. to 6:00 p.m.), individuals are advised to relax, meditate, and generally take it easy. That is, we are asked to do the opposite of "movement." When pitta, which is fiery, peaks in the world (from 10:00 a.m. to 2:00 p.m. and 10:00 p.m. to 2:00 a.m.), we are asked to avoid overheating the body and

mind and choose coolness in environment and thoughts. And of course when kapha is peaking in the world (from 6:00 a.m. to 10:00 a.m. and 6:00 p.m. to 10:00 p.m.), we are advised to move the body, breath, and mind and to never remain sedentary—or worse, fall asleep. Isn't that clever?

In terms of time and our daily activities, this is another application of the Ayurvedic principle "like increases like; opposites decrease each other." To keep a dosha in balance, invoke its opposite.

While I teach these laws, my students greet them with great excitement. There are some people, of course, who still find it difficult to wake up early when kapha time begins at 6:00 a.m. I find this unfortunate. Those who choose to remain asleep, even after receiving this life-changing knowledge, remain imprisoned under the heavy cage of self-imposed kapha, with hard-to-break habits and inner resistances.

Fortunately, the wisdom tradition of Ayurveda continuously reminds human beings of our true place in Nature and why it serves us to work with Nature rather than to defy her at every opportunity. Ayurveda is perhaps the first medical science to declare a union between the individual (*purusha*) and the universe (*loka*), a concept called *loka purusha samya*.[2] Here, *samya* means "equality." In this relationship, the individual unit can be anything: a tiny ant, a blade of grass, or the most evolved thinking, feeling animal of all, the human being. Yet, all living creatures are obliged to exist under the same law of macro- and microinterconnectedness. We are bound by the same physical and spiritual laws, and in fact, these laws exist on a continuum, which spans from the largest to the smallest form of creation. The individual living unit is a miniature replica of the universe. Hence, we humans will benefit immensely if we learn to follow Nature's cues and take action accordingly.

It is my hope that the beautiful wisdom of Ayurveda will awaken in you the desire to align with Nature and her rules. Your life is an extension of Nature. You are invited to use Nature to your advantage. I have found that the more I embrace Nature's laws, the more I find myself embraced by her compassion.

The followers of Ayurveda lifestyle wisdom begin to discover the deep nurturance that is available in Nature and to gradually become one with the great cycle and rhythm of Nature. It all begins with respecting Nature and understanding the basic truth that we and Nature are one; we are each other's extension, and disrespecting or disregarding one leads to abuse and injury of the other.

Time and the Three Gunas

The human mind has a unique relationship with the light of the sun. The scriptures that inform Ayurveda say that the sun is the source of our human life.

While we can take the sun and its gift of illumination for granted during the daytime, at night, we miss it. We may not be aware that we miss the sun, but the absence of light does something to our minds: we experience fears that we did not know lurked in our subconscious. We may not demonstrate or verbalize our inner experience, but in the dark hours, we are more easily swayed by self-doubt, hesitation, and dread.

Far from the bravado we experience during our daytime socializing and professional engagements, deep inside our hearts at night we can feel abandoned and anxious. We surround ourselves with artificial light, and when we go to

bed and switch off the electric light, we hope to fall asleep quickly and remain suspended in slumber until morning. As the Earth cycles from light to shadow and back, so too does our own mental state cycle.

The Vedic sages inform us that all of Nature is composed of three types of fundamental vibrations or qualities that weave the cosmos, known in in Sanskrit as *gunas*. The three gunas are *sattva*, *rajas*, and *tamas*. Imperceptible to the human senses, the gunas are like what modern physics describes as the phenomena of matter and antimatter. Gunas are the ultimate and irreducible entities that operate at the subtlest level of this universe.

According to the Vedas, rajas represents energy; tamas represents mass, inertia, or resistance to this energy (equal and opposing force); and sattva is the stabilizing force, the essence or intelligence that manifests itself as existent and brings about manifestation in spite of the presence of opposing forces. Varying quantities of intelligence (sattva), energy (rajas), and mass (tamas), in varied groupings, act on one another, and through their mutual interaction and interdependence, a world of diversity and matter, from subtle (space) to gross (earth), is born.

Thus, the gunas are the primal qualities of Nature and the mode through which Rta or cosmic intelligence operates. Clearly the gunas are not qualities in the average sense of the word. An entire galaxy—a speck of dust and a tiny amoeba to a full-fledged human being—comes under the purview of gunas.

In the human being, the gunas are witnessed through the workings of the body because they influence the doshas; they are even more subtle than the doshas, and in fact, drive the doshas themselves. Rajas (quality of motion) influences vata dosha, and tamas (quality of inertia) drives kapha dosha. Finally, sattva, or the quality of cosmic intelligence, drives pitta dosha. Additionally, the human mind—from imagination to ideas to expression of complex beliefs and concepts—is influenced by gunas, and the mind expresses itself through the interplay of the three gunas. The descriptions below clarify this point further.

Sattva Guna: Sattva guna is expressed in the cosmos through the luminosity of light, power of reflection, harmony, balance, goodness, knowledge, and purity. When sattva emerges in our minds, we experience inner clarity, pleasure, purity of being, contentment, intrinsic peacefulness, and a desire to be noble, good, and godly and to share and to care for others. Sattva has a special affinity with truth, and hence, those with sattvic minds are receptive to spiritual learning and can access inner wisdom with ease. Light, especially the pure light of the sun, or of a lamp or candle lit on an altar, is a beautiful symbol for sattva.

Rajas Guna: Rajas guna is the principle of motion. When in excess, it produces pain, both physical and emotional. Restless activity, feverish effort, and nonstop stimulation are its manifestations. It is mobile and energizing. Rajas expresses itself in the bold strokes of passion, action, change, movement, activity, and compulsion, not to mention agitation and turbulence. In the mind, it expresses itself as restlessness, changeability, addiction to activity, and the undertaking of excessive activities fueled by a multiplicity of desires with underlying selfish interests to advance. Constant change and rapid speed are characteristic of actions with rajas behind them. Changing, shifting light is indicative of rajas.

Tamas Guna: In tamas, both light and movement are absent. Tamas literally means darkness; it is the principle of inertia. It produces apathy and indifference. Ignorance, sloth, confusion, bewilderment, passivity, and negativity are its results; it is heavy (*guru*) and enveloping (*avarna*) and as such is opposed to sattva. It is also opposed to rajas as it arrests all activity. Thus, darkness is a special feature of tamas. It is often associated with nighttime in the macro sense and ignorance in the human mind in the micro sense. Ambiguity, lack of initiative, incomprehension, and the inability to see through mental confusions and emerge from self-delusions (sometimes in spite of counseling, teaching, and handholding) are characteristics of a tamas-dominant mind. Due to lack of inner movement, there is often an experience of psychological paralysis in the tamasic mind, leading to great inner frustration. Naturally, it is difficult to access wisdom and knowledge in this type of mental state.

 On one of our many trips to River Sarayu, Baba explained to me that the rising sun is an important event that the entire universe prepares to greet. The plants and tress wait for it; the birds, bees, beetles, and cows bow to it. Everyone is ready to greet the rising sun's majestic appearance in the sky. However, because humans have a choice, many of us simply stay lost in sleep.

"Why?" I had asked him. Baba explained that while it may be daytime for birds, roses, and buzzing bees, who are off to work being their spiritual best, the human mind is filled with the mist of tamas. So people can feel defeated even before the day has started. "But," Baba reminded me, "this defeat can turn into success by simply resolving to wake up. Fight this one battle with yourself at brahma muhurta, Shunya. Wake up at any cost, and all other battles in life yet to come will simply fade away." ✒

The Dance of the Gunas across the Sky

All three gunas—rajas, tamas, and sattva—play a role in Nature. When tamas peaks in the cosmos, darkness takes over. Nighttime falls and envelops everything, including the minds of all living creatures.

This is why, at night, when we are under the influence of tamas, we often feel uncertain, less courageous, and we may postpone decision-making until the next day. In the evening hours, we seek the solace of friends, family, food, and finally, sleep. This is not to say that tamas is a bad thing. We need all three gunas in our lives. Without tamas, this world and its creatures would never take a break, relax, let go, or fall asleep.

When the sun is out, bright and shining during much of the day, we have a natural abundance of sattva. Of course, our individual minds may be tamasic or rajasic, firmly entrenched in its pattern, but Mother Nature, from her side, shines sattva on us through the agency of the luminous sun, giving us each repeated opportunities every day to literally clear our head of excessive sloth (tamas), as well as distracting thoughts (rajas), and get centered and focused with a more balanced state of mind (sattva).

The junctures between night and day—sunrise and sunset—and the times leading up to them are both dominant in rajas because this is a time of transition and change. It is a cosmic light switch of sorts.

While both of these periods are dominant in rajas, they have very different effects on the human mind. The three hours prior to sunset is a period of rajas that tends to evoke restlessness, even anxiety. This is because sattva will soon disappear and be replaced with the shroud of nighttime tamas.

In contrast, between 4:00 a.m. and 6:00 a.m., everyone is naturally infused with the right kind of rajas, the positive kind, which leads us gracefully and ineluctably toward a full-blown encounter with sattva, both outside of us and, importantly, within us, in our own minds.

As the sun sets and darkness spreads in the macrocosm, so, too, does our ignorance of Self rise forth in our minds, and our courage plunges, bit by bit, in our mental landscape. The sight of the setting sun is exquisite, no doubt, but who can ignore an inexplicable disquiet that clutches our being at this time of the day? We can ignore it, but if we are being honest with ourselves, we cannot deny this foreboding. Tears, sadness, old memories, and even depression often follow sunset.

Fortunately, thanks to the big cycles in Nature, we won't drown in the smaller tamas waves of our mind. The rajas period that begins around 3:00 a.m. and peaks one and a half hours before sunrise is quite the opposite in its quality. It is as if, in this part of the cycle, Mother Nature is lending our minds majestic wings of rajas to fly above the slumbering Earth and meet the rising sun halfway across the sky. The tamas accumulated over the night ends with the sunrise and the scattering of the brilliant vibrations of sattva. It is no wonder that, when we wake up at this time of the early morning, we feel reenergized, expansive, creative, and nobly inspired.

It is important to remember that while sattva is associated with light or illumination, it is not the same as the particles of physical light. Sunlight is a mode of delivery for cosmic sattva—the qualities of peace, balance, and purity. Sattva is by no means limited to the rays of the sun. Rather, think of sattva as the sun's subtle quality, the original source of life for all beings. A burning ghee lamp or eating certain pure and rarefied foods can also transmit sattva. We could say that the ghee lamp and the food are really just altered forms of the sun's original fire.

Catch That Extraordinary, Expansive Time

The period from 4:00 a.m. to 6:00 a.m., when rajas is moving to sattva, is considered the best time for nurturing activities that require both inner movement and purity. Self-study and learning with a guru who gives us spiritual knowledge are traditionally recommended during this time. Yoga and meditation during this time of day reap the best results.

To absorb any subject, whether material or spiritual, we need a clear mind and also the inner movement that takes us from ignorance to illumination. For countless centuries, students in traditional Vedic gurukulam would gather around their teacher's home in the early morning, the time of sattva, to meditate together, join sacred worshipping rituals, connect with the rising sun, and then study Vedic texts. In contrast, during periods of rajas, the student's mind is often distracted, and in periods of tamas, the mind is often prone to dullness and even unconscious fear of the knowledge being presented.

In my own gurukulam, at Vedika Global, I have noticed that it is very different when I teach in the early morning. At other times, especially at night, I have students begin by chanting several sattva-evoking Vedic mantras, especially the Gayatri mantra (a Vedic prayer for illuminating intelligence), and by lighting ghee lamps. The lamps brighten the nooks and crannies of my school and also evoke sattva in my students' minds. Vedic altars in the school are adorned with fresh flowers and radiate all sorts of vibrations of blessing, so this, too, creates a sattvic microenvironment.

All of this does work a kind of magic. While the teacher and the students feel blessed at each class, the activity of teaching and learning is still harder work in the evenings.

In the early mornings, Sanskrit verses that were difficult to memorize the night before are effortlessly recalled from memory. The knowledge of Self and the reality of divine oneness is revealed beyond doubt in the student's psyche. Universal compassion arises as if spontaneously in the student's heart. Knowledge of principles of Ayurveda become established and naturally known. And discourses on the science of Ayurveda that were received in previous days—from me, the teacher—are converted in the student's mind from facts to convictions.

Something of this sort can happen in your life, too, in relation to your own spiritual journey and study—if you begin awakening in brahma muhurta.

Brahma Muhurta and Modern Science

At times, I like to point out some observations of modern science that corroborate what the divine science of Ayurveda discovered thousands of years ago.

Modern science has identified two separate chemicals that are secreted by the brain, serotonin and melatonin. Serotonin's secretion is triggered by sunlight, and once triggered, it automatically arrests the secretion of the other chemical, melatonin. After sunset, serotonin stops being secreted, and melatonin begins to take over.

Both chemicals perform different functions, and in Ayurveda language, serotonin assists rajas because it supports the experience of wakefulness, and melatonin assists tamas in the brain because it slows us down in general and helps us sleep. The modern scientists are explaining the circadian rhythm with the help of these chemicals and by monitoring the human, animal, and plant responses to exposure to light and dark environments.

Thousands of years prior to these discoveries, the Ayurvedic sages were talking about inner clock functions and how the mind reacts to light and dark signals from the environment. It is important to clarify, however, that I am not advocating reducing the spiritual modes of rajas and tamas to the chemicals serotonin and melatonin, which are but a material demonstration of the universal spiritual principle in action.

Many of us with night-shift jobs, who have to stay up rather than sleep at night (that is, willfully evoke rajas instead of tamas), will attest to how hard it is to go against the modes of Nature. And seasonal affective disorder (SAD) is a well-known condition that arises from inadequate exposure to sunlight, a deficiency that leads to depression (tamas).

The Best Antidepressant

Those living in lands that are deprived of sun for large parts of the year can be susceptible to depression or sadness that sometimes sets in due to absence of adequate sunlight. If they practiced the Ayurveda lifestyle, they would not rely solely on the sun for their necessary dose of sattva. Rather, they would evoke sattva through other methods mentioned earlier, such as sitting and gazing at a lit ghee lamp or chanting Vedic mantras or prayers (in any language), connecting to the inner contemplation and image of a rising sun.

In fact, an Ayurveda lifestyle can be the best antidote to depression and even a preventative measure to ward it off. Each lifestyle practice that I introduce in this book promotes healthy rajas and sattva in large measures. And certain nighttime practices promote healthy tamas so that we can have a good night's sleep.

There is something about watching a sunrise with our eyes directly and literally perceiving the phenomena of change from tamas (the pitch dark of night) to rajas (the shifting of darkness to light) to full-blown sattva (the risen sun) that is deeply healing to human consciousness.

The act of seeing a spiritual phenomenon through our human eyes, is called *darshan*. Through witnessing this cycle of change, from darkness to light, deep-seated inner wisdom can be evoked. This inner knowledge illuminates our entire being and reassures us frail humans that the light is the only truth, and darkness is but a passing phase. This is an important lesson to remember: light is the only truth.

Ayurveda thus teaches peace with the internal elements that regulate body and mind and a peaceful relationship with the external elements that comprise our environment. Ayurveda is indeed based on remembering, reconnecting, and celebrating the eternal harmony and sacred connections between living beings and Nature.

Waking Up Early Helps Us Sleep Better

It naturally follows that the earlier you wake up, the earlier you will want to go to bed. It's not just the physical fatigue that sets in earlier when we start our days earlier. There is a subtler point. The sooner the human mind perceives light through the sense organ of the eye, the sooner it activates the "awake" cycle. Think of the times you switched on the bedside lamp for a drink of water or took a bathroom visit in the middle of the night. These actions can end up waking us up more than we had intended and lead to our tossing and turning throughout the rest of the night.

While all light can send us a signal to wake up, there is something about our exposure to the early morning sunlight that is special. By exposing our senses to sunlight right after sunrise, we can regulate our inner biological clock and provide it with the most natural time-to-awaken signal. Thus, the timing of our first exposure to light for the day is critical. Early morning light has a greater effect on good, timely sleep than does exposure to sunlight at any other time during the day. If we wake up late and greet the sunlight late, our time for sleep is also being pushed later. Hence, to counteract this forward glide of the circadian clock, it is best to expose the brain to sunlight during brahma muhurta.

And while any source of light can have its effect on us, all light sources are not the same. The ancient Veda recognizes light from the original source, which is the sun. All other light sources, even special light boxes or high-tech lightbulbs that simulate the sun, are functioning on borrowed light. These types of light may activate rajas, but they cannot impart the sattva of the rising sun, which we require in order to be happy and productive for the rest of the day and to get a timely, balanced sleep the following night.

Ayurveda's sun-powered lifestyle is a twenty-four-hour cycle of living. When we wake up at the right time, sleep follows at the right time. From this perspective, the best cure for insomnia is waking up at brahma muhurta.

When Early Sunlight Is Not Always Possible

The Earth's angle and rotation around the sun create dramatic variation in sunrise and sunset patterns. At our planet's poles, the sun rises and sets only once each year. In surrounding areas, short distances below the poles, there are extended periods of phenomena such as the midnight sun (sun shining at night), white nights (twilight during night), and polar nights (sun below the horizon, even in the daytime).

What should you do if you live in such a location? Can you follow an Ayurvedic lifestyle? Yes, but to a limited extent. If you're in Alaska over the winter, when the sun rises at 3:00 p.m., you should spend an hour and a half before sunrise watching the sun come up. This will lessen the effect of the late sunrise; it will not counteract it.

The Ayurvedic concept of *desha* pertains to the impact of our geographical location on our health. Understand that not every location on Earth is an equally healthy environment. From the standpoint of Ayurveda, the area at or near Earth's poles is not a natural environment for human beings. For most of the year, the weather is forbidding. We humans have employed technology to triumph over Nature, rendering these places habitable, yet it remains to be seen who has triumphed over whom.

Those who live in areas where the sun does not set often report having sleep difficulties, raging insomnia to hypomania with persistent elevated or irritable moods. In Ayurvedic terms, this is all due to an excess of rajas. In places where the sun does not rise, inhabitants are often plagued by deep gloom and depression, due to the buildup of excessive tamas. If I were to travel to an area with dark days, I would take along my ghee lamp, and several times a day I would gaze at its bright flame for stretches of five minutes. I would also chant Vedic mantras to ignite some much-needed sattva. Although Ayurveda can offer some relief to people living in such conditions, it cannot fix a condition that is not, in and of itself, ideal for human habitation.

How to Wake Up at Brahma Muhurta

Before closing your eyes for the night, make a firm decision to wake up at a chosen time the next morning. In Sanskrit, there is a word for a decision that you make with your highest Self; it is called a *sankalpa*. Each sankalpa you make carries its own spiritual power, or shakti, and each invokes sattva. Every time you keep your

sankalpa, you generate more spiritual power, and that helps you maintain the practice.

Not everyone has the ability to automatically awaken at a determined time. It's a good idea to set an alarm to make sure you don't sleep beyond dawn. Make sure, however, that your alarm isn't so shrill or jarring that it jerks you abruptly out of sleep. When the alarm sounds, do not press the snooze button and let yourself doze off again as this simply reinforces procrastination (tamas). Once you hear the alarm, this is your cue to wake up and get up. You must battle with the inner enemy of laziness. Plan to not entertain second thoughts. Wake up simply by waking up. Make your actions swift to overcome any weakness that arises in your mind.

The vibration of inertia (tamas) cocoons our consciousness for several hours. It casts a spell over our minds and holds us paralyzed with dreams fueled by the memories and desires of the subconscious. To take full advantage of the restfulness of sleep, upon awakening you can quietly watch your breath. Become aware of your softly rising and falling chest. Once your attention has become mindfully established on your breath—it will take only a few seconds—then you are ready to take more energetic action. Employ your breath to activate movement. Swiftly move aside any covers and simply stand up. Once you are awake, if it's needed, switch on a bedside lamp. Do not continue lying in bed once you've awakened. It's too easy to fall back into sleep. Now is a time for action. During the colder months, keep some warm clothes and slippers next to your bed so that feeling chilled doesn't give you an excuse to get back into bed.

In this way, slowly and steadily, you can circumvent your own mind by teaching it a new wake-up routine. In this pause between the complete inertia of sleep (tamas) and the total activation of an awakened state (rajas), you can begin to awaken with poise and mastery of the moment through embracing the illumined quality of your mind—sattva.

By following the lifestyle practices that assist sleep (provided in chapter 7), your sleep will become predictable as well as deeply nourishing. This, in turn, will ensure that you will be able to wake up fresh and rejuvenated at brahma muhurta.

Auspicious Encounters upon Awakening

Soon after waking and rising from your bed, deliberately look at something auspicious or pleasing to the senses. This could be fresh flowers, a mirror, an image of something sacred to you, or a lit ghee or oil lamp. If you have access to an open-mouthed urn of ghee, one traditional suggestion is that you simply glance at the yellow mass of ghee, which will serve as a mirror to look at your own Self as a temple of divinity.[3]

My mother loved to grow a variety of jasmine flowers in pots on the terrace of our home in Ayodhya. Jasmine was her favorite flower because of its fragrant aroma. Every morning before I opened my eyes—it could have been hours or minutes; I never knew—my mother would place a bunch of freshly picked jasmine flowers at the altar of Hindu goddess Durga in the room where my sister, our little cousin, and I slept. Sometimes when I awoke and my eyes fell to the northeast corner of the room, I would look at the flowers placed at the tiny bedroom altar. There lay a splendid sight for me to absorb through my senses. To this day, when I smell jasmine, I am instantly transported back to my childhood home.

At our altar, the Durga deity was smiling. She looked like a heroine in her blazing red sari with its gold border and her dark, flowing tresses that fell below her knees. The goddess sat astride a lion, a symbol of her personal power—and a reminder to me of my own power. The fresh flowers that decorated the altar perfumed the entire room and blessed me on behalf of Mother Nature. Often, the image of my mother picking these flowers for my room would bring comfort to my heart. The lamp burning on the altar, which my mother lit while I was still asleep, would display a beautiful and unwavering flame, reminding me of everything beautiful and steady in my life.

On the other walls hung mirrors and depictions of gods and goddesses as well as my mother's paintings of flowers and birds. On the southern wall hung the photos of my ancestors. I especially loved looking at Baba's father, a Hindu saint himself, who had such a kind face. In his lifetime, Paramatman Sadhu Shanti Prakash (as Baba's father was called) had undertaken great spiritual and socially uplifting projects and had started a spiritual movement in my hometown of Ayodhya. What a wonderful feeling it was to wake up to these walls, where every inch was shining with beautiful symbols of upliftment, symbols with auspicious meaning for me.

Whatever we see, smell, or hear when we first come out of sleep sets the tone for the rest of our day. Consider the difference between waking up in a mindfully arranged space that supports inner well-being versus waking up to see a room where the closet door is only halfway shut and clothes are strewn here and there—or worse, looking at the screen of your smartphone to get news of the latest accidents and atrocities.

If you were to think of your home as a temple, the temple of your being, how would you arrange your personal space? What gifts would you give yourself every morning? Think about visual and aromatic gifts and even auditory gifts like beautiful music to greet your ears as you wake up!

Start Your Day with Purification

As soon as you are up and your eyes have taken in something pleasant and auspicious, it's time for elimination of your body's wastes. Do not, for any reason, suppress the urge to evacuate your bowels, as this can lead to a number of health issues.

Once you have evacuated, drink eight handfuls of water, a ritual called *usha-paana*. In Sanskrit, one handful is called *prasriti*, which is a normal-sized adult hand. You can measure the eight handfuls into a glass, as the volume varies per person, but do not translate eight handfuls as eight glasses, as that, of course, would be far too much water to consume at one sitting.

Ayurveda sage Bhava Mishra notes that, aside from aiding digestion, drinking this amount of water at brahma muhurta helps balance all three doshas. This practice also reduces the incidence of hemorrhoids; edema; chronic fever; indigestion; skin diseases; pain in the ears, throat, head, and pelvic region; and diseases of the eye.[4]

In winter, drinking warm water is advised, so heat your water on the stove or electric kettle before drinking it, or heat water the night before and put it in a thermos so it's waiting for you at brahma muhurta. In summer, room-temperature water is preferred. Refrigerated or ice-cold water is never advised in Ayurveda, under any weather condition. Ice water leads to a number of maladies, including digestive problems and skin conditions.

For added benefit during the summer, store water in a clay, copper, or silver pot overnight. Storing the water in this way is not mandatory, so don't give up the entire practice because you do not have a special pot. Water consumed at this time is an elixir, regardless, so the pot is only offering a secondary benefit.

Ideally, you would brush your teeth before drinking the water. You can read more about dental hygiene in chapter 4.

Create Your Own Sacred Morning Flow

Waking up during brahma muhurta not only allows you to savor the sattvic sunrise, it also gives you time to perform valuable lifestyle practices before you go about your regular day. Ayurveda is comprised of countless practices that impact all dimensions of your being.

There are a variety of spiritual practices to follow upon waking up during brahma muhurta. There is no specific order in which these practices must be followed. You can choose the practice or practices that most appeal to you. To start, select one that is realistic to implement and that makes the most sense to you, one that will impact the particular dimension of your being that you wish to nurture.

What is vital is that in the first moments you are awake, you must not start thinking about your to-do list for the day. Your first thought should be to bless yourself. Let me first explain the reason behind such a blessing.

We are not merely biological entities of flesh and blood. Nor are we merely a psychological phenomenon, a randomly emerged cognizance of thoughts, ideas, fears, and doubts that remains mostly confused about its own purpose and finally succumbs to death.

According to the ancient Vedic tradition, each one of us is a spiritual entity with a body and mind that act as our instruments. We are eternal and infinitely powerful beings. We are connected with a universal spiritual source, both outside and within us, and it is important that each day we remember our divinity. We are advised to reach into our hearts every morning, and grab a handful of divine powers to recall the truth that we are not beggars of well-being, but royal beings infused with the spiritual power to be always abundant, knowledgeable, and healthy, and always in an authentic "inner power seat."

The Ayurveda lifestyle prescription includes the chanting of mantras at every occasion. The Sanskrit word *mantra* comes from two root syllables: *man*, referring to the thinking mind, and *tra*, meaning "to protect." A mantra protects us when we meditate on it. It is a specific grouping of sound vibrations that, when verbalized mindfully or when its meaning is meditated on silently, creates a sound-based frequency that protects the mind from its own conflicting emotions, desires, and thought vacillations. A unique concentration or single-mindedness is naturally manifested in the mind upon the chanting of a mantra or even, for that matter, upon just hearing one.

So a mantra is a sacred utterance that protects and frees our minds. Ayurveda encourages that we chant mantras even while conducting the simplest of everyday activities, such as while waking up, first putting our feet on the floor after a night's sleep, taking a shower, and before partaking a meal.

What is the significance of such a practice? It is simply that we remember at all times that we are spiritual beings having a temporary physical experience in the body, that we are one with a higher spiritual presence that is not only all around us but also dwells within us. This spiritual truth goes beyond religion to touch our hearts, to spark our awareness of oneness, and to give us joy and enthusiasm for realizing our highest Self on a daily basis.

The Vedas, which are the spiritual and philosophical bedrock of Ayurvedic medicine, attest that the infinite and inexhaustible creative force has entered the creation and enlivens it with divine potential from within each form in the universe. Each of us can feel secure in this assurance that the divine truth exists within us. The Vedas tell us that each and every form, whether large or small, whether living or inanimate, is charged with the same divinity. This is why the supreme truth is sometimes known as *antaryami*, "the one who moves inside us." This truth is our innermost divine Self.

So this is all a great reason for offering blessings to oneself. Throughout the rest of this chapter and elsewhere in the book, I share some of my most beloved mantras, the mantras I learned in my family's home. The simplest of these mantras can be repeated by almost anyone.

Chanting Sanskrit mantras is a practice. In the beginning, you may have difficulty with it, especially with the obligations and distractions of modern life. With a little repetition, however, you will soon find that these mantras are emerging spontaneously in your heart and that invoking them transforms mundane life into something harmonious and sublime. Mantra vibrations can help you overcome any tendency toward repetitive thoughts and anxiety and can also help you become fully present to every moment of your day. Once you begin incorporating mantras, the most banal events will transform into self-affirming, self-honoring sacred rituals.

With the morning mantras, your intention and quality of consciousness—that is, whether you are connected with the meaning of what you are chanting—is more important than the diction itself. A perfect chant cannot replace a heartfelt, genuine sentiment. So do not hesitate to dive into these practices, even if the mantras are in a language that may not be familiar to you. Sanskrit is considered a divine language, and mantras are powerful utterances that deserve your wholehearted attention.

Daily Self-Affirmation

Ayurveda's lifestyle begins each day with an ancient ritual of positive affirmation. In my own traditional school, Vedika Global, over the last ten years, incoming students have reported a leap in their consciousness within days of learning this ritual of self-affirmation. These students thank me for the gifts they have received through this prayer, but I offer thanks to my teacher, Baba, who showed me the way.

At any time of day, a positive affirmation will raise our mental energy. When such a ritual is done during brahma muhurta, however, the rising sattva in the macrocosm mirrors its golden reflection in our own minds and tunnels a great pathway to the source of our very beings, connecting us to our divine potential.

 Through this morning ritual, Baba taught me how to access my inner divinity and its limitless powers. "Yes, little Shunya," Baba said to me, "the divine exists in the depths of your own being. Evoke it daily from the depths of your being through this ritual, and once connected with your inner divinity, recognize the same divinity in the Self of every being you encounter. Your day will be lit up with the light of a thousand suns by this recognition. Move through the living present with this constant divine awareness guiding you."

As I would chant the special mantra that accompanies this ritual, a little shiver would go up and down my spine. I was remembering, through this prayer, that the divine powers of the universe, known as Lakshmi, Saraswati, and Durga (the goddesses of abundance, wisdom, and personal power), dwell in my own being, literally accessible in the palms of my own hands. ✒

How to Perform the Ritual of Positive Affirmation

Bring your hands together and look at the palms with gentle focus. As you perform this action, repeat aloud or silently in your mind the following traditional Vedic mantra. Gaze first at your fingertips, contemplating that these are the divine abode of cosmic abundance. Then look at the hollow of your palms and acknowledge these as the abode of cosmic knowledge. Finally, pay attention to your wrists, acknowledging these as abodes of personal power emanating forth from your own heart.

TABLE 11   Mantra for Daily Self-Affirmation

Sanskrit Transliteration	Sounds Like
Karaagre vasate Lakshmi	kuar-AA-gre vasa-TEY Luck-SHMEE
Karamadhye Saraswati	kara-MADH-yai SARAS-watii
Karamoole sthita Gouri	kara-MOOLE sthi-TAA Gow-RII
Mangalam kara darshanam	MUM-galum kara DAR-shanum

Simple meaning: In the morning, I observe that at the tips of my fingers resides Goddess Lakshmi, in my palms resides Goddess Saraswati, and in my wrists is Goddess Gouri, or Durga.[5]

Deeper meaning: On my fingertips, dwells the divinity of abundance. With her blessings, I can create all forms of personal wealth for myself with ease. In the hollow of my palms dwells the divinity of knowledge and wisdom. I am literally holding all the knowledge I will ever need to be successful, balanced, and spiritually aligned with the highest truth. It all sits right here, in the hollow of my own palms. And the divinity of personal power, health, courage, and noble deeds dwells in the root of my hands (wrists). She is blessing me with infinite personal power. Through this chant, I am taking into account all my divine powers upon arising so that the rest of my day will be blessed and productive.

Thank Mother Earth

Ayurveda's oral tradition recommends chanting a hymn of gratitude to Mother Earth as soon as you first place your feet on the floor or shortly afterward. You can also chant this hymn at any time of the day, whenever you wish to connect with Earth as your cosmic parent. Through this ritual, you will be able to offer your love and respect to our living and breathing planet.

Ayurveda conceives a dynamic and animated model of our universe, where all objects, beings, events, phenomena, and experiences are interconnected and vitally linked to each other. In such a mutually interactive state of affairs, human will and human gratitude impact not only the immediate state of mind, but also the condition of the environment, and actually extend to influence the entire cosmos.

Most of us stumble out of bed, reach for our laptops or handheld devices, and make our way to the coffee machine with no consciousness of the Earth and the environment. By chanting this mantra the moment our toes first touch the floor, a unique intimacy of the Self with the universe begins to manifest. You are acknowledging the union of the Self with the universe. This sense of oneness ends the abuse and misuse that is possible from a perception of separation. The limited ego with its desire to exploit natural resources for its own selfish ends is submerged in the ocean of unity consciousness that makes us take care of a random rock from the river in the same way we would take care of our own bodies.

When this mantra becomes part of our daily lifestyle, we have the potential of becoming deeply respectful beings, dwelling in profound harmony with all of Earth and her creatures. This is true health, the universal health espoused by the sages of Ayurveda.

TABLE 12 **Mantra of Gratitude to Mother Earth**

Sanskrit Transliteration	Sounds Like
Samudra vasane Devi	samu-DRA vasa-NEY day-vi
Parvata stana mandale	PAR-vata stana MUN-duley
Vishnu patni namastubhyam	VISH-nu pat-NI na-MAS-tu-bhi-UM
Paada sparsham kshama-svame	PAA-da spar-SHUM sha-MA-sva-MAY

Simple meaning: (O Mother Earth) who has an ocean as her garment and mountains as her breasts, please pardon me for touching you with my feet.

Deeper meaning: Salutations to the Earth who is the fullness of Goddess Lakshmi, the deity of abundance, creativity, and fertility. As I rise to begin this day, please forgive me for touching you with the base of my feet. May I imbibe from you your humility and generosity.

 I heard this mantra repeatedly from the time I was a baby in my mother's lap. She would say it as she got up from her bed holding me. And I was uttering the mantra as a toddler in my baby voice. I loved the morning ritual of talking to Mother Earth and how she would respond by sending back some earthy blessings through my feet, reaching all the way up to the crown of my head. When I asked Baba about this, he did not reply, but the sparkle in his eyes told me everything I needed to know. I hope that you, too, will consider incorporating a morning practice that connects you with Mother Earth and, through her, to this entire magical, generous, and ever-abundant universe. ✦

The Gayatri Mantra—Sun Worship

The Gayatri mantra is known as the mother of all mantras and emerges from India from the *Rig-Veda*, the world's oldest body of spiritual knowledge.[6] The Gayatri mantra is actually known as the Savitri Mantra in the *Rig-Veda* and in Ayurvedic texts. It is typically chanted during brahma muhurta all over India today, especially on the banks of holy rivers. Baba and I would chant it together every morning.

The Gayatri mantra directly connects us to the power of the sun, which is sacred to nearly all indigenous peoples. In the Vedic tradition, the sun is a perceptible divine manifestation of celestial light, representing the infinite power, splendor, and magnitude of the supreme truth. Thus, Gayatri mantra connects us to the concealed spiritual reality that lies beyond the physical sun and is immanent in it yet transcendent to it.

The Gayatri mantra thus reveals to us the spiritual truth of our own interconnected existence, and the common spiritual presence that throbs and pulsates through everything and every heart, as its innermost underlying truth. In short, through the chanting of Gayatri mantra, our individual minds are immediately connected with the great universal truth.

By meditatively contemplating continuously on the rising sun through the chanting of the Gayatri mantra, we see revealed all the secrets of the Ultimate Reality that lie beyond human senses and human reasoning. And chanting it on a day-to-day basis purifies our thinking and emotions and plants seeds of greatness, courage, and nobility in our consciousness.

TABLE 13   **Gayatri Mantra to Connect to the Sun**

Sanskrit Transliteration	Sounds Like
OM	OM
bhur bhuvah svaha	bhoor bhu-VAH sva-HA
tat savitur varenyam	tut savi-TOR vare-NYUM
bhargo devasya dhii mahi	bhara-GO DEVA-asya DHI mahi
dhiiyo yo nah pracodayaat	DHI-yo yoo NAH pracho-da-YAT

Simple meaning: We meditate on that sacred, effulgent Sun God that activates all our intellects.

Deeper meaning: We meditate on the spiritual effulgence of that absolute, supreme Ultimate Reality, the source or projector of the three phenomenal experiential planes of existence: the gross, the subtle, and the causal, while it itself remains unchanged. May that limitless, nameless, formless supreme truth (worshipped through the manifest Sun God) guide our intelligence so that we, too, realize the state of supreme truth.

My own life has been blessed with the Gayatri mantra from childhood. Every brahma muhurta (except when it was raining), I would walk to River Sarayu holding Baba's hand firmly. Five warmhearted street dogs named Bhura, Kalu, Lali, Munna, and Chottu would always accompany us as we walked in total silence. We must have looked like a formal procession.

I remember being intently focused on each step, treading swiftly yet softly. This was because Baba told me that all the grass on our path was actually a colony of people like us, just in different bodysuits. I would focus on being extra gentle so as not to disturb the "grass people."

For a short part of our journey, Baba and I traveled on a *tanga*, a small horse-driven carriage that is still used in some smaller towns in India today. We rode the tanga to the *ghat* (riverbank), with the procession of dog friends trailing excitedly behind us and our sweet horse galloping along like a happy breeze, as if in a hurry to greet the sun himself.

Upon arriving at the river, when I got down from the tanga, I would slow my steps in sheer admiration. River Sarayu was always alive. Her immenseness and grandness never ceased to captivate me.

Baba would enter the river, wading in much farther than I. He would cup his hands to hold water and raise them to the east. He would then chant our lineage mantra, the Gayatri mantra.

I always heard the river chanting the mantra back; only the river's voice was booming and thunderous, while Baba's voice was quiet and filled with reverence. I, too, would raise my own little cupped palms, filled with water, look toward the eastern sky, as Baba had taught me to do, and chant.

Before I could even speak, Baba taught me the Gayatri mantra by chanting it to me repeatedly. I knew the mantra in my mind even before I could utter the sounds. Though I lived inside a toddler's body then, he said I was still as wise as the whole universe, as that is the true nature of the Self.

On many mornings, as I chanted the Gayatri mantra by River Sarayu, I noticed how the sky seemed to stoop in closer to hear me, as did the Earth and wind. I felt so blessed to be awake at this hour. I knew that God knew little Shunya was wide awake. ✒

How to Perform Sun Prayers

Do this beautiful spiritual ritual outside on days when weather permits. Each time you perform it, you will be filled with spiritual power. If you live near a body of water, perform the ritual beside the water, or even better, wade into the water.

1. Fill a clay or copper cup with water. Be sure to set aside a cup just for your sun worship ritual. Do not use it for eating or drinking.

2. Go outside and face east, the direction of the rising sun.

3. Raise your hands above your head and, with both hands holding the cup, slowly and reverently pour water downward to the Earth below.

4. Keep your gaze turned upward toward the open sky, where the sun is about to rise.

5. As you pour water from the vessel, you can, if you wish, chant the Gayatri mantra, or you can simply chant OM throughout.

You can shower or bathe either before the spiritual ritual or afterward. In India, when this ritual is performed immersed in a body of water, such as in the Ganges River, that takes care of bathing. Many people, however, also choose to return home and take a full shower. For tips on Ayurvedic bathing and a special pre-bath massage ritual, see chapter 5.

Other Mindfulness Practices for Brahma Muhurta

Once you have recited mantras, you can undertake asanas (yoga postures) and pranayama (breathing exercises). The order in which you perform these is up to you, but ideally, poses are done first, followed by pranayama, and lastly meditation. Whatever the order, however, these must be performed on an empty stomach, preferably before breakfast.

Surya Namaskar (Sun Salutation)

The yoga postures I most heartily recommend is an asana series known as the sun salutation (surya namaskar), with accompanying chants. These practices have been passed down through many generations and have been finely tuned to be most effective during brahma muhurta. The sun salutation benefits all doshas.

The sun salutation is a spiritual ritual and not simply a set of physical exercises. Though it is rarely taught in this way in modern hatha yoga classes, I feel it is important that you learn and understand the meaning of the twelve chants that accompany the twelve postures in sun salutation. Each of these twelve chants connects you ever more deeply with the power of the cosmos that radiates through the sun. As you synchronize your breath perfectly with each chant and posture, your entire being will come alive with energy and spiritual joy.

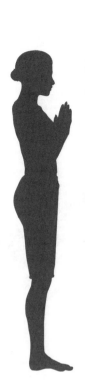

ॐ मित्राय नमः

om mitrāya namaḥ

Prostration to Him who is affectionate to all.

ॐ रवये नमः

om ravaye namaḥ

Prostration to Him who is the cause for change.

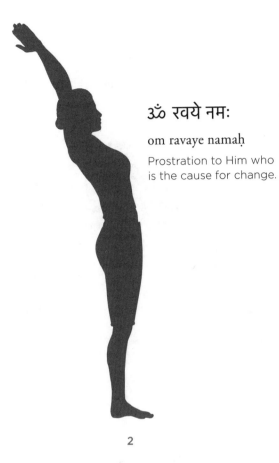

1

2

ॐ सूर्याय नमः

om suryāyā namaḥ

Prostration to Him who induces activity.

ॐ भानवे नमः

om bhānave namaḥ

Prostration to Him who diffuses Light.

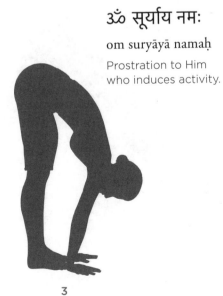

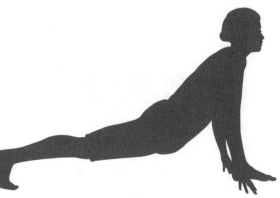

3

4

ॐ खगाय नमः

om khagaya namaḥ

Prostration to Him
who moves in the sky.

ॐ पूष्णे नमः

om pūṣṇe namaḥ

Prostration to Him
who nourishes all.

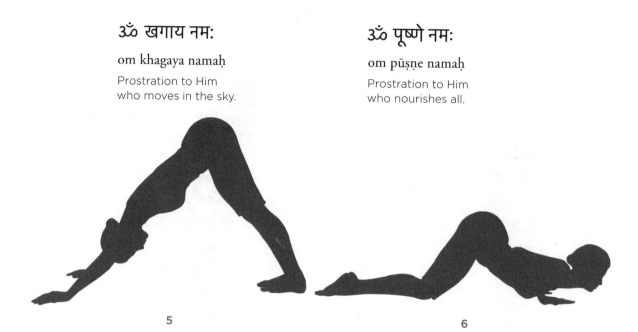

5

6

ॐ हिरण्यगर्भाय नमः

om hiraṇyagarbhāya namaḥ

Prostration to Him who
contains everything.

ॐ मरिचये नमः

om marīcaye namaḥ

Prostration to Him
who possesses rays.

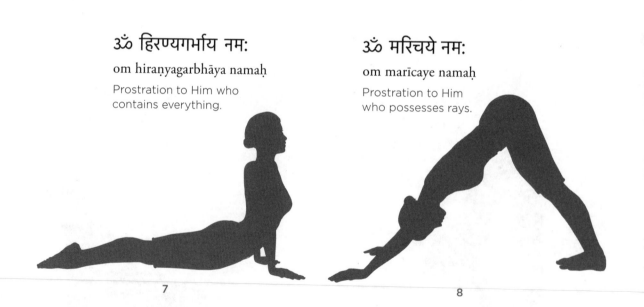

7

8

ॐ आदित्याय नमः

om ādityāya namaḥ

Prostration to Him
who is God of gods.

ॐ सावित्रे नमः

om savitre namaḥ

Prostration to Him who
produces everything.

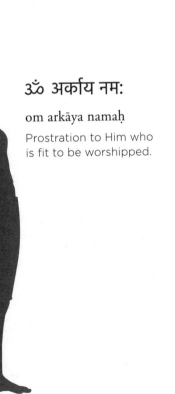

9

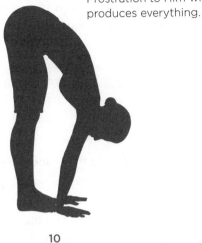

10

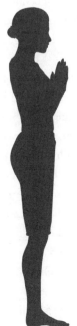

ॐ अर्काय नमः

om arkāya namaḥ

Prostration to Him who
is fit to be worshipped.

ॐ भास्कराय नमः

om bhāskarāya namaḥ

Prostration to Him who
is the cause of luster.

11

12

Pranayama (Breathing Practices)

In the Ayurvedic tradition, *prana* is the life-sustaining force that pervades all living organisms. This life force flows through the body along a series of channels known as *nadis*. As the prana quantity and quality ebbs and flows, it impacts the general health and the quality of the mind and consciousness. In fact, prana is critical to life itself. We are alive only as long as prana continues working inside us. The moment the prana stops working, we die. When our prana becomes unbalanced, we fall sick. This imbalance can be corrected through the conscious practice of an ancient process called pranayama, which—because *prana* is also defined as "breath"—means "prana expansion through deliberate breathing exercise."

 One spring morning many years ago, when the weather in Ayodhya was particularly sweet, and the air was filled with smells of springtime and sounds of the river, Baba taught me pranayama by the banks of the river.

"Breathe in deeply, all the way to your belly," Baba instructed. "Prana is divine, invisible healing energy that is always around us. But, at special times of the day, like at brahma muhurta, you can breathe it in effortlessly. As prana enters your body, it makes you healthy, and you will feel especially happy for no reason."

That day, I understood that at brahma muhurta, the universe is charged with sattva as well as prana. At that divine time of day, the universe generously gives prana away to anyone who cares to be awake during this cosmic event and breathes it in deeply and mindfully. This time of the morning is like a prana buffet. The question is: Are you up and ready to enjoy it?

As a little girl, I loved imagining and experimenting with closing my eyes and breathing in all this divine prana into my entire being. I liked how my body felt light and energized from head to toe. I liked how, when I exhaled, my breath would make the flowers bloom in the garden and my mother look less tired with her daily chores. I felt I was having a supernatural effect on my immediate environment, and I sent people I loved all this prana I had inside me. Baba said, "Why not? So be it." ✒

It is important to craft a daily discipline of pranayama. One type of pranayama that has an especially wonderful and transformative impact on us during brahma muhurta is humming bee breathing, which I describe below. Other types of breathing exercises—and there are many—along with some dos and don'ts for creating a stable pranayama practice, are discussed in other chapters. I hope you will be inspired to dedicate some time for your pranayama practice right after waking up at brahma muhurta.

Humming Bee Breathing

The timeless practice known as *brahmari pranayama* is what, for obvious reasons, I call humming bee breathing. There are numerous benefits of this pranayama, especially when it is done in brahma muhurta. Instantaneously, the rajas and tamas in your mind will be replaced by sattva. Any anxiety will end. All your senses will become rested and rejuvenated. As for the rest of the benefits, simply do it and know for yourself.

To do this, simply sit in a comfortable posture or on a meditation cushion with your spine softly erect. You can also sit on a chair with legs uncrossed. The hands can be in *jnana mudra* to begin, as shown in the box, "Jnana Mudra (Wisdom Seal)."

Close the eyes and relax the whole body for a minute or so by breathing normally. Now raise both arms and bring them toward your ears. With the index or middle finger of each hand, plug your ears gently. If you wish, you could press the flaps of your ears over the opening without inserting the fingers. Now, bring your attention to the midpoint between your eyebrows. This is the place of the *ajna* chakra. Breathe in deeply, inhaling through the nose. Then breathe out through the nose, making

Jnana Mudra (Wisdom Seal)

The Sanskrit word *mudra* means "seal"; a mudra is a means in hatha yoga to hold in prana so that it doesn't leak out. The jnana (wisdom) mudra is associated with meditation.

To do it, touch the tip of the forefinger to the tip of the thumb so that the finger and thumb form a complete circle. Continue in this position for the full duration of your meditation. This hand gesture increases inner focus and calms the mind.

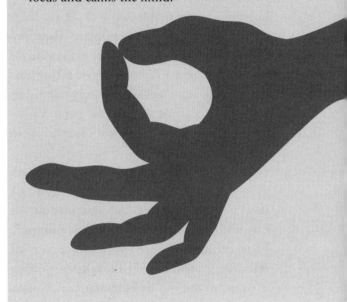

a humming sound like the buzzing of a bee (OMMMMMMMM). Exhale slowly, smoothly, and in a controlled manner while making this deep, steady humming sound. There is no requirement to raise your pitch. This completes one round. The inhalation and exhalation should be smooth and controlled.

Continue, performing at least three rounds of breath—or longer, if you wish.

After a while, you may notice that not only your skull but your entire body is reverberating with the humming sound. In reality, cosmic energy, or prana, is flowing through your entire being. The body becomes like a live wire conducting prana electricity. There are no contraindications. The only side effect is health and happiness!

Surya Dhyanam (Sun Meditation)

One form of meditation Baba taught me was called *surya dhyanam*, or "sun meditation." This is an original spiritual practice within my lineage. It's very simple and will fill you with delight. To perform it, sit in a place where you can be alone, with a view of the eastern sky. If you do not have a direct view, sit facing that direction in any quiet spot inside your house. Sit upright, do not slouch, and remind yourself that you are sitting down consciously to conduct a spiritual ritual.

With your eyes closed, observe your breath in its natural state for a few moments. As you slowly inhale, imagine the sun sending its first rays into your being through your breath. Then, exhale slowly. Do not rush. Repeat until your entire body feels as though it's glowing like the sun and you are humming with golden, sattvic energy.

With your eyes still closed, do a scan of your body, as if you were observing your body from the inside. Observe what you're feeling in your body without trying to make any changes in it. Start at your toes and work your way up the entire body to the scalp, noticing whatever is going on in your body. Be aware of places you're tight, loose, or neutral. Send each part of your body light and radiance. Let each part light up from inside, as you turn your attention to it. Soon your entire being will be glowing with the light of the sun, from inside.

Thoughts may arise. Notice these thoughts. Know that you are the pure, neutral subject observing the thoughts in your mind. You are not questioning, editing, criticizing, or controlling your thinking. You are observing your thoughts without judgment. Continue this as long as you can. As the thoughts become quiet, turn the focus of your attention inward and begin observing the "observer," the one who is watching, the true Self. Your Self is the witness that shines like the sun in your heart.

After a while, you will encounter a silence. This is not a negative silence. It's not what is left in the absence of physical speech. It is a positive silence because it is the womb of all speech. In this silence, there is nothing missing. It is a state of fullness. After dwelling in this supreme solitude for some time, you will naturally emerge. Your ears will begin to pick up sounds from the world around you. The thoughts in your mind will no longer seem to be miles away. Allow yourself to slowly emerge from deeper layers of your being that lie beyond your mind, coming back to the superficial mind and its everyday consciousness. When you are ready, open your eyes and slowly integrate back into the world. Each time you meditate, keep it simple, heartfelt, and truly inspirational!

Atmabodha Meditation: My Lineage Practice

There is another form of meditation I want to impart here, the *Atmabodha dhyanam* that is one of the primary practices of my *parampara* (lineage). The word *Atmabodha* means "awakening to the truth of our spiritual nature," also known as "self-realization" in English.

When I was a child, Baba and I often sat by the bank of River Sarayu to meditate. Baba told me that meditation is simply being one with our own highest Self, without paying heed to anything else.

Filled with anticipation, I would leap into Baba's lap, unmindful of his posture of contemplation on the riverbank. Baba would immediately make room for my little body and snuggle me into his warm blanket so I could sit for meditation with him.

The stillness of Baba's body, the silent music of his breath, and the peacefulness of his being would then envelop me with a different kind of blanket. Soon, all I could hear was the river.

Baba's face, body, skin (which was translucent, since it was always exuding so much inner light), slim wrists (though he could carry such heavy weight), and long, bony, slender fingers (which became extremely gentle when he patted the head of a suffering person) were all familiar to me. Baba's blanket was also something I had nuzzled into, by now, at least a thousand times since birth.

Yet, within the familiarity of Baba's body and blanket was now an unfamiliar Baba, a deeply special and almost changed Baba. This was a Baba who did not seem to hear, speak, touch, smell, or see, yet seemed to be fully present and apparently one and the same with me, River Sarayu, the river rocks, all the big and small river creatures, the sweetly blowing wind, and the spreading rays of the sun. Everything and everyone meditated alongside Baba, or so it felt to my seven-year-old self. ✒

These meditation moments were my first-ever lessons in sweetly dwelling with the Self, in what Baba called Atmabodha dhyanam, which means "meditation (*dhyanam*) to know (*bodha*) one's own higher Self (*Atman*)."

I have never resonated with an intellectual approach to meditation, one that requires me to explain what happens in the brain and neural circuits. My way of teaching meditation is to lead you down a path from the heart. Meditation is simple, and I feel that we should keep it simple. Jargon can only complicate the experience of meditation, which is essentially being in touch with your true nature, your natural state of being.

You can enter into the state of meditation any time you have a few moments to be with your own Self. As a matter of common sense, you won't want to meditate while you're driving a car or conducting—or even just attending—a business meeting. But you certainly can meditate after parking your car or once the meeting has ended. You don't need any of the rituals or paraphernalia associated with meditation. You don't need incense and altars and special silk pillows for meditation. Nor do you need to be religious, vegetarian, or least of all, Hindu or Buddhist.

You need to be with yourself for a period of uninterrupted quality time. That is all. To begin,

I think a five-minute slot is great, but even three minutes or just one minute will do. Gradually, you will find yourself wanting to meditate more often and longer. The people around you may think you are resting, contemplating, or being moody. You, however, will know that you are meditating. You have dropped in—inside—to say hi to your own abidingly beautiful, blissful, and peaceful Self.

Don't get me wrong. You *can* have the trappings. If you have a meditation altar or a meditation room or a meditation garden in your backyard, that is wonderful. But don't worry if you don't. Any clean corner of your home or room will do. Welcome to the bare bones meditation tradition I grew up with and that I now teach!

As a child, I meditated all the time and everywhere: atop trees, inside lotus ponds (where we plucked lotus for Mother), beside rushing rivers, on my bed (before sleeping and upon awakening). When I was ten, I even meditated next to my mother's body as it lay cold and inert because her Self had that day accomplished the final act of meditation and merged with the universal Self.

To begin meditation, simply ensure that you are sitting comfortably, either on a cushion or a chair. You may close your eyes so you are not distracted. Then take a few moments to relax your body and mind. Make sure that you are sitting comfortably, with your spine gently erect. Rest your hands loosely in your lap and fold your fingers in jnana mudra, wisdom seal (refer back to the box on page 79). Or simply place them gently on top of each other with the palms facing upward.

Now breathe normally and allow yourself to relax. You will know that you are relaxed when you begin to lose awareness of your body. Your body will not be rigid nor your muscles tight. Everything will begin to feel soft.

I define meditation as "awakening to the truth of our spiritual nature." I remember my Baba telling me that by meditating, I am making an appointment to meet my own spiritual Self. I remember this when I sit to meditate.

I also remember certain affirmations. Here are some to help you embrace meditation. Read through the words I suggest below a couple of times. Then allow them to become thoughts and allow these thoughts to lead you into a deep inner silence.

I am opening a door to the center of my being.
Deep inside my being dwells a silent presence,
My true Self
I acknowledge this presence as my divine Self
I AM
Stillness, Peace, Tranquility.
I AM
Limitless Existence, Infinite Knowledge,
Unbounded Bliss.

These meditation-initiating thoughts will enable you to rest in your witness consciousness mode.

Words can help a great deal to take us to the state beyond words. In meditation, we find that our thoughts may come and go, but we are at peace because we are witnessing those thoughts from a distance; we not participating with our thoughts; we are not identifying with them.

Atmabodha Meditation is based on Vedanta, the ancient science of Self. The philosophy is founded on the premise that you are not your day-to-day personality, but merely its witness, its observer. Whatever you can observe—your breath, your body, and your mind and its thoughts, ideas, beliefs, memories, opinions—you are not that. There is a difference between the observer and what is observed.

"May it be known, Shunya," said Baba, "you are the source of consciousness, not the objects illumined in consciousness. You are the witness alone. Know it that you are Sakshi Chaitanyam; *Sakshi* is the nonjudging, nonparticipating, unattached witness, and *Chaitanyam* refers to the Self, which is pure consciousness. Pure awareness is the invisible background in which everything arises. Like a cloudless sky, it has no form. It is eternal space; it is infinite stillness; it is the essence of being. Objects appear, exist, and disappear in awareness, yet this awareness, the Self, remains unchanged. Know you are not the breath, the mind, the body identified in a personal story of planet, race, gender, age, class, religion, family, profession, sorrows, and joy. All this, your personality with all its labels, dissolves in the presence of the sheer awareness of the divine Self that you are.

"Set your personality aside, Shunya, and sit in your own divine awareness."

I heard this great call from master to disciple, and I followed it. Again and again I dwelled in my own divine awareness, until the great, indescribable, absolute spiritual presence beyond conceptions and perceptions revealed itself to me. "You are that divine presence, which eyes cannot see and which words cannot describe," Baba said to me. "You are pure spirit, none other."

"Yes, I am that, the indescribable Self," I said to him quietly and without an iota of doubt. ✐

If you wish, try these lines of thought during meditation:

This body, I witness; therefore, this body, I am not. I am the witness alone.

Ask yourself: *Am I the body?* Spend some time observing this material container called body, in which your awareness appears to dwell. Observe your own body. The observer is always different from that which is observed.

This mind and its contents I witness; therefore, this mind, I am not. I am the witness alone.

Ask yourself: *Am I the mind?* Spend some moments observing your mind, watching the mental events—the feelings, thoughts, perceptions, memories, ideas, sorrow, pleasure, fear, anger, grief, excitement, and all such emotions. Are you the mind? The observer is always different from that which is observed. You witness the mind; therefore, the mind you are not. Your mind may be jumping around like a monkey. So let it jump around. With knowledge that you are not what you observe, you can view the monkey mind with dispassion. And then you can shift your attention. Becoming aware of the observer, you may note a whole different silent presence within, the infinite, indivisible, inexhaustible, spiritual Self. This encounter with the Self is known as Atmabodha (Self-knowing).

This is the true meditation from the sages, known as dhyanam, or attention to what is truth (spirit) and to not what appears like truth (mind). Imagine if we were trying to control a battery-run flashlight. We wonder to ourselves: *Why is it flickering so much? Why is it coming on so strong? Why can't it be this way or that?* And we fidget with it. And then suddenly we become aware of a sun, with the light of million galaxies, shining right inside us. Does the silly flashlight and its peculiarities matter anymore? Treat the mind like a mere instrument or tool. Our true concern with meditation is whose instrument it is.

Until you are aware of the Self, a divine presence within, it is only an academic concept, and you mostly experience darkness, fear, anger, and restlessness in your inner world. And then, with the help of knowledge such as what I am providing through the pages of this book, you begin to—first intellectually and then emotionally and then, finally, with full conviction and experience—identify with your true Self; you will experience a natural resolution in all your sufferings—of body and mind. You would have experienced God because that is what you are.

Baba told me that in reality there is no sin, no hell to fear, and no heaven to yearn for. Rather, each moment here on Earth is an opportunity to use our free will and perhaps make a momentous discovery of inner divinity, the Self. As previously mentioned, the discovery of the inner unbounded, all-powerful Self is known as self-realization in English and Atmabodha in the sage tradition. This Sanskrit word literally refers to that moment in which our fragile ego self-encounters our indestructible, unlimited, all-powerful Self within, from beyond the mind.

The human who was seeking and searching for God here and there comes home to the God dwelling within. This is a momentous experience.

The transcendent practice of Atmabodha Meditation will have a beneficial impact on your mind and body. Anyone who practices meditation in this way will find that this single lifestyle choice is the greatest possible propeller of positive change. It can fill you with joy and renewed abilities.

Throughout this chapter, I have been asking you to be physically present to witness the actual phenomena of the rising sun. This will change your consciousness. Why does the mere viewing of gigantic ball of fire do that? Technically speaking, the sun is nothing more than a gaseous mass aflame in the sky. But here we are stepping away from the rational world, with its measurable parameters, into the realm of spirit, where we may witness the emergence of an inner sun gifting us inner radiance and inner illumination.

So I implore you to entertain the idea of a pure, splendid, eternally healthy Self present within you, in spite of any health challenges you may have, in spite of any problems you may experience with your mind and your moods. This Self is your friend, and if you are willing to connect with it, your guide. You can access the Self through meditation—not after long years of practice, but immediately, right now, within minutes! Once you have connected with the Self, you will benefit all the more from Ayurveda lifestyle wisdom. This is, in fact, the way I teach: through my soul, from a script of fierce spiritual living, ignited with vivid moments of personal transformation.

As you begin to meditate, you may simply spend a moment with yourself. Do that. You may feel directed to place a hand on your heart.

That may be enough. Do not be surprised if what comes up initially does not feel like peace or enlightenment but rather a sadness or an awareness of ways you betray your own Self by accepting feelings of shame, guilt, or powerlessness. Accept this insight. It too is a gift to you from the Self.

As you continue to meditate, the self-delusions and games your mind can play on you will lie exposed every morning. But when you keep returning to the center of your being, these difficult reality checks will be replaced by knowledge, insight, wisdom, and unconditional love. Claim it. This is yours. It's who you truly are, your own joyful Self.

If I had not touched my own authentic Self through awakening early and meditating daily, my life as I know today, as a source of inspiration and comfort to many, and this book could not have manifested. I thank my Self and rest, always, in its infinite grace. And I invite you to claim this same freedom by awakening in brahma muhurta and then evoking the Self through my teachings on Atmabodha Meditation. Let me reassure you. The Self is true—it is truth—and it does not require much digging around for you to encounter it. Look for it in the ways I suggest, and you will meet it face-to-face—Atmabodha.

My Own Little Rebellion

My family has been following the tenets of Ayurveda lifestyle every day for the last several hundred years. As a child, I would happily follow along with the routines my elders set. As a preteen and teenager, however, coming into my own sense of life, I sometimes resisted the routine of waking up early, especially on school holidays. In my adolescence, I challenged many

things I had taken for granted as a child. My elders dissolved this youthful angst quite efficiently, not by lecturing or forcing me into compliance, but by continuing to be cheerful role models.

During my childhood, my mother always woke up very early. As she went about her morning chores, she would croon songs and ancient verses, collectively known in India as *hitopadesha*. These songs, sung in my mother's sweet voice, were brimming with life wisdom and were subtly planting seeds in me to always wake up early, to not give in to the temptations of laziness and self-indulgence.

Some days in my teens, I languished in bed well past 7:00 a.m., my body curled up in defiance, my eyes tightly shut. My conscience, meanwhile, was fully awake, and I now feel was watching me with dry amusement, asking, "Are we really going to sleep in? Why are we doing this? It is becoming tedious already!" I wondered if my beloved grandfather, Baba, was waiting for me at the banks of River Sarayu, peacefully performing sacred rituals, meditating, and meeting with his devotees.

As I lay in bed, my family was awake, my beloved animals were moving about, and I could hear Baba's students (*shishyas*) chanting mantras. For several years at a time, my grandfather's students lived at our home to study and apprentice with him. In the early mornings, they were always chanting a section of the *Rig-Veda* or some Upanishad that was to be committed to memory.

These chants reverberated throughout my home, setting into motion energizing vibrations. The mantras invigorated my tamas and soothed my rajas, clearing the way for my natural sattva. On the days when I heard Baba leading a new chant, his powerful, peaceful voice would enter my ears and pierce my heart. When such chanting as this was happening, how could I stay in bed with my eyes shut?

Baba never said a word to me on the subject of my sleeping in. Perhaps he understood that it was merely a phase I needed to go through in order to fully own this knowledge. Fortunately, Baba and my higher Self were both wiser than my noncompliant teenage mind.

Hence, I soon cast off the desire to prove some trivial point by sleeping late and returned to those blessed early morning practices.

Forty years later, as I write these words from my home in California, the memory of my adolescent rebellion brings a smile to my face and mist to my eyes. Now I wake up gently, with ease, and at the right time; I have no distress, confusion, or questions in my mind about the importance of rising in the brahma muhurta. Sometimes, I feel that the golden-lit sky is gently crooning my mother's morning songs. One of these translates roughly in this way:

Wake up, O Traveler,
Dawn has broken into the sky.
Where is the night that you still continue
to sleep?
The one who sleeps
Loses out on every type of wealth.
The one who is awake
is the one who receives the wealth
worth receiving.

In this song, it's understood that we are the traveler, the ones who have gone through many lifetimes; the "sky" is the infinite space of our own minds, "night" is our illusions and lazy indulgences, and "wealth" includes not only material abundance but also good health and spiritual wisdom.

My mother's morning wake-up song planted questions in my consciousness, and I, at the age of nine, took these questions to my grandfather.

 In our community, Baba was an important person, sought after by hundreds of people every day for both spiritual guidance and Ayurvedic medicine. So I naturally felt he was the best person to ask about this so-called "wealth" that I would potentially stand to lose if I were to remain asleep each morning.

Baba looked at me very seriously and chanted a sentence in Sanskrit: *sharira madhayam khalu dharma sadhanam.* He then explained the phrase, saying that we inhabit only one body in each lifetime and that we must use this body not only to fulfill our desires but also to serve others. This God-given body is a divine instrument for each soul's worldly and spiritual aspirations. For this reason, it is important for us to take care of the physical body with mindfulness and regard for natural laws. ✒

Blessings from the Sun

By waking before sunrise, you take charge of your life. As the sun rises in the macrocosm, you will experience a sun of pure consciousness manifesting within your own being. This inner sun will fill you with power, and you will find yourself able to meet your material, relationship, social, and professional goals with abundant clarity, vitality, and joy. You may find that you have more and more energy for yourself, as well as for others, as you increasingly become a gift to this universe.

Ultimately, I honor the sages who have given us Ayurveda. True well-being dwells within each one of us, enfolded like a fresh bud, ready to awaken, awaiting the morning of wisdom and the magical rays of sweet sunlight. Allow this bud to open, petal by petal, and intoxicate you with the pure bliss of your own existence.

A good morning to you. A very good morning!

CHAPTER 3

The Importance of Elimination

As I was growing up, Baba told me many times that the Vedic concept of internal and external purity (*shoucham*) was important in the journey of Self-realization. Nowhere does the concept of purity come to life more concretely than in the science of Ayurveda. In the physical realm, Ayurveda is a perfect mirror of the inspiring and transcendent Vedic ideal of purity.

Decades later, I find myself echoing Baba in so many ways. Though I now live halfway around the world from India, I hear myself explain again and again to my earnest students that by not waking up on time, they will not only miss out on the predawn sattva I talk about in chapter 2, they will also delay elimination of the impurities the body has gathered overnight. This delay of a bowel movement may seem minor in the larger scheme of things, but starting late each day drags the body down, bit by bit.

Ayurveda underscores the importance of physical purification, especially through the regular elimination of the body's wastes. To ensure this daily physical cleansing, elimination must happen without fail every twenty-four hours. To help maintain this balance, the Ayurveda system of health and healing recommends following a particular diet, doing special types of detoxes when needed, and further cleansing the digestive system with spices, home remedies, and herbal medicines—but only if needed.

Biological wastes (urine and feces) must leave the body. It is a natural law, and a law is something that must be followed. If we do not uphold this law, we leave poison in our bodies, and this poison will, sooner or later, take the form of serious disease—an incurable and untreatable disease. If you wish to avoid disease, then as soon as you wake up, you must attempt to purify your body through a regular elimination practice. Remember, the sooner you wake up, the easier it will be to let go of whatever needs to be eliminated!

Sadly, many people wake early now not because they feel excited to greet the sun and naturally purify themselves but because they must get to work early or because they have to make a long, dreadful commute. On the days these people don't have to report to work, sleeping in late feels like something they've earned, waking up whenever they please is a respite from their daily grind. Natural laws, however, do not take into account a person's reasons for breaking them.

There are students who have come long distances to study with me and wonder, *So, this is it? I've come all this way just to hear that I have to use the toilet on time? All creatures go. What's the big deal?*

It *is* a big deal. That is why I am dedicating this entire chapter to the practice of eliminating physical waste. I call it a *practice* because I am not describing elimination of waste merely as an urge. Due to our busy lives, many of us have learned to suppress our urges. We must now learn to be disciplined in them and to *practice* purifying ourselves in the Ayurvedic way. Many of my students, after learning first-hand about the importance of elimination, will not eat a morsel of food unless and until they have had a good bowel movement.

The Best Prescription: A Natural Way of Life

One student I will never forget had read deeply on Hindu and Buddhist philosophy, chanted mantras, and meditated several hours a day while studying to become an Ayurveda *vaidya* (healer). This man came into Vedika Global's volunteer-run clinic with some problems: his skin was prone to rashes, and he was prone to depression. I understood why when he informed us that he eliminated only once a week, if that.

This man also said that he had an inability to "feel the bliss." Despite his daily spiritual practice and his understanding of bliss on an intellectual level, he wasn't doing the physical practice he needed. His physical body was filled with toxins that kept him from experiencing the bliss that was, clearly, within him.

As I listened to this student, Baba's teaching came rushing back to me: the body and mind are intricately connected. They must be purified simultaneously. If you purify just one, the other will inevitably pull it down. Without tending to both mind and body, you will have no real transformation in your life experience.

This is the kind of message I heard Baba give again and again to those who sought his advice. One man who came to see Baba was suffering from hemorrhoids, a colon condition that developed from his chronic constipation, which responded completely to my grandfather's surprising prescription.

 This prosperous middle-aged man arrived in a new and expensive car that he had driven all the way from Jaipur, almost five hundred miles away—a long road trip in the India of the 1970s. He joined the queue to see Baba, his face a study of physical discomfort. He could not even sit peacefully. When it was his turn to speak to Baba, this man said in a lowered, almost embarrassed voice that he was suffering from painful piles—hemorrhoids that have become inflamed. Piles can cause sharp, severe pain in the rectum, as if you're carrying a nail there.

This man had visited various doctors and had taken every medicine suggested, even Ayurvedic medicine. When he heard about Baba, he drove to Ayodhya as fast as Indian road conditions (and his sore bottom) would allow.

Baba told the man he would help him. "But first," he said, "you have to give something to me." The man looked relieved. It is customary in India to make holy men gifts of money or land, and he obviously had the wherewithal to do this. Little did he know that Baba had never in his life asked for a single rupee, that his work was wholly motivated by his compassion for all living beings, whom he served selflessly day and night.

"This is what I want from you," Baba told the man. "Go home, and on half of your land, instead of cash crops, grow *aparajita*." This is a common garden plant, a fast-growing climber known as the butterfly pea, or *Clitoria ternatea*.

Butterfly pea is well-known in traditional Ayurvedic medicine and has been used for centuries as a mind tonic. It enhances memory, reduces stress (acting as an antidepressant), and normalizes sleep patterns. And it was obvious, even to a child like me, that stress relief was what this man needed. His face had a pained expression, and his eyes had lost their light.

Butterfly pea also has anti-inflammatory, analgesic, and local anesthetic properties and is used by Ayurvedic healers specifically to control the bleeding and pain of hemorrhoids. Dozens of scientific studies have now confirmed its efficacy in hemorrhoids. In such treatment, the piles are cleaned with the decoction of the whole dry plant (root to seeds), and a fresh paste made from the dried plant is applied over the area to relieve pain and staunch the flow of blood.

I expected Baba to tell this man how to prepare and use the herb, but to my surprise, he did not. He said, "Do not consume any of the herbs yourself. Do not even taste it. The medicine must all be given away. That will be my *dakshina*." *Dakshina* is a Sanskrit term to describe the offerings made to holy men not in payment but in gratitude.

My grandfather did, however, give this man specific directions regarding the changes in his lifestyle. "You must spend two to four hours in the fields every day, digging and hoeing—get your hands dirty as you grow this beautiful flower. Spend time in Nature. Let your garden be filled with butterfly blessings."

Then, Baba gave the instructions that made the greatest change in this man's life: "Take a one-year break from your business pursuits. Live in your farmhouse, either with your family or—even better—alone. Spend time with your animals, especially your cows; take care of them. Keep your life simple.

Wake up with the sun and go to bed with the sun. Consider this a one-year retirement."

Baba told the man to continue planting and harvesting the butterfly pea through the year. Several crops of this herb will mature in that time, as they blossom from seed within five weeks. Baba told him to dry the plants in the sun and then grind them—root, stem, flowers, leaves, and seeds—into a fine powder. "Bring me the powder," Baba said, "and I will make sure it is distributed to the poor people who cannot afford to buy medicine."

The man looked confused. "But if I don't use this medicine myself, then how will I get better?"

"Giving this herb to those who are sick and have no resources will, itself, be your medicine," Baba responded with such finality in his voice that it seemed to put an end to questions. Then Baba turned to give his attention to the next person who was waiting.

One year later, this man returned, and this time, he was smiling. He looked happy and younger; he had lost weight. His arms were loaded with sacks of butterfly pea powder, and his wife and two daughters, who also had big smiles on their faces, carried marigold garlands and sweets.

"I am healed," the man reported with childlike glee. Baba nodded his head, looked at the man with compassion pouring forth from his eyes, and blessed him quietly by repeating a mantra under his breath. This man, who had been so ill, touched Baba's feet, which is, in India, a deeply traditional demonstration of reverence and gratitude.

Later, Baba told his students that hemorrhoids are a complication of constipation, with mental stress as the cause in hard-to-cure cases. For this reason, it was important, first and foremost, to relieve this man of his stress by eliminating the root of his problem—preoccupation with himself and his business.

Taking time to relax healed him. By living in Nature, following the sun's course through the sky, and eating seasonal food, this man was living the true Ayurvedic prescription. The body is a self-healing entity; our job is to provide it the right environment and to change our behaviors so that they work in harmony with, rather than in opposition to, Nature. Health will blossom if you plant the right seeds and tend them in the right way. Contrary to popular belief, regaining your health can actually be a simple and straightforward matter. ✒

Indeed, my Baba declared the spiritual truth that our health is intricately and ceaselessly bound up with our whole life. Therefore, in order to reclaim the health of our bodies and minds, restoring well-being and balance to our entire lives is necessary.

Looking back, sometimes I am amazed at how bold Baba was with people who sought his advice. As a spiritually inspired healer, he worked not to merely pacify the patient, not to provide yet another herbal medicine. He clearly wanted to end the patient's suffering by alleviating the patient's ignorance. Baba invited his patients to join him at a level of higher consciousness—where anything is possible.

Baba's prescription to the stressed man to take a break from the very lifestyle that was giving him disease and to rest and nurture his mind with fresh air, the sun, and the moon was truly a prescription for restoring life.

As for the other part of Baba's prescription, I never asked him why he told the man with hemorrhoids to give away the healing herbs he had grown. It wasn't for many years that I understood. At that point, I was studying the Hindu scripture Bhagavad Gita at Baba's feet, chanting it in a group every morning with his other students, and then intently listening to his explanation of each verse, word by word. When we got to the passages on karma yoga, the path of spiritual action, I understood the depth of Baba's spiritual prescription to that patient.

Karma yoga converts our actions (karmas) into a yoga, or spiritual discipline. Ordinary action becomes extraordinary action when we work for the benefit of other creatures. Karma yoga is not about the monetary amount on a check we write for donation, but the attitude and spirit behind the action. If we truly offer an action to uplift others, it becomes karma yoga.

Karma yoga lifts us above ego-motivated consciousness into a blessed, selfless state. When this higher energy circulates throughout our minds and bodies, we generate karmic merit. This merit is spiritual in nature and, while it cannot be seen, it begins to heal us with inner growth and elevated consciousness. I believe that this is what happened to the businessman. When this man, who had worked only to generate income for himself and support his family, began to grow herbs for the benefit of others, he was helping to heal the world. With the karmic merit (*punyam*) he received from this action, he himself was healed. It is a Vedic spiritual law that by helping others, we heal ourselves.

Watching Baba at work later emboldened me in my own work to truly alleviate the suffering of those who sought my help by listening from my heart. And because my heart is filled with the conviction that was instilled in me over the decades by my Guru, I am able to influence many lives.

So my "prescriptions" include not only making diet changes and consuming herbs with discipline, but also quitting toxic jobs and ending abusive relationships without further delay or indulgence in self-destructive guilt. At my suggestion, one seeker of health returned to her family home, which was in another state, so she could care for her aging parents. The journey back home to her duty and pledge to fulfill her spiritual responsibility (dharma), even at the cost to her own comfort, became a unique spiritual path for regaining her lost health and peace of mind. Within weeks, her blood pressure normalized, she began losing the weight that she had been unable to lose for the prior nineteen years, and her recurrent nightmares ended. With little else but her faith in Ayurveda's prescription for a wholesome life—and not just for overcoming a specific disease—this woman was able to reclaim a deep, abiding state of well-being in her body, mind, and soul.

Traditional teachers and healers like my Baba and myself often prescribe karma yoga for hard-to-cure disorders that are resistant to other treatments. Ayurvedic texts call these disorders *karmaja*, "born from karma"—that is, from the negative karma in one's current or previous lifetimes. These disorders require a selfless spirit and positive karmas in the present moment to heal. No medicine can resolve such problems because, in cases like these, taking medicine is no more than self-gratification. Such individuals are still taking from the universe, not giving back. With karma-induced suffering, no matter how terrible they feel, this is the time to forget their own pain and to wipe away another's tears, to throw themselves wholeheartedly into caring for others.

Everyday Steps You Can Take

You may not all be able to move to a farmhouse, take a yearlong break, or grow herbs for charity, but anyone can return to Nature—that is, to the natural human state—by adopting Ayurveda's principles in your day-to-day life. Those who follow the disciplines of Ayurveda approach life with enthusiasm, energy, and joy find that the wisdom of Ayurveda begins to take root in their consciousness.

Many people ignore constipation. People can go days without eliminating and still continue to eat large amounts of food without giving it a thought. Either they skip going to the bathroom in the morning—unless they feel an urgent need—or they are oblivious to any sense of routine and go whenever the urge strikes them. In my organization's charitable clinics,

my students and I have met countless people who, when asked about their bowel habits, look at us with a completely blank stare. They cannot remember when they had their last movement!

One person who sought counsel on this had been constipated for eleven days! Laxatives were not helping. But this isn't why she came to the clinic. She didn't care about why her bowels weren't moving; she wanted to lose weight. When we spoke further, I learned that her lower abdomen was distended and causing her discomfort, her tongue was heavily coated with toxins, and she burped often—an indication that she was filled with toxins and gas.

This woman saw burping as "normal enough" and said she had been constipated for even longer periods than this in the past. "Oh, *that*!" she said with a smile when I asked about it. "I know," she added as if she'd been through this before. "I need to drink more water. I am bad about drinking water!"

To give this woman credit, her medical doctor had told her not to worry about her constipation. He suggested that she drink more water and take over-the-counter laxatives when the need arose, but then he told her, "It's going to come out sooner or later." The doctor didn't think constipation was a big deal, so why should she? Everyone she knew was often constipated—her sisters, her mother, even her darling pit bull went only occasionally and with no set pattern of elimination.

I instituted changes in her diet, and these had an immediate effect. Up to that point, this woman had eaten mainly raw salads, dry foods like raw carrots, lots of snacks, and clogging foods like cheeses. Despite her feeling that she needed more fluids, she'd had an excessive water intake and also drank a lot of coffee and soda. We will explore foods in chapter 6, but for now

I will say that this woman's diet was focused on foods that created a drying, cooling action in the colon—foods that led to a vata disturbance, which resulted in constipation.

To counteract this, I recommended she eat warm, cooked, light, and easily digestible foods—specifically, I told her to eat *khichadi* and drink *takra* (see appendix 4, "The Ayurvedic Diet Resource Guide" for these recipes). Instead of soda or cold water, I also recommended that first thing in the morning she drink hot water boiled with ginger root—fresh ginger is a mild laxative.

I gave her other instructions as well. I said that every morning, before eating, she should massage her lower abdomen and lower back with warm castor oil and, afterward, place towels soaked in hot water on that area.

Within two days, this woman's constipation was relieved and her accompanying pain and discomfort was gone. Her first bowel movement came in the form of hard, dry black pellets, but later the stools became easier to purge. In time, this woman developed greater insight into her digestive problems, noticing that constipation was a pattern that came for her when she would overeat or snack on overly processed foods made with white flour or white sugar.

Over time, I was able to show her ways to ensure daily elimination, including following a vata-balancing diet, eating only at fixed mealtimes (no snacking), and developing a regular practice of hatha yoga postures to regularize elimination.

The main point that I made was that it is necessary to take steps before day one and not to wait, suffering as she had, until day eleven. The constipation was her body's way of speaking to her, telling her there were things about her lifestyle that she needed to change. As far as I know, she is doing much better now: her chronic constipation and all of its uncomfortable consequences—weight gain, bloating, lethargy, and malaise—are all gone.

Are you listening to your own body and hearing its message?

Respect Nature's Call

All creatures are conditioned to purify themselves. Typically, the urge to eliminate comes in the early morning hours, almost as if the body were on autopilot. That is why, at this time, when parents are still slumbering, babies lie happy and fully awake in their own productions—smiling and cooing with pride. This is why puppies beg to go outside when dawn has not even broken, making owners wonder if it was really such a good idea to have brought a puppy home.

Human adults can, of course, train themselves, their children, and their pets to sleep in and to subdue this natural urge by ignoring it. But if you ignore it long enough, the urge will be more than subdued; it will be suppressed. We will no longer be aware that we have to go at all. At this point, our preferences have disrupted this natural process to such an extent that half of humanity does not go, cannot go, or goes way too many times in a day. This has happened because we ignore the call of Nature.

According to Ayurveda, early morning elimination that is timely, unprompted, and comes without much effort or straining is a sign of good health.[1] Becoming mindful of this vital physiological activity will promote your longevity, keep you free from abdominal heaviness, and protect you from attacks of intestinal gas.

In other words, ignore the call of Nature at your own risk because, before long, Nature will stop calling, and imbalance will call instead.

Ask Yourself, "Am I Regular?"

Asked if your bowel movements are regular, you might answer yes. If, however, you rely on laxatives or if you void your bowls at random times of day, don't be lulled into a false sense of security. Ideally, elimination should occur naturally (without the aid of habit-forming medications), and it should happen once or twice a day, generally very early in the morning, almost right after waking. The second urge is often felt late afternoon, after lunch is digested. Too many movements or too few is not a good sign.

Like everything else in the body, the bowels are connected to the doshas (which were discussed in earlier chapters). Each human being has a genetically determined dosha constitution or body type—often a dominant dosha and subordinate dosha. The purpose of this book is to explain basic principles of Ayurveda lifestyle wisdom in a way that helps all doshas. There is, however, quite a bit of difference between the doshas regarding problems with elimination, and if you have trouble in this area, you might find table 14 helpful.

The Colon and Immunity

For thousands of years, Ayurveda has addressed problems associated with a condition that is known today as leaky gut syndrome. Instead of moving toxins out of the body, the colon absorbs these harmful substances and creates inflammation and disease. The colon cells' absorbing function and these especially sensitive, super-absorbent, permeable membranes are known as *kala* in Sanskrit to Ayurveda scientists.

Research in recent decades has shown that disturbances in the colon can lead to inflammation. The diseases linked to this inflammation—arthritis, Crohn's disease, ulcerative colitis, irritable bowel

syndrome (IBS), and inflammation in various organs—are generally regarded as anomalies of the body's immune system.

Such conditions as constipation, chronic loose stools, and other disturbances in the colon are usually considered "nonissues" in mainstream medicine, and doctors often recommend over-the-counter medications for such complaints. Ayurveda, on the other hand, does not take disturbances of this nature lightly and recommends measures to deal with the problem at its root. One primary consideration of an Ayurvedic healer is always the doshas.

The three doshas circulate throughout the body, but each has an area in the body where its influence is most strongly felt. This is the dosha's "seat," its area of predominance. For kapha dosha, this is between the heart and the top of the head. Pitta dosha's seat is between the heart and navel. Vata dosha's seat is between the navel and the lower extremities. In regard to our organs, we can say that kapha dominates the heart, lungs, and brain; pitta holds the stomach, liver, gallbladder, and small intestine; and vata pervades the colon, kidneys, bladder, and organs below.

From this perspective, any adverse events in the colon impact vata dosha, and any vata imbalance affects the colon. If vata dosha increases in the rest of the body, or even in the mind, its impact can be seen in the colon.

The Colon and Toxins

Ayurveda holds that sometimes the intestinal mucosa absorbs not only what the body needs but also what the body does not require—what the digestive system has rejected in earlier stages of digestion. These unwanted substances are toxins (which means they are harmful, even

TABLE 14   Dosha-Based Bowel Characterstics

DOMINANT DOSHA	HEALTHY BOWEL CHARACTERISTICS	UNHEALTHY BOWEL CHARACTERISTICS
Vata	One bowel movement per day at a minimum; well-formed; may be slightly hard, but not dry; voids with ease.	Bowel urge may skip a day or more, or urge may manifest at fluctuating times; bowel is very hard, dry, and difficult to void with accompanying pain at times or gas and flatulence.
Pitta	One to two bowel movements per day; softer in consistency, oilier, and yellower in color; voids with ease.	Excessive bowel movements; bowel is almost too loose or diarrhea-like at times; oily and sticky bowels; can irritate anal area; gas and burning sensation can be present, along with excessive foul odor.
Kapha	One to two bowel movements per day; bulkier; soft, but well-formed; voids with ease.	Bowel urge is often sluggish and a sense of partial clearance remains even after eliminating; can be entirely constipated at times, or bowel is too bulky, sticky, and sometimes pale-colored.

poisonous) or autotoxins (which means they are formed within the body), and their name in Sanskrit is *aama*.

When excrement is mixed with toxins, it does not float but sinks to the bottom of the toilet bowl quickly and smells even more foul than usual. Naturally, all waste has an unpleasant odor, but when toxins are present, the smell is excessive. Other signs that your body may contain toxins include a coated tongue and flatulence, unpleasant-smelling gaseous emissions. With chronic constipation, the toxins are reabsorbed into the body and, ultimately, disturb healthy tissues.

Aama is associated with what Western medicine calls inflammatory, degenerative, or atrophic mucosal damage from plaque, debris, or deposits in the body. Ayurvedic science describes how the body with an impaired digestive system creates and stores these toxins. The ancient texts note how aama obstructs a channel, coats a membrane, or in some way binds with the blood or the skeletal or nerve tissues. We have all witnessed the devastating effects of aama in coronary arteries, which can result in heart attacks, and in damage to the nerve tissue, which is linked to multiple sclerosis. In the form of plaque, aama is also responsible for the premature aging of cells and, as mentioned earlier, for many inflammatory conditions. It's just a matter of vocabulary: what Western medicine calls plaque, Ayurvedic medicine knows as aama.

As I've mentioned, constipation or an occasional diarrheal-type condition are often low priorities in Western medicine, but Ayurveda sees them as conditions meriting our timely attention since aama is at their root, and aama is a cause of disease.

It is commonly said, "You are what you eat"; in Ayurveda we say, "You are what you can digest." If your food choices are important, no less important is the understanding of what your body can adequately and efficiently digest and metabolize—and what it cannot. Eating more than your body can digest leads to aama. In chapter 6, I describe how to eat on a daily basis in such a way that you don't manufacture aama.

Prevention is always the best strategy, and anyone who follows Ayurveda lifestyle will never become constipated. Those who suffer from chronic constipation or diarrhea due to previous lifestyle and dietary indiscretions need not lose heart. Ayurveda offers a restorative protocol. Once you regain balance and follow Ayurveda's lifestyle teachings, and you will never become a victim again.

What Is Healthy Elimination?

Most of us pay no attention to what comes out of our bodies or the frequency with which it comes. Glance through this list of ten qualities of good elimination to determine whether your elimination is healthy:

1. The urge to evacuate bowels is experienced once or twice every day.

2. The urge to evacuate the bowels is experienced at the same time every day (ideally in the early morning, before 6:00 a.m.).

3. In shape, the stools are generally well formed and cylindrical.

4. In density, the stools are soft and dense, not too loose or runny.

5. In color, the stools are yellowish-brown and not dark (black, green, and red are not healthy colors).

6. Stools typically have a foul odor, which is due to metabolic processes and bacterial breakdown, but healthy bowel movements are somewhat earthy in odor and not extremely offensive.

7. The stools float in water and do not sink to the bottom of the toilet bowl.

8. The stools are oily but not with so much fat that they're sticky.

9. In quantity, the bowel movement is neither very large nor very small. One sign that the size is right is that you feel satisfied after a full evacuation of the bowel.

10. The bowel movement happens easily, without discomfort, though a sensation of very mild pressure in the lower abdomen is normal.

Constipation Prevention Protocol

Many believe that constipation has very little to do with what we eat and how we choose to live our lives. In Ayurveda, however, constipation is a sign that your whole life needs to be brought into order—what time you go to sleep and wake up, what time you eat, and what you eat during the twenty-four-hour cycle. Constipation signs and symptoms include the following:

- No urge to pass stool

- An urge to pass stool at random times and intervals

- Difficult passage of stool; straining

- Dry, small, and hard fecal formation

- Abdominal bloating, cramps, and uneasiness in abdomen

- Bad breath with coating of mouth and tongue; loss of appetite (sometimes)

- Feeling lethargic with miscellaneous physical aches

- Slow digestion

There are many potential complications of constipation. These include fecal incontinence (generally defined as the inability to control bowel movements, causing stool to leak unexpectedly from the rectum), fecal impaction (hardening of stool inside the rectum), rectal prolapse (protruding rectal tissue), and of course hemorrhoids and anal fissures (tearing in the lining of the lower rectum or anus) cannot be ruled out.

What follows are tips to support the daily ritual of elimination, to prevent constipation from occurring or, if it has already begun, to bring your system back into balance:

- Bring no cell phones, reading material, or coffee cups with you to the toilet.

- Maintain silence and concentrate on the physiological act. This helps the entire process, as both your body and mind are involved in elimination.

- Resist straining or actively applying force to evacuate your bowels, as this can lead to complications (such as hemorrhoids), though it is fine to apply some concentrated muscular effort to stimulate the urge to evacuate.

Disadvantages of Relying on Laxatives

The laxative market is growing worldwide every year! Laxatives move the bowels, but—as any laxative label will inform you—there can be serious problems when you rely on such solutions, even herbal solutions, long term. Unfortunately, laxatives are often habit forming and cause dependency instead of resolving the root problem. On top of that, laxatives have a diminished effect over time because the body becomes resistant through extended use. Further, new symptoms can emerge, such as bloating, gas, cramps, and abdominal pain. Another potential complication of laxatives is that they can cause diarrhea.

Six Rules to Help Overcome Constipation Naturally

Here are some simple and extremely efficacious ways to handle constipation.

1. Say No to Irregular Mealtimes and Snacking

One aspect of a modern lifestyle is to eat whenever we want to. There is a trend, sometimes called "grazing," that promotes snacking throughout the day. The only one getting healthier through this grazing is the formidable ready-to-eat snack industry. Our bodies, sadly, struggle with the overload.

Snacking disturbs the body's metabolic processes. If you eat breakfast and then, before it is digested, eat a snack, the recently eaten food mixes with the partially digested food. Together, they generate toxins. One predictable outcome is constipation. The next time you open your mouth to pop in one between-meal grape, ask yourself: Will this grape make its way out anytime soon? Or will it get stuck in my digestive queue?

2. Do Not Eat Very Heavy or Very Light Foods

Very heavy foods are meats, processed foods with added sugars, and foods laced with cream, butter, and nuts. Very heavy foods take a long time to digest. If our digestive fire, agni, is not at an optimal level, we may not have the capacity to benefit from these heavy foods. If we don't, our systems will reach an impasse, and autotoxins will be formed.

Very light foods, on the other hand, such as puffed rice, popcorn, barley, lentils,[2] raw vegetable salads, and fruit, are easy for the body to break down and digest quickly, but they also lack natural fats so they add to the inherent dry quality of vata dosha. A trace of oil or fat is needed with every meal. This might mean eating certain foods that contain oil—wheat or nuts—or it might mean drizzling warm ghee over foods like popcorn, salads, and cooked lentils.

An important tenet of Ayurveda is moderation, and accordingly, we are instructed not to eat foods that are either excessively heavy or excessively light. We need a judicious mix. Food rules are covered at length in chapter 6.

3. Avoid Excessive Fasting and Dieting

Extreme diets or fasting protocols, such as water fasts, can be brutal on the body and, by creating an absence of food, aggravate vata dosha. Hence, fasting and dieting must be approached with extreme caution. The aim is to ensure that the body's channels are purified and that, at the same time, vata dosha doesn't become aggravated.

Signs of aggravated vata dosha during dieting or fasting include such symptoms as constipation, physical aches, dry skin, cracking joints, fatigue, irritability, moodiness, and even depression. Some of us may think we are meeting our bodies' requirements with calorie-controlled shakes, bars, or packaged foods. These do not, however, also meet all of the body's requirements for nutrients and foods—life energy (prana), for instance, and the requisite warmth and fats to balance vata dosha.

Ayurveda does recommend occasional detoxes, and the approved detox guidelines are described in appendix 4, "The Ayurvedic Diet Resource Guide."

4. Consume Only Warm Foods and Drinks

Today, it's conventional wisdom that the lower a food's temperature, the more it challenges our metabolism to work hard, so the greater the number of calories that are burned. So, in California at least, chilled water is the rage!

In contrast, Ayurveda teaches that cold increases vata dosha and dulls the digestive fire agni. In fact, agni benefits from the deliberate intake of warm, or even hot, foods and drinks.

Remember, cold is an intrinsic quality of vata dosha, just like wetness is a dominant quality of water, and heat is a dominant quality of fire. Therefore, due to the natural law of "like increases like," all cold-temperature foods increase vata dosha—the dosha that governs the colon and, therefore, the most significant dosha for elimination. This is one reason Ayurveda recommends eating foods that are hot or warm.[3] Refrigerated foods, including fruit, should be allowed to warm to room temperature before being eaten.

What does the temperature of our food have to do with the purification process? Everything! First, it's important to understand that Ayurveda envisions the human body as a creation of natural substances (the five elements) interlaced by pathways, channels, and pipes, gross and subtle. These conduits are called *srota*. The srota serve the physiological functions of transportation, circulation, and elimination. Some srota are large and visible, namely, the esophagus, veins, arteries, and intestines. Other srota are smaller (like the tiny intestinal villi that pass nutrition to the cells and help eliminate waste), and some are subtle. The mind affects each and every srota through its own srota, which are spread throughout the body—everywhere except our nails and hair. This is why when our nails and hair are cut, we do not have a mental sensation of pain.

From all of this, it should be obvious that if we want to be healthy, then all the srota in our body need to be open and unrestricted.

The basic principles of physics state that cold constricts while heat expands. If what you consume is cold (that is, cooler than room temperature), it will constrict your body's channels, a metabolic liability. If you are already experiencing irregularity or constipation in the eliminative pipes, cold water is disastrous. Ice-cold water and food extinguishes the fire of your digestion and leads to vata disturbances, such as constipation. Pumping freezing cold water, iced drinks, or frosty smoothies into your stomach—especially if you are trying to purify your body—is inevitably counterproductive.

Drinking water and eating foods that are warm or hot in temperature will, on the other hand, keep all the srota open.

Many late-night infomercials these days are selling the latest fat-burning smoothie recipes. These commercial messages are cleverly crafted, with miraculous weight-loss success stories delivered, as scripted, with big smiles. Each time I even glimpse one of these commercials, my heart hurts for all of the gullible viewers who are desperate to lose weight or purify their bodies and think that loading up on crushed ice and frozen fruit will help!

If you drink cold smoothies or ice water, ask yourself whether such a diet could possibly be natural for the human body. Have you ever seen any animal—other than the human animal—consuming such things as crushed ice? Such a thing wasn't even known to humanity until the invention of refrigeration and ice-making technology.

Today, without any awareness at all, we consume cold water, cold drinks, and cold foods. This modern habit is, I believe, one of the contributing factors to obesity, which is becoming a global epidemic. I say this because cold foods and drinks consumed in quantity are a liability. The excessive and unseasonal cold quality in foods and drinks not only disturbs digestion and excites vata dosha, but it also aggravates kapha dosha. This is a double whammy, because when kapha dosha becomes aggravated, one of the ways it manifests is as weight gain—slow, continuous weight gain. To refresh yourself on the qualities of doshas, and what happens when they become aggravated, refer back to chapter 1.

A study assessing the effect of temperature on gastric emptying was conducted in 1988 by introducing a temperature sensor into the stomachs of six men.[4] They then drank orange juice at three temperatures: 4 degrees Celsius (cold), 37 degrees Celsius (the control group), and finally, 50 degrees Celsius (warm). These men's mean intragastric temperature returned to normal ten minutes sooner when they drank warm juice as opposed to cold. A later study by the same team demonstrated that both warm and cold liquids could suppress gut motility (the contracting and stretching of muscles in the gastrointestinal tract) for thirty minutes after ingestion, but that with cold liquid, the muscles showed greater inhibition.[5]

Those who need to lose weight or are suffering from toxicity or elimination challenges should begin by removing cold beverages and foods from their diet. It's that simple. A daily intake that is vata-aggravating and agni-extinguishing must be stopped if a person is to make any headway in the goals of regular elimination, detoxification, and weight loss.

5. Incorporate the Right Kind and Quantity of Fiber in Your Diet

It is unfortunate that Western concepts largely endorse a totally mechanical view of the human body. Constipation is viewed as a case of "plugged up bowels." Hence, those suffering from constipation are asked to add more fiber to their diets, typically through an increased intake of raw vegetables. The question I want to raise here is this: How much is too much, and at what point should a person stop adding fiber?

As we've said, in Ayurveda, constipation is inexorably linked with digestion. A healthy bowel movement is possible only when healthy digestion happens. As Ayurveda sees it, to throw into your digestive system something that is highly fibrous and not easily digested can only further compromise your digestion. Fiber is not a solution for constipation; it is a cause!

The properties of fiber lead to bloating and digestive distress. The colon's native bacteria act on fiber's indigestible carbohydrates, which leads to further bloating and—thanks to the production of gases such as methane, hydrogen, and carbon dioxide—to flatulence. If the digestive fire is already compromised, then every ounce of additional fiber becomes dead weight to the body. Sadly, if someone who only occasionally suffers from constipation begins to focus on a fiber-rich diet, their constipation will inevitably become even more pronounced.

For a number of years, there were trends toward low-fat cooking that caused people to stop using oil in their cooking, even though oil is needed to lubricate the colon. Their focus on low fat combined with the added dryness of fiber, worsened constipation for many. Fiber acts like a sponge, absorbing water and oil content from the colon, and this renders stools even drier than they otherwise would be. And the solution suggested by many modern health mavens is to drink more fluids. Now, you've added water to an already "clogged" system, one that's already filled with fiber. How is the digestive fire, agni, to survive this? In some cases, diarrhea may occur within hours of consuming fiber.

The media continues to sing the praises of fiber, and we continue to see its commercial promotion: fiber supplements, high-fiber candy bars, books promoting fiber-rich diets, Internet

A Doctor Asks, "Do We Need So Much Water? Really?"

Heinz Valtin, a professor of neurobiology and physiology at Dartmouth College's medical school, debunked the "8 x 8" myth (that everyone should drink eight eight-ounce glasses of water a day) in a scientific review published in the *American Journal of Physiology* in 2002.[6]

Dr. Valtin was inspired to undertake this project, he writes, because he found it "difficult to believe that evolution left us with a chronic water deficit that needs to be compensated by forcing a high fluid intake." In fact, he found "no scientific proof" to support the recommendation that everyone needs eight glasses of water a day. He adds that there are many ways drinking too much water can be harmful—including possible water intoxication, kidney failure, potential exposure to pollutants, and the expense.

The author suggests that the "8 x 8" myth might have arisen from a National Research Council report that recommended "approximately 1 milliliter for each calorie of food," which would amount to roughly two or two and one-half quarts. In the next sentence, the report stated that "most of this quantity can be found in prepared foods," but it seems that this explanation was missed.

sites dedicated to the "fiber miracle." Humanity seems to have made fiber some kind of god!

In recent years, this situation—colons jammed with stools and minds jammed with pseudoscientific claims—has prompted many to contact Vedika Global's clinics. We've broken the news that the fiber-plus-water approach is not all it's cracked up to be, that the duo is taxing to digestion. This news has not yet gone viral, but its fans are growing in number.

Fiber, of course, is a natural part of various human-friendly fruits, vegetables, and cereals. The soft, soluble variety of fiber is amply present in dried beans and legumes, oatmeal, oat bran, barley, and citrus fruits. The hard variety, usually referred to as roughage, includes the woody or structural parts of plants, such as wheat bran and whole-grain cereals. Ayurveda doesn't discount these foods, but suggests them for only those who have a capacity to

digest them. There is never a one-size-fits-all recommendation in Ayurveda.

Cooking these fiber-rich foods in light oil or ghee with the addition of digestive spices, like cumin or mustard seeds, makes them easier to digest. These adjustments make fiber much more palatable as an anticonstipation diet strategy!

Take the example of the guava, a tropical fruit that contains ample soft fiber and, more important, also has natural oils to balance vata. I suggested guava to a person who had off-and-on constipation. Since she was of Latino heritage and familiar with this fruit, I asked her to consume one fresh, ripe guava fruit at breakfast each day. She liked that prescription and smiled when she received this guidance. The home remedy to make it even more effective and digestion-friendly requires sprinkling some fresh-ground black pepper, rock salt, also called Himalayan pink salt,[7] and grated ginger on the

TABLE 15   Effects of Chilled Drinking Water on Doshas

COLD WATER QUALITIES	PHYSICAL IMPACT	LIKE INCREASES LIKE PRINCIPLE IN ACTION	IMPACT ON DOSHAS
Fluid	Moistens the palate	Fluid quality of water increases the fluid, or drava, quality of kapha and pitta.	Increases pitta Increases kapha
Smooth	Removes dry texture of tongue	The smooth quality inherent in cold water increases this same quality, which is inherent in kapha.	Increases kapha
Cold	Antiheat effect	The cooling quality of cold water increases through likeness the cold quality of vata and kapha.	Increases vata Increases kapha
Heavy	Gives sense of a heavy belly	The heaviness of water aggravates through likeness the heavy quality of kapha.	Increases kapha
Ayurvedic Conclusion	Benefits accrue in natural thirst	All three doshas are aggravated when consumed in excess. So consume with caution.	Aggravates all three doshas simultaneously!

slices before eating. I also reminded her that when we consume fruit in Ayurveda, we do not mix it with dairy or other food items.

I always smile when I recommend this recipe. Any person who grew up in the countries in which guava is a native plant will tell you that of all trees, the guava is the easiest to climb. Guava branches are low, smooth, and slippery—a natural play structure of sorts, as kid-friendly as a tree can be. While the tree trunk and branches are slim and not very substantial, the inner oiliness makes the wood strong. It's great to swing and hang from. The guava tree branches also remind me of the way healthy intestines look—when we take the time to eat well, exercise, and purge daily.

Within a few days, my Latino friend e-mailed me to let me know that everything was "moving along," happily and regularly.

6. Drink Only When You Are Actually Thirsty

Since when did we start requiring a minimum eight glasses of water each day in order to have

Water Q&A: The Ayurvedic Perspective

Q: *Does anyone benefit from naturally cooled water?*

A: There are, of course, physical problems that can be addressed by drinking cooled water. In any heat-generating condition, cooled water is prescribed. This includes pitta aggravation, dizziness, heat exhaustion, burning sensation of body, poisoning, alcohol intoxication, blood-related conditions, excessive strain (including strain due to exercise), and nose bleeds. The water should be cooled naturally (see chapter 6).

Q: *For what conditions does Ayurveda prohibit cooled water?*

A: If possible, cold water should be avoided any time the digestive fire is compromised. This includes constipation, diarrhea, indigestion, abdominal bloating, flatulence, loss of appetite, anorexia, irritable bowel syndrome, and conditions associated with vata and kapha doshas such as hiccups, colds, coughs, asthma, recent fever, or pain in side or lower back. Under all such conditions, any water should be first boiled and then cooled to a drinkable warm temperature (see chapter 6 for more about boiling water before drinking).

Q: *When should water intake be reduced or measured?*

A: Excess water is very harmful according to Ayurveda in conditions such as nasal discharge, weak digestive power (impaired digestion), dropsy, consumption, excess salivation, enlargement of the abdomen, eye diseases, fever, ulcers, and diabetes mellitus. A person with any of these conditions should sip water from time to time (but not immediately after meals) and in a carefully measured quantity. This water should be boiled and then cooled to a drinkable warmth.

Q: *How much time is required to digest water?*

A: Natural, room-temperature water is digested in six hours. Water that has been previously boiled and then cooled to room temperature is digested in three hours. Water that has been boiled and consumed when still warm (but not piping hot like tea) is digested in one and one-half hours. Essentially, the hotter the water (through the process of boiling), the less time it takes to digest the same.

a bowel movement? Today, nutritionists, personal trainers, articles in trendy health magazines, and even many responsible physicians prescribe drinking water as a solution for constipation and as a panacea to a variety of health problems—even when the person is gagging at the thought of taking in even one more drop of water.

It may be a coincidence that the fad of drinking water parallels the rise in brands of bottled water, but I think otherwise. Research has shown that too much water can kill you. Water intoxication is known medically as hyponatremia, and it is a serious consequence that occurs when the body is flooded with fluid, which upsets the delicate balance of salt and other electrolytes. This condition stresses various organs, including the kidneys and brain, and stresses nerve impulses, and can cause rapid brain swelling that can lead to coma or death.

From an Ayurvedic perspective, we see that drinking too much water aggravates not one or two but all three doshas—in other words, not some people but everyone! Following the law of "like increases like," let us examine the impact of drinking too much refrigerated or ice water. The heart of this analysis comes from the classical Ayurveda text Ashtanga Hridayam, recorded between the fifth and sixth centuries CE.[8]

Remember that each dosha has its inherent qualities and additions and subtractions to these qualities make for increases and decreases of the individual doshas. Cold, dry, rough, and mobile are the qualities of vata dosha. Fluid, hot, light, and sharp are qualities of pitta dosha. Smooth, heavy, slow, dull, and cold are intrinsic qualities of kapha dosha. Table 15 demonstrates that drinking water, especially cold water, aggravates all three doshas simultaneously. Hence, ideally, chilled water must not be consumed. Cool water is advised at times,

but only in the autumn or when the body is undergoing heat-related challenges (see more on this in chapter 6).

Because this is the effect drinking water has on the doshas, drinking too much water would escalate these effects. Besides, extra water—that is, water the body does not need—becomes a liability to digestion. This extra water dilutes the digestive enzymes, blocks the bio-channels of circulation (srota) and, in general, taxes the digestive system.[9] The body now must spend precious energy processing each extra swallow of water.

If, after a health-inspired water binge, you become bloated, feel heavy, and lose your appetite, then you and your digestive fire are most likely drowning in the water you have consumed. Rather than causing a so-called flushing of toxins and stools, this excess fluid actually causes toxins to increase in the body because it obstructs the channels and aggravates the doshas.

While millions lap up their ice-cold water, and the bottled water industry thrives, weight gain is epidemic. Excessive water intake can make your brain fuzzy through hyponatremia, and perhaps this is why masses of educated, intelligent people never stop to ponder the research on the harmful effects of water drinking. Few pause to reflect on whether drinking the supposedly requisite eight glasses a day might be just a fad or a myth, with no basis whatsoever in science.

Newborn babies instinctively know when they are hungry and when they are not. Why don't we just listen to our own bodies? We live in strange times, when someone else tells us what to drink, how much to drink, when to drink, and which brand we should buy.

Of course, adequate hydration is important, especially during increased physical activity, during the summer, at the warmest part of the day, or while experiencing certain illnesses. What I find distressing is the arbitrary, one-size-fits-all prescription of at least eight glasses of water a day. It just doesn't work. Even the apple-a-day proverb can lead to indigestion in those who have a vata disturbance in the digestive system; it's clearly not *always* a way to keep the doctor away!

Ayurveda never imposes arbitrary dictates of foods, fluids, or behaviors on a group of people. Each of us differs widely in our dosha constitution, physical strength, digestive power, level of aama (toxins) in the body, status of bodily tissues, age, and health history. How could it be possible to prescribe one optimal diet for all? Ayurveda's customized, specific, and detail-oriented system celebrates that we are, each of us, one-of-a-kind. The human body's ingenious design, with the integrity of its complex systems and those systems' needs, should never be tyrannized by the latest health fad.

Let me assure you that if you wait until you are thirsty to drink, you will not have become dehydrated! That is a myth. Every animal I know makes its way to the best-known source of water—and slowly!—when it's thirsty. Sometimes, in the wild, this can take hours. Nature has built us with much more resilience than water industry experts would have us believe. Ayurveda restores to us our power to drink only when thirsty. And fear not, it will be a long, long while before our thirst becomes life threatening.

Diarrhea Prevention and Restoration Protocol

Diarrhea—excessively watery stools due to increased motility of the intestines—is a debilitating digestive extreme that many face on an almost daily basis. This condition results in an increased amount of excrement, sometimes with accompanying discomfort or pain. It manifests due to accumulation of doshas, mainly vata and pitta, in the large intestine, along with impaired agni, which lead to hypermotility and hypersecretion.

Once you decide that you no longer want to live out of control, you can heal your tendency toward diarrhea using Ayurvedic lifestyle and diet modifications, as well as home and herbal remedies.

Correcting Lifestyle vs. Battling Bacteria

For those who suffer from diarrhea, the Ayurveda system of health and healing recommends selecting foods that are gentle to the digestive system (for instance, lentils, Ayurvedic buttermilk, white rice—for recipes and a list, see appendix 2, "Healthy Elimination Resource Guide"). Restorative activities like yoga stretches (see appendix 2) are helpful, and abstaining from activities that aggravate vata and pitta doshas is also important. In most cases, I don't recommend medications. Why take chalky antacids or pills that momentarily curtail the problem? Why not instead look for lasting relief through lifestyle habits and food?

My recommendation may baffle those new to Ayurveda, particularly those who are used to blaming diarrhea on pathogens that invade the body. Some may wonder why it's necessary to modify eating and lifestyle habits to correct their weeping bowels when it's so simple to just take a series of antibacterial pills.

Let me warn you: Ayurveda's expectations of you are definitely more demanding than those of most Western medical doctors. If you visit a modern medical facility for help with your diarrhea, you will likely walk away with a prescription for an antidiarrheal and perhaps an antibiotic—and nothing else. At an Ayurvedic clinic, you would be asked to take stock of your entire lifestyle and be ready to make some changes in it.

If healing were as simple as taking a pill, there would be no need for this book. Allopathic remedies for diarrhea may provide immediate respite, but this relief will not be long lasting. Without lifestyle and dietary corrections, you'll once again find yourself in the doctor's waiting room. Some types of bacteria have virulent strains, so multiple prescriptions are becoming necessary to destroy the pathogens. In the meantime, you, the unfortunate victim, remain unaware of your role in the loose bowels that deplete you every morning, continuing to make the same choices of food and lifestyle that are the root of your problem.

Weeks later, you may feel guilty that your body—weakened from yet another round of antibiotics—seems to be experiencing an obstinate, rare, unique, perplexing, or unresponsive pathogen. The doctor has told you, with a professional smile, "Sorry, we killed the wrong pathogens and some good guys, too, in the process. But, don't worry; this *new* antibiotic will kill the one we want to get. This time it's sure to work!" Sound familiar?

In modern Western medicine, there is often a failure to evaluate the whole picture when determining the cause of a particular effect. You, the patient, have diarrhea. Isn't it possible that what you eat could be one of the reasons? Yet once a patient has a particular ailment, Western medicine practitioners tend to look mainly at the symptoms and how to assist in symptom management. While this is important, too, allow Ayurveda to address the big picture or the root cause.

The Ayurvedic sages encouraged building immunity and creating a healthy environment inside the body by virtue of a healthy lifestyle from the very beginning. Such a lifestyle incorporates a healthy diet, regular exercise, thinking pure thoughts, and reining in excess emotions. This holistic view of health, which has been adopted by forward-thinking Western physicians, ensures that the body is not vulnerable to germs. When a person's immunity is strong, even eating rotten food and living in unsanitary conditions (as are seen in much of the world) will have a much less damaging effect.

Food Choices to Combat Diarrhea

I offer specific suggestions of foods (with recipes) for the dietary treatment of active diarrhea in the appendix 2, "Healthy Elimination Resource Guide." Here, I focus on the general qualities in foods that anyone who is prone to diarrhea should avoid. Notice the word *overly* in these suggestions. This indicates that someone combating diarrhea should avoid these types of foods in excess and instead eat foods that will in no way be a shock to the digestive system. The goal is to find a happy balance between the diverse qualities of dry and oily, heavy and extra light. In anyone with a tendency toward loose stools, the gastric channel has become hypersensitive, and just about anything can set it off. So, try to avoid foods on this list of seven:

1. Avoid Overly Heavy Foods (*Atiguru*)

Closely examine your eating habits to weed out foods that are heavy in quality, which are more difficult to digest. From an Ayurvedic perspective, these foods are typically dominant in the water and earth elements. Be especially careful at night, when your agni technically "falls asleep."

Heavy foods include beef, nuts, pastries, cheesy pasta dishes, thick-crust pizza, and anything that causes difficult digestion. Bear in mind that "overly heavy" is a subjective designation. One person may experience difficulty in digesting even one slice of thin-crust pizza, while another is able to digest the entire pie without any trouble. It is up to each of us to evaluate what feels "heavy"—that is, what foods leave an uncomfortable sensation in the abdomen after you've eaten them? And, of course, which foods give you, shortly thereafter, loose stools?

2. Avoid Overly Oily Foods (*Atisnigdha*)

Avoid consuming anything overly oily, as it will excite pitta dosha. On the "avoid" list are fried foods of almost any kind, oily curries, pickles in oil, and cream- or cheese-based pasta dishes. A compromised agni has a difficult time breaking down fat. And whatever a digestive system in this condition cannot break down, it will literally throw out—often with discomfort and accompanying sound and fury. Even a beneficial fat like ghee should be consumed in only very small quantities until diarrhea is no longer an issue.

3. Avoid Overly Dry Foods (*Atiruksha*)

Overly dry foods, which aggravate vata, include chips, crackers, popcorn, pretzels, breakfast cereal, and rice cakes, as well as most salads and raw vegetables. Those with the tendency toward diarrhea have to be especially careful to avoid vata buildup. Instead of eating drying salads, you can steam your veggies and serve them with a small spoonful of ghee.

4. Avoid Overly Hot Foods (*Atiushna*)

While warm food is preferred over cold, it should not be at an excessively hot temperature. While some degree of heat will enhance the digestive fire, which is typically compromised when we experience loose stools, too much heat will overstimulate it and expand the bodily channels, the srota. The heat of spices is not suitable in dealing with diarrhea either—spicy hot food can also overstimulate agni—so you'll want to avoid wasabi, jalapeños, *sriracha* sauce, and so forth.

5. Avoid Overly Cold Foods (*Atisheeta*)

Eating food that is cold has a double liability: it dulls an already compromised digestive fire and aggravates vata dosha in the digestive tract. This means that you should avoid cold cuts, frozen yogurt, ice cream, and ice cubes. During the flu and bouts of diarrhea, it is popular advice for the patient to stay hydrated by sucking on popsicles, drinking chilled lemon-lime sodas, or eating Jell-O. This entirely mechanical prescription is counterproductive. It sees diarrhea as a one-to-one ratio of "liquid out" to "liquid in." Instead, we need to consider the properties and temperature of the liquid, and what the body requires.

6. Avoid Excessive Water Drinking

Doctors often advise drinking plenty of water and fluids or eating watery foods like soups, fruits, and vegetables to a patient with diarrhea so that they may avoid becoming dehydrated. It is true that a person loses fluids during bouts of watery stools. But taking in too much fluid can exacerbate this condition—and besides, drinking too much extra fluid means your digestive system cannot rest. Water, too, is digested, and a compromised digestive system cannot withstand a constant influx of fluids. To combat diarrhea, Ayurveda prescribes restorative foods, which deliver results every time (see recipes in appendix 2, "Healthy Elimination Resource Guide").

7. Avoid Incompatible Foods

Fortunately, Ayurveda makes a point of identifying food combinations that are incompatible and, therefore, cause gastric distress. Any number of these food combinations (see chapter 6) can result in loose stools.

The Power of Choice

Even if you were not born with good digestion, you can achieve it by consuming the right foods and making the right lifestyle choices. It's important to pay attention to your body's wisdom. Certain extremely commonplace and seemingly benign practices—drinking ice water, eating a cold breakfast—can undermine your digestive power and set you up for serious health issues in the future.

It all seems like minutia, I know, but the hundreds of tiny choices we make, minute-by-minute throughout our day, determine whether the magnificent apparatus we call the body is able to digest food and eliminate toxins—in other words, whether it can continue to function. The choice is up to you!

CHAPTER 4

The Art of Naturally Sparkling Smiles

Only Ayurveda can conceive of oral health as not only cleaning the teeth and rejuvenating and protecting the gums and mouth but also as a support of speech and of our ability to discern flavors. We explore all of these topics in this chapter, but first I want to point out that, of course, Ayurveda's oral hygiene supplies and practices are completely natural.

From my earliest years, I was told, "Chewing on a neem twig is the best way to clean your teeth." The neem chew stick is a tender twig of the evergreen neem, or margosa tree (*Azadirachta indica*) that grows throughout India and Southeast Asia.

 When I was a child, everyone I saw walking around in the morning had a chew stick in their mouths. So as a child I, too, chewed on a stick. My mother would give me a smaller twig to suck and chew on, the right size for my gums and baby teeth. Neem tastes quite bitter, which shocked me at first, but I soon became accustomed to the flavor, and each cleaning session left me feeling refreshed.

As a child, I would climb the well-anchored neem trees to play and hang from the branches. A local neem tree was one of our favorite hideouts. While playing, we kept an eye out for the straight, smooth, and somewhat delicate twigs. The best twigs had very few knots. Baba taught us to honor the neem tree by chanting a mantra before taking anything, even just one twig, from the tree. The first line of the mantra was *yaam drushtwa muchythe rogai* by which we addressed the divine presence (*vanaspataya deva*) that surely dwelled in the heart of the tree. Through this mantra, we asked for permission to take parts of the tree, the twigs, so we could use them for our own purposes. We asked that each twig be blessed by the spiritual presence of that tree—the same presence that blesses my heart and yours too. My sister and our cousins and I would often return home with our arms loaded with fresh green twigs.

Baba impressed on us how important it was to be respectful of the tree. I remember him telling me, "Shunya, you have to approach

Nature with humility and reverence as Nature has the solutions for us. Bow to her wisdom. You must never, ever think that you can plunder Mother Nature, hoard her gifts, or manipulate her for your benefit alone. If you do this, then in the end, you are the one who will lose. You will be robbed of all health and joy."

I always felt that my beloved neem tree was a friendly soul, much like my Baba in the way she gave her gifts selflessly, without asking for anything in return. Before climbing the tree, we always said *namaste*, "the One in me bows to the One in you." We offered our friend, the tree, ample water in case the monsoon was delayed and lots of natural manure thanks to our obliging cow, Nandini. We were careful to never pluck leaves or twigs or disturb the tree after sunset, as Baba warned us that the tree needs its sleep to be its best. I would often touch her trunk and feel something like love for this tree. ✐

My young intellect could not formulate words for my feelings, but today I might say, "Thank you, for being a supreme healing being whose each and every part is medicinal." Another name for the neem tree is *arishtha* (reliever of sickness), for in Indian villages, it is regarded as an all-in-one medical dispensary.

Baba used to explain that neem is naturally antimicrobial and helps fight infections of all kinds. In our home, we applied neem oil to fungal infections and washed any wounds with decoctions of neem leaves. Due to its blood-purifying and cooling properties, Baba suggested neem rinses for hot and painful mouth ulcers. Also Baba wanted us to apply neem sticks to our gums, as gums are a fertile field for microorganisms. Even as a child I understood this and knew that every part of the neem has medicinal value.

The beneficial properties of the neem, known by Ayurveda for thousands of years, have been recognized by the U.S. National Academy of Sciences.[1] More than 135 useful compounds have been isolated from various parts of the neem tree and identified, variously, as antiarthritic, antibacterial, anticarcinogenic, antifungal, antihyperglycemic, anti-inflammatory, antimalarial, antipyretic, antiulcer, antiviral, diuretic, immunomodulatory, and so on.

Neem oil and the bark and leaf extracts have been therapeutically used in folk medicine to control leprosy, respiratory disorders, rheumatism, syphilitic sores, and indolent (nonhealing) ulcers and also as a general health promoter. Neem oil controls various skin infections. The neem bark, leaf, root, flower, and fruit together have been used to treat blood and biliary afflictions, skin ulcers, and itching and to alleviate burning sensations.

The tremendous international interest in neem can be gauged by the number of patents filed on the various properties, active principles, and their extraction and stabilizing processes in the United States and Japan. More than thirty patents have been granted.[2]

The Generosity of Nature

 As a young child, I remained fascinated by the whole array of homemade preparations my family used for oral care. They had beautiful aromas, textures, and colors and ranged from the herbal pastes we used to brush and polish our teeth to the fragrant oils with which we gargled and also massaged our gums. We would harvest the herbs in their various seasons, and then my mother would dry them and pound or grind them by hand into fine powders. On the stove in our kitchen, she also cooked the herbal oils that promoted our dental health and relieved our tooth pain.

For many years, I took for granted my family's reliance on the abundance and generosity of Nature, and I thought everyone lived as we did. Then one day in a local shop, I saw plastic tubes of toothpaste and colorful plastic toothbrushes. These little packages looked so strange to me—as if someone had thought we could seal and lock Nature's goodness in a tube with a cap and an expiration date. Over time, I watched the people of my small and not-very-modern hometown stop using the tender neem twigs or, in guava season, the guava leaves to clean their teeth and stop roasting fresh turmeric root or pomegranate peel to make the tooth-polishing agents Baba recommended. The people of our own culture were slipping into cultural forgetfulness, so they could buy factory-manufactured toothpaste, far removed from Nature's wholesomeness!

At nine, I was kind of a natural health activist. I was well intentioned, certainly, but a bit immature. At school, with the self-righteous indignation of the very young, I glared fiercely at the children whose father had opened Ayodhya's first general merchandise shop. I had determined that it was because of this shop and all its fancy goods that many people had been seduced by bright lights and fancy packaging and were forgetting the gifts of Nature.

When I told Baba, he laughed at my fears. "A forgetting of the way is necessary to truly find the way," he said. "Once you've done this, you will choose never to forget again."

While I didn't understand Baba's words, his heartfelt laughter and gentle demeanor told me this was a nonissue, and I should let it go. I did let go of my anger. But I addressed this "nonissue" in my own way.

Hanging upside down from the branches of my beloved neem tree, I demonstrated with loving pride to the same children, the ones whose father had opened the sundries shop, how to chew on a neem twig. I told them about the many dental benefits this would confer on them. When my mother called me inside for dinner, my new friends took home loads of the neem twigs we had collected that day. I even loaned them my scarf, so they could carry more twigs home. ✒

You see, that day I changed my strategy. I was no longer going to shove and push for what I wanted to see happen in my little world. I was going to teach and educate the souls who had forgotten the way. I was going to try my best to stay on the path myself and patiently wait for others. After all, souls returning home to Nature do need to be handed a sacred neem twig, do they not?

It was on this day, I think, that the teacher was born in me. My heartfelt love of our noble neem tree, my firsthand experience of how the tree's gifts had helped me and my family, and my deep reverence for the philosophy my own teacher had imparted to me—all of this instilled in me the sentiment that health is our birthright and true nature. I will never forget the day.

Now, when I go online and read thousands of articles and blogs protesting the imposition of dangerous chemicals in items we use every day—toothpaste, soap, and shampoo—I feel grateful that my teacher, my Baba, never forgot his way, no matter where the world was heading.

Our well-being is a precious goal indeed, and I believe it is not supported by manufactured pharmaceutical drugs or what is found in the tubes on supermarket shelves. Above all, well-being does not emerge from synthetic-based toothpastes and mouthwashes that are produced from mixing artificial fragrances, flavors, and colors with detergents, preservatives, surfactants, film-forming agents, and even (with a prescription) antibiotics.

Our well-being is right inside us, ready to sprout forth when we make calm and nurturing choices that are tempered with wisdom. This notion is especially relevant today in the face of the proliferation of synthetic dental products that can subtly harm consumers. You are, I know, faced with an array of conflicting choices.

With appropriate knowledge, you can decide to follow a more natural path of self-care. Armed with Ayurveda's wisdom, you can transform your morning oral routine into a self-loving, self-healing ritual that is blessed by Nature.

Yes, we *can* take the aid of technology and, of course, electricity; we can make our brushes fancier and speedier, but has that reduced the incidence of cavities or gingivitis? Has it gotten rid of the foul smells from our mouths? Generations of elaborate brushes, flosses, and dental appliances later, we are still defeated by the staggering growth in oral and dental challenges that are besetting younger and younger populations. Fluoride has become a household term; this dangerous chemical is in our toothpaste and tap water, a seemingly harmless presence in our lives, though in reality, it is a semihazardous substance that poses serious health risks.

Routine visits to the dentist for professional cleaning and cavity prevention are surely marvelous. Yet, in the name of protecting their teeth, we make young children submit to annual x-rays and fluoride gargles. What about protecting the whole child? The fluoride that laces our water and is used in dental hygiene products is synthetic and has been shown to have an adverse effect on cognitive development in children.[3] This means that fluoride affects the brain! Studies are beginning to link these same effects with Alzheimer's disease,[4] a life-destroying condition that is growing to epidemic proportions in our population. Perhaps it is time we explore some natural options for dental hygiene.

I suggest that you not consider this to be a choice between modern and ancient. I see it as a choice between synthetics and the all-natural Ayurvedic agents that have delivered excellent results over thousands of years. Why not consider taking a conscious pause in your current oral care routine so that you can demonstrate a growing self-awareness and sense of responsibility toward your own health by adopting the holistic Ayurvedic method I am describing? Choosing Ayurveda in this way would be a righteous experiment, a way of coming out of autopilot and taking back your own power.

Remember that all nutritional nourishment comes into your body through your mouth. Having a clean mouth at the start of the day can impact your overall health because your perception of tastes will be enhanced, and this, in itself, will have a positive impact on digestion and the conversion of this food into life-giving nourishment for your tissues and energy for your body. Baba used to say, "*It is all connected—the perception, experience, and ultimate transformation and benefit.*"

Ayurveda's Three Oral Hygiene Steps

Ayurveda sages began promoting the practice of toothbrushing in ancient times, with textual references as early as the second century BCE. In fact, these texts describe elaborate oral hygiene practices, making Ayurveda perhaps the first medical science to introduce a systematic practice of complete oral care specifically to prevent destruction of dental structures and gums by microscopic pathogens (krimi). The source texts discuss invisible organisms that target the dental structure called *danta krimi*. *Danta* means "teeth," and *krimi* refers to pathogens that are either blood-borne (*shonita krimi*) or invisible to the ordinary eye (*adrishya krimi*).[5]

Thus, Ayurveda sages were developing strategies to deal with microorganisms centuries earlier than Louis Pasteur, and toothbrushing

with botanicals identified as antimicrobial agents (*rakshoghna ghana*) was one such strategy. In ancient days, these botanicals were also put to use to fumigate the environment and for sterilization of Ayurveda hospital rooms, medicine labs, kitchens, and so forth.

Along with the knowledge of counteracting microscopic pathogens, what I find most fascinating is Ayurveda's attention to detail. The morning oral hygiene routine is three easy steps, and with each of these steps, you are invited to engage Nature with increasing mindfulness. The three steps, which are to be completed in the order given, are as follows:

1. Toothbrushing (with botanicals)

2. Tongue scraping (with specialized scrapers)

3. Gargling (with rejuvenating and protective substances) in one of two ways: (a) oil pulling: swishing a small amount of liquid in the oral cavity; or (b) oil pooling: holding to full capacity a large amount of fluid in the oral cavity

Step 1: Toothbrushing (Dantadhawan)

The seers of Ayurveda gave the world what I consider the most advanced and eco-friendly method of caring for teeth and gums. They recommend cleaning every tooth carefully with a soft botanical brush.[6] The Ayurvedic toothbrush is known as a *koorchaka*, a soft brush made of natural plant material. What can be closer to Nature than using a natural substance like an herbal chew stick to brush our teeth? In Ayurveda, brushing your teeth is an art, and anyone who masters this art reaps long-lasting dental health, indeed. The method is described below, but first, I will talk about the tooth-cleaning implement itself.

Nature's Disposable Toothbrush

The primary implement for dental care is the neem chew stick. Most Indian villagers have never visited a dentist in their entire lives, yet they enjoy a full set of healthy teeth until their eighth or ninth decade. How is this possible? My Baba use to say, "*Why would you ever need to visit a doctor if you have a neem tree at your house?*"

In addition to the advantages of neem twigs mentioned above, this herbal chew stick has natural bristles, so it is totally biodegradable. This is a toothbrush you can throw away with a clean conscience. In fact, if you wish, you can eat it!

The word *toothbrush* is not entirely accurate in Ayurveda's context, as the word *brushing* does not describe Ayurveda's approach to cleaning teeth. Ayurveda prescribes an entirely different approach to dental hygiene. In cleaning your teeth, you use them to do what they always do: bite and chew. What's different is that you are biting and chewing on herbal stems, which polish the biting surfaces, encourage salivary secretion, and assist in plaque control. The plaque control happens because the herbal stems have a demonstrated antimicrobial effect on oral bacteria. The chewing and biting action also exercises the gums. Because the plant fibers are soft, the gentle pulling and tugging actions that the stem demands before expressing its juice further support dental health.

A modern nylon-bristled toothbrush mechanically massages the teeth and gums, helping dislodge stuck particles and plaque on a daily basis. The natural neem twig accomplishes the same purposes but with less abrasion and with the added advantage that the herb's pharmacological benefits are immediately transmitted into the mouth via the tongue. The bitter taste of the neem twig carries with it all of this herb's inherent bioactive potential. As mentioned, it has antiarthritic, antibacterial, anticarcinogenic, antifungal, antihyperglycemic, anti-inflammatory, antimalarial, antipyretic, antiulcer, antiviral, diuretic, and immunomodulatory properties, among others.

The bitter taste of neem is said in Ayurveda to help remove toxins (aama), foul odors, and subtle waste (mala) from the teeth, tongue, and mouth. This leaves the mouth refreshed and receptive to the next meal.

How to Select an Optimum Chew Stick

Not every wood makes a good chew stick, and those that do have some varying effects on the body—meaning that some are better for one dosha than for another. Fortunately, neem works for every dosha type. Here is a list of options to consider if you know your dosha:

Vata: Neem tree, licorice roots (not the candy!), wattle tree (known in India as the *cutch* tree)

Pitta: Neem tree, guava tree, arjuna tree (grows primarily in India)

Kapha: Neem tree, mainly, along with sewak, or miswak, (*Salvadora persica*), known as *arak* in Ayurveda

As you can see, neem is the first choice for every dosha type.

Chewing sticks have been used traditionally not only in India but also throughout Asia, Africa, and South America, and there are a number of other trees and shrubs that are popular for this purpose around the world. A few of the others are *Fagara zanthoxyloides, Randia uliginosal, Streblus asper Lour,* and *Achyranthes aspera*.[7] In fact, chewing sticks have been so successful in maintaining oral health and preventing disease that the World Health Organization also supports their use as effective tools for oral hygiene.[8]

In selecting a chew stick, it's convenient, of course, to live near the right kind of tree or shrub. If you do, it's ideal to obtain a fresh stick every day. The twigs should be healthy and soft, without leaves and knots, and they should also be green and moist. The stick should be about one centimeter in diameter (about the size of your small finger) and twelve centimeters in length. If the twig is not soft and supple, if it's somewhat dried out, then soak the end you will chew in water for twenty-four hours before using it. If the twig is woody and completely dried out, then it cannot be used as a chew stick, for it has no juice to impart.

Most of us, of course, do not have ready access to an appropriate tree. Fortunately, it's easy to find and order hygienically processed, vacuum-packed chew sticks of neem, licorice root (*yashtimadhu*), and miswak online.

An order of chew sticks usually arrives with a dozen or, most economically, several dozen. Store those not in use in a dry, hygienic place.

When to Use (and Not Use) a Chew Stick

The primary times to use a chew stick are right after waking up and right before going to bed. Since chewing neem wood is a preventive health practice, you will receive the optimal benefit from your chew stick if you also use it after every meal. Some people from India also chew the purifying neem before their prayers.

Is a Chew Stick as Effective as a Nylon Toothbrush?

A clinical trial comparing the effectiveness of the chew stick and the toothbrush in gingival health published in the North American Journal of Medical Sciences found that the chew stick is as effective and, at times, is even more effective. The study also showed that the chew stick is an effective method of removing plaque from the teeth.[9]

Each of us is, of course, unique in our needs, and there are times when we should intentionally pause, modify, or slow the pace of our disease-prevention strategies. Do not use a chew stick when you have symptoms of a cold or flu, which includes a fever, sore throat, inflammation of the mucosa, bronchitis, and vomiting. Also, you should refrain from using a chew stick if you have any disease involving the throat, palate, lips, tongue, or teeth, or if you have difficulty breathing.[10]

Further, Ayurveda cautions not to use chew sticks when you're feeling weak or exhausted (whether this is due to excess work or alcohol intoxication) or when you have indigestion, hiccups, or a headache or are thirsty. Nor should you use a chew stick if you have a heart condition, if half of your face has been paralyzed (facial hemiplegia), or if you have pain in an ear or a disease of the eye (since doing this will instantaneously aggravate vata dosha).[11]

Under such circumstances, the best way to clean your teeth may be by gently rubbing herbal tooth powder or an Ayurvedic toothpaste with your regular toothbrush.

How to Use a Chew Stick

Before you begin, you can presoak the end of the stick you will put in your mouth. Using about half an inch of water, soak the stick for ten minutes if possible. This step is optional and has the advantage of making the wood softer.

Remove outer bark: Using your teeth, nibble the bark off a half-inch piece of the twig. Or if you prefer, use a kitchen knife to shave off the bark.

Begin to chew: Begin chewing on the inside softer, or less woody, fibers until they become frayed and stand out from each other almost like bristles. Your "brush" is now ready to use.

Build up saliva: Continue chewing on the frayed end. Gradually, the juices from the fibers will mix with your saliva and saturate your mouth. If you have a lot of saliva, spit out the excess. There is, however, no harm if you do end up swallowing the saliva. It will taste bitter, but it's highly medicinal. Some of the neem juice will be absorbed into your body directly through the soft tissues of your mouth, providing an antibacterial effect.

Use the Brush: With the brushlike end of the stick, clean your teeth with vertical movements. Use the brush to remove food deposits in the crevices between your teeth. Also, use it to gently scrape your tongue. This will reduce any white coating on your tongue and also improve your breath.

Continue for Five Minutes: Keep up this biting, chewing, and brushing for at least five minutes. By the time your teeth feel clean, some natural foam may have formed. Simply rinse your mouth several times with fresh water. You are done.

How to Store a Chew Stick Between Uses

People in most ancient cultures found ways to clean their teeth. The idea of using nylon bristles in toothbrushes comes from the early use of animal hair, especially the horsetail and hog bristle. In most of Europe during the Middle Ages, it was a common practice to rub a rag with soot and salt over the teeth. Any of these practices are susceptible to moisture retention and the growth of bacteria.

With neem, whose stem fibers are naturally antibacterial, this problem is avoided. This is why it's possible to continue using the same chew stick. And if you order them online, you will certainly want to reuse your chew sticks.

You can prevent the growth of mold on a used chew stick by cutting off the part last used. Simply trim that end with a dedicated clipper. The important point here is to keep the stick dry. Any organic substance, like wood, if kept damp, will eventually mold. You can also dry your chew stick with a paper towel after use and keep it in a hygienic and well-ventilated place. A clean bowl works well. Do not store this bowl near the bathroom sink.

Alternatively, you can purchase a single stick holder, called a miswak holder. This holder, which looks like a pen, keeps the stick dry and fresh, inhibits mold, and makes it more portable, which is handy if you travel.

Replace the twig every few days to ensure freshness.

A Two-Thousand-Year-Old Ayurvedic Tooth Powder Recipe

A chew stick is a complete dental care agent unto itself. It does not require a cleaning powder or paste to be effective. If you wish, however, while carefully using the twig brush, you can also apply herbal tooth powder for additional benefits.

The recipe I have for tooth powder dates back to the second century CE and is found in the Sushruta Samhita, one of the source texts that form the great triad of classical Ayurveda literature.[12] This traditional concoction is easy to put together, and you'll probably have most of the ingredients in your own kitchen or garden. The ingredients are also readily found online.

The various herbal powders come together to create a potent antibacterial cleaning agent that counteracts both tooth decay and gum disease. Sesame oil nourishes the roots of the teeth, anchors them more firmly, and with regular use, can prevent early loss of teeth.

AYURVEDIC TOOTH POWDER

INGREDIENTS

1   part cinnamon powder

1   part powder of toothache tree, also known as prickly ash bark[13]

⅛   part ginger powder

⅛   part ground black pepper

⅛   part ground Indian long pepper or *Piper nigrum*

⅛   part ground rock salt, or Himalayan pink salt Raw, organic sesame oil—enough to blend powder into a paste at each use.

METHOD

1. Mix together all the dry ingredients and keep in an airtight container. Ideally this container should be glass or ceramic rather than metal or plastic.
2. Immediately before cleaning your teeth, put about ½ teaspoon of the mixture in your palm or in a separate ceramic bowl used only for this purpose. Add two drops of sesame oil and mix into a paste with the

bristles (either natural or nylon) of your toothbrush.
3. Use this paste for brushing your teeth. The taste will be salty, slightly bitter, and pungent, and will leave your mouth feeling refreshed and awake.

Step 2: Tongue Scraping (Jihva Nirlekhanam)

Ayurveda's total dental hygiene includes cleaning the tongue—a part of the mouth ignored by Western dentists until quite recently. The tongue is literally scraped. According to Ayurvedic texts, tongue scraping removes food debris, any bad taste, stickiness, or staleness on the tongue (caused by the deposit of toxins or any foul smell from the mouth).[14]

Look at your tongue in a mirror and you'll probably see that it has deep pockets. As we sleep, the toxins (aama) our body is trying to eliminate collect in these pockets. In this sense, your tongue acts like an organ of elimination. This is why it's important to scrape away this waste and, in this way, rid your body of these toxins. Because the mouth is a warm and moist environment and the tongue has a rough texture and deep pockets, this area becomes a breeding ground for microorganisms (krimi) and biological waste. When you scrape away these toxins daily, using an antimicrobial metal scraper, you keep your mouth fresh and limit any infections.

The tongue scraping that has been practiced in India for thousands of years is gaining attention now in the West. The American Dental Association has declared that cleaning the tongue has the potential to successfully reduce breath odor and tongue coating,[15] and the Journal of the American Dental Association has published several favorable articles on tongue cleaning. In

TABLE 16   Benefits of Tongue Scrapers

Metal	Sanskrit Name	Impact on Doshas	Special Attributes
Gold (can be plated)	*Swarna*	Three-dosha balancing	Nontoxic; antipoison; rejuvenates eyes (vision), heart, memory, intelligence; aphrodisiac
Silver (can be plated)	*Rajata*	Mainly vata and pitta balancing	Nontoxic; strengthens all seven tissues; antiaging agent
Copper	*Tamra*	Mainly pitta and kapha balancing	Nontoxic; heals ulcers, obstinate skin disorders
Brass	*Pittala*	Mainly pitta and kapha balancing	Useful mainly for eyesight (not available in today's market)
Tin	*Vanga*	Mainly kapha balancing	Mainly alleviates kapha and fat; promotes vision (not available in today's market)

an article published August 2005, the author concludes that tongue cleaning can help prevent some dental problems, and he advocates the use of specialized tongue cleaners.[16]

Online research indicates that in the United States, dentists are now increasingly recommending routine tongue cleaning to lower the number of microorganisms in the mouth and to prevent periodontal disease.

The Practice of Tongue Scraping

Tongue scraping is a practice you can easily master. It is, however, important to invest in the right tool. Ayurveda recommends using an instrument that is curved in a U-shape. The blade of the scraper should be gently blunted, without sharp edges, so that it does not hurt the tongue. Tongue scrapers are inexpensive and can be found at most natural food stores and from many sources online.

Today, the market is flooded with plastic and stainless steel tongue scrapers. Stainless steel will mechanically dislodge deposits on the tongue's surface; however, the classic texts do not mention this metal, of course. They speak instead about the medicinal properties of gold, silver, copper, tin, and brass.[17]

I have listed these in their order of efficacy and advise using copper at the minimum. Glance at table 16 to understand why Ayurveda sages wanted us to benefit from metals like gold, silver, and copper.

I will focus here on using copper tongue scrapers, which are more affordable than those made of gold or silver (even gold- or silver-plated ones). For more details on using copper, silver, and gold tongue scrapers, see appendix 3, "Oral Health Resource Guide." Similar to gold and silver, copper contains toxin-removing properties (*lekhana*). Copper tongue scrapers are readily available in the United States, as are those that are gold- and silver-plated.

According to the science of Ayurveda, copper is sweet, astringent, and bitter in taste and cool in potency. Hence, it becomes a powerful pitta-balancing agent. Since copper also has the quality of being light, it counteracts kapha's natural heaviness.

Copper also heals mouth ulcers and tongue sores on contact. Ayurveda calls this quality *ropana*, a word that means something that "fills in" or "seals together." I personally use a copper tongue cleaner; I like knowing that a beneficial metal is touching my taste buds.

Please understand that the benefits of the metals listed in table 16 do not mean that it's recommended for you to ingest these metals.[18] Let me repeat this: *Do not swallow gold, silver, or copper in any form.* For external use, such as with a tongue scraper, it can make a difference which metal you use.

Should You Analyze Tongue Patterns—Or Not?

There are some healers and also Ayurvedic students who like to analyze the patterns toxins make on the tongue to diagnose the health conditions indicated, but I do not suggest this, nor do the Ayurveda source texts (this is a practice prescribed by the Chinese medical tradition, not Ayurveda). When you see a white coating on your tongue, immediately clean this coating off by applying your tongue scraper. This is what I recommend to my students and clients, and it's what the sages recommend. Why spend time analyzing the pattern? If the tongue is coated,

this means toxins are present. And these toxins, according to Ayurveda, circulate throughout our entire system. They do not come to rest on only one organ. Mapping out where these deposits appear on our tongue will not truly tell us in what other organs toxins are located.

If you feel that you need to rid your system of pernicious toxins, what the sages recommend is that you fast for a reasonable period of time. Fasting gives your own digestive fire (agni) the opportunity to metabolize or process the toxins you may have in your body. After a fast, your tongue will automatically look cleaner; the circulating toxins will be reduced in quantity. For details on a special detox protocol, see appendix 4, "The Ayurvedic Diet Resource Guide."

Step 3: Ayurvedic Gargling (Gandush or Kaval)

Ayurveda's most innovative contribution to preventive dental hygiene is its concept of gargling. Ayurvedic mouthwashes are, of course, completely natural and have been studied for centuries. They are made with select medicinal oils and herbal decoctions that act as dental tonics. These ingredients contribute to maintaining excellent oral health and support the healing and development of teeth, gums, and connective tissue. Not only are these mouthwashes rejuvenating for the mouth and throat, they can impact the health of the entire body. You can make many of them in your own kitchen, using, for the most part, what grows in your home garden. See appendix 3, "Oral Health Resource Guide" for recipes.

In contrast, popular commercial mouthwashes are simply antiseptic. Their one purpose is to fight germs. Our society's phobia with germs is, I feel, a fear-based response to health

Questioning the Unquestioned Ingredients

Marketing tactics to promote products that are good for your teeth and gums can be misleading in regard to the potential these products have to damage other, more critical aspects of health. Table 17, adapted from information found on the *The Ecologist* website, lists ingredients commonly found in over-the-counter mouthwashes, what they do in the product, and their possible unintended side effects.[21]

Another study, published in 2013 in the journal *Free Radical Biology and Medicine*, states that popular commercial mouthwashes that contain chlorhexidine, a powerful antiseptic and disinfectant, can actually increase blood pressure, and if used daily, the risks of heart attack and stroke.[22]

conditions we cannot understand or control. This fear has become a collective delusion that the world is unsafe and its inhabitants are unclean and unsafe. This has resulted in wholesale disinfecting of our planet in which we wipe and scrub our environment and ourselves. We have declared a war against germs, but even so, diseases haven't been eradicated or even significantly reduced. What we have done, instead, is create an imbalance. By attacking germs, we are also killing protective bacteria, and doing this allows for more harmful and complex germs to proliferate. So my suggestion is that you pour your antiseptic mouthwash down the toilet!

I am not alone in this assessment. C. Norman Shealy, an American neurosurgeon whose focus is holistic medicine, spoke strongly against commercial mouthwashes on national television, saying, "Antiseptic mouthwash is among the more damaging things people do to themselves. They kill the essential good bacteria in your mouth. Yes, just as in the entire digestive system, your mouth is loaded with good bacteria."[19] Shealy went on to say that these good bacteria are responsible for converting nitrates into the life-essential nitric oxide, which is itself critical in maintaining blood flow, cell energy, blood pressure, and a strong immune system, adding, "I wonder how many of the 40 percent of Americans with hypertension use killing antiseptic mouthwashes."[20]

Ayurvedic Alternatives to Antiseptics

I am grateful that Ayurveda has given me options that have no harmful side effects, and for gargling, Ayurveda's main choices are sesame oil and water. That's right, oil and water: completely natural, completely effective!

Ayurveda's strength has always been in treating each person as a whole. We are more than just one part of our bodies and more, too, than just the sum of our parts. Ayurveda recommends gargling with either water or oil, depending on the challenges you're addressing. Whatever challenge is happening in your mouth is a reflection of other challenges in your body—and these challenges express an imbalance in one or more of the doshas. Just as there are three doshas, there are three options for gargling.

Gargle with cool water: Gargling with cool water is especially helpful when you are suffering from an aggravation of pitta dosha; in

TABLE 17 Purpose and Effects of Common Mouthwash Ingredients

Ingredient	Purpose	Potential Side Effects
Alcohol	Antiseptic, antibacterial	Dries and denatures mucous membranes in the mouth; changes mouth and throat pH; promotes mouth and throat cancer
Sorbitol	Sweetener, tartar control agent	Mostly safe, but can cause bloating, diarrhea if swallowed
Poloxamer 407	Surfactant, detergent, film-former	Potentially contaminated with impurities linked to breast cancer
Benzoic acid, sodium benzoate	Preservative, antibacterial	Allergic and hypersensitive reactions; urticaria, asthma, rhinitis, and anaphylactic shock reported following oral, dermal, or inhalation exposure to both substances
Sodium fluoride	Antibacterial	Leads to spotting, mottling, and yellowing of the teeth, especially in children; leeches calcium from the bones, possibly leading to osteoporosis; allergic and hypersensitive reactions; nausea, vomiting, epigastric pain, and diarrhea if ingested
Menthol	Fragrance, antiseptic	Irritants to skin, eyes, and respiratory tract

which case, your mouth will feel hot and dry. Cool water eliminates toxins and alleviates any tendency toward chronic thirst. It makes the mouth cavity feel fresh and light.

Gargle with lukewarm water: Warm water gargling is helpful in balancing a kapha imbalance, which manifests in the mouth as a feeling of heaviness or stickiness. Gargling with lukewarm water relieves a gummy, sticky feeling on the tongue, and it also clarifies your sense of taste and eliminates any feeling you may have that

your mouth has muck in it. Warm water gargling gives the sensation of lightness in the oral cavity.

Gargle with sesame oil: Ayurveda recommends organic, raw, cold-pressed sesame oil as a gargle for anyone dealing with an imbalance of vata dosha, which might manifest as pain or soreness in the jaw. This kind of pain disappears with regular sesame oil gargling.[23] Gargling with warm sesame oil is also especially useful for people who sing or speak in their professions—teachers, for instance, or salespeople—as one major benefit from gargling with oil is that the practice strengthens the jaw muscles and mandibular joint.

There are, obviously, additional alternatives available for gargling. I give a number of recipes for gargles with diverse natural ingredients, taught to me by my Baba, in appendix 3, "Oral Health Resource Guide." I recommend that you invest the time to read about the benefits of these homemade herbal gargles. Try them, and see the difference. Rather, taste the difference! You may never want to buy another antiseptic mouthwash again.

The Efficacy of Sesame Oil as a Gargle

Sesame oil is known in India as *tila* oil. The sages of Ayurveda consider this to be the best strength-promoting oil. Sesame oil endows the body with enduring stamina.[24]

I have said that sesame oil is an excellent—actually, the best—balancing oil for vata, and now I want to add that sesame oil does not aggravate kapha and only slightly increases pitta. This makes it a wonderful oil for gargling. While most oils and fats dampen the agni in the oral mucosa, sesame increases agni, heightening the body's metabolism and offering the mouth natural protection from harmful microbes (krimi).

All Ayurvedic body treatments use only organic cold-pressed sesame oil. Some things to bear in mind: do not use oil that is more than a year old, never use rancid oil, and do not store it in the refrigerator.

Get ready to say good-bye to commercial chlorhexidine-based antiseptic mouth rinses and welcome Ayurveda and its original, organic, all-natural mouthwash. Raw sesame oil gargle will strengthen your gums, your voice, and the muscles of your face. That is right, sesame oil gargle is, in and of itself, a complete antiaging, beauty-imparting package.

As for bacterial control, sesame oil works against bacteria and reduces both tooth decay and plaque buildup.

Two Techniques of Ayurvedic Gargling

Ayurveda recommends two distinct approaches to gargling, either of which, when done routinely, rejuvenates and protects the oral cavity. The names in English are so much alike that it's easy to confuse them. They are *oil pooling* and *oil pulling*.

Oil pooling (gandusha): Oil pooling involves filling the mouth totally with the gargling liquid—enough so that the cheeks are fully expressed—and then holding the liquid there until the eyes begin to water. It's usually about three to five minutes, and don't worry, you're not actually weeping. It's just that the retained fluid puts pressure on the lachrymal ducts, bringing tears to the eyes. While the liquid is being held (pooled) in your mouth, do not swish it around and definitely do not swallow it. Because it is filling the mouth, the liquid penetrates the oral mucosa and gums, with great healing effect.

Oil pulling (kavala dhaarna): Oil pulling involves taking a comfortable dose (1 to 2 tablespoons for adult mouths and 1 to 2 teaspoons for children) of liquid into the mouth to gargle. As you gargle, make intentional swishing and pulling movements so that oil touches all surfaces inside the mouth and also penetrates between the teeth. Make this dynamic but keep it gentle; don't work too hard. The oil will have its effect. Gargle long enough for the oil to become frothy and lighter in color (which happens when oil particles mix with saliva and air bubbles)—typically one to three minutes. Gargling any longer is not so easy because fatigue builds up, and in any case, the extra time investment is unwarranted. It is the consistency, the daily practice, that is emphasized, not the length of time in any one session.

Both of these are simple techniques and can be practiced even by children as long as they are old enough to follow parental instructions.

The gargling liquid can be sesame oil—which, as I've said, is highly recommended—or it can be any other fluid recommended by Ayurveda. The liquid's temperature can be room temperature in the warmer months or slightly warm during the cooler months. With oil pulling, be sure that you're comfortable with the size of the dose you take. You can always build up over time.

If your jaw and mouth muscles become fatigued sooner than you expected, spit out the oil. Do not push yourself beyond your capacity. And if you experience a gagging sensation at any time, again, you must immediately spit out the oil.

As for when to gargle, if you're going to do it once a day, then gargle upon awakening. If you can gargle twice a day, then do it at bedtime as well. Gargling must be done on an empty stomach or at least three hours after eating. You can drink water before gargling if you need to, but don't eat immediately before.

Note that in Ayurveda's three oral hygiene steps, gargling follows brushing your teeth and scraping your tongue. The three are always to be done in the order given: brushing, scraping, then gargling. The simple reason for this is the same reason you would clean cobwebs from the walls, then dust the furniture, and finally vacuum the carpet. The earlier processes dislodge dirt that the later processes can clean. So, gargling is always the closing practice for dental hygiene.

One important thing to remember is that you should *not* swallow the gargling liquid. It will contain the toxins and germs you have just removed from your oral cavity.

Also, after gargling with oil, briefly gargle with tepid water to remove oil residue completely. This is important for the same reason that you shouldn't swallow the oil.

Once you've washed out your mouth with water, you can eat at any time. You'll probably notice that the food tastes wonderful!

Not everyone can gargle, and none of us can gargle all the time. Ayurvedic texts say that gargling is not recommended if you have a fever or an infection in any part of the body, including times when you have a sore throat, cold, or flu. Gargling is also contraindicated for anyone who has ingested poison, who has fainting spells, a bleeding disorder, eye inflammation, or constipation. Once these conditions have abated, of course, gargling can continue.[25]

Gargling is not, however, at all dangerous. In the thousands of years of Ayurveda's history, no one has died or even suffered harm from oil gargling. So do not worry. If the dos and don'ts are followed, this is a safe, nontoxic practice, with no known side effects and amazing results!

The Amazing News about Oil Pulling

Recently, the practice of oil pulling has become incredibly popular. Like all health practices that become fads, oil pulling too has gathered its legion of fans and adversaries.

Do a cursory online search on "oil pulling," and you will find hundreds of sites that eulogize this ancient technique as a cure for just about every ill mankind has ever faced. Naturally, you will also find an equal number of adversaries—at least some of whom would mechanically dismiss any solution that isn't pharmaceutical.

I don't know about oil pulling being a cure for *everything*, but I do know from my own experience that it's powerful. I'm going to cite just two of the scientific studies that support this. First, in 2009, in a randomized, triple-blind study with a control group—I won't define these terms here, but they're important to scientists—the researchers found that oil pulling with sesame oil was just as effective as chlorhexidine mouthwash in reducing the count of microorganisms, plaque, and plaque-induced gingivitis in a group of adolescent boys.[26]

In 2011, some of the same researchers carried out a study to evaluate the antibacterial efficacy of sesame oil and—once again—found it to be just as effective as chlorhexidine mouthwash.[27]

Of course, what the researchers did not go into was the long-term differences between the overall health of the boys using sesame oil and those who were given chlorhexidine mouthwash.

The germ theory and how it has played out in traditional Western medicine versus how it has been to put to use in Ayurveda are examples of one truth explored and put to human use differently; one in harmony and acceptance of the truth, and the other through separation with the truth. Germs are an intrinsic part of the universe. Ayurveda focuses its attention in strengthening the individual immunity rather than identifying and destroying classes of pathogens.

The Ayurvedic vaidyas R. H. Singh and J. S. Tripathi put it this way: "One of the therapeutic strategies in Ayurvedic medicines is to enhance the body's overall natural resistance to the disease-causing agent rather than directly neutralizing the agent itself. Here lies the difference between the fundamental therapeutic approach

of Ayurveda and modern medicine, which emphasize on direct attack on the disease causing agents using chemotherapeutic drugs."[28]

Nature always has the last word.

Ayurvedic mouthwashes and the practice of gargling and mouth rinsing is an immunity-enhancing event. This morning ritual of gargling has given me many gifts. I am a full-time teacher and public speaker, and as you can tell, I have firm convictions. I need a strong voice. There are days when I speak for ten to twelve hours non-stop, and still, my voice never fails me. Not only this, I also have a healthy set of teeth. I attribute both of these benefits to gargling with sesame oil every morning.

But don't take my word for this. I invite you to conduct your own study on yourself to experience the benefits firsthand.

The Ayurveda system of health and healing ensures that the body does not become a barren landscape and a host to side effects and secondary conditions that can sap vitality and life essence. Of course, germ annihilation may become necessary in an emergency situation, but generally, Ayurveda advocates a change in relationship with germs rather than eradication.

Germs do not exist without a reason; they are Nature's helpers and recyclers, not to be venerated but not to be feared either. Recognize them, know them, and identify them (as Ayurveda also has) but then leave the germs to their own devices, and work, work, and work on your inner immunity through optimum foods and optimum lifestyle practices. This is the teaching of Ayurveda from the shastra, the scriptural sources.

Benefits of Daily Gargling

The Ayurvedic gargling regimen is both preventative and curative, and it's so simple that it's an easy habit to adopt and sustain. The benefits of this practice listed below are from Ayurveda texts.[29]

- Eliminates any foul smell in mouth—removes bacteria and freshens the oral cavity with natural ingredients.

- Benefits teeth—roots teeth strongly, protects them from cavities, and alleviates any oversensitivity to hot or cold.

- Strengthens jaw—helps to prevent temporomandibular joint (TMJ) disorders.

- Strengthens voice—prevents hoarseness or loss of voice and has a beneficial impact on both volume and pitch.

- Strengthens facial muscles—prevents wrinkles!

- Improves taste perception—increases the ability to relish subtler tastes and is helpful in dealing with anorexia.

- Prevents dryness—moistens both throat and lips.

- Improves immunity—protects from future diseases.

Full-Spectrum Dental Health

Now that we've gone all the way through the three steps for oral hygiene, we're going to take a step back and look at the big picture. More than just oral hygiene, Ayurveda is concerned about oral health, and more than oral health, it is concerned with the health of the whole person.

I'm going to present two additional steps to put oral health into the big picture. Seeing that the causes for tooth decay are more than a pathology localized in the mouth, that they are systemic, Ayurveda recommends adding two additional steps to support oral health. And because I feel that the first three steps are vital, I'm going to repeat them here before adding the two additional steps:

1. **Toothbrushing, or biomechanical cleansing:** This is, of course, step 1 of the prior list—vigorous mechanical cleansing of teeth and gums using herbal twigs for removal of food debris.

2. **Tongue scraping, or aama elimination:** This, step 2 on the prior list, involves specific treatments for dislodging deposited aama via tongue scraping and the use of bitter tasting (anti-aama) botanicals such as neem, which eliminate toxins on the spot.

3. **Gargling, or immunity escalation:** This is step 3 on the prior list and a means to improving the ability of the oral cavity to withstand microbial colonization by boosting its immunity through a variety of healing and soothing gargles.

4. **Rectifying digestion:** This means doing whatever you need to do to correct or maintain the digestion process in an optimum condition so that you can prevent production of aama. Throughout this book there are recommendations for doing this—especially in chapters 2 and 6.

5. **Eating strategically:** This means choosing every meal carefully, with consideration to the season, your dosha imbalances, and the rules of food combining so that you can prevent indigestion and aama formation. This is covered in-depth in chapter 6.

What's new, of course, are the final two items on the list. While chapter 6 is devoted to addressing these two issues, I want bring up just a few specific points here.

Aama and Oral Health

Ayurveda declares that we are not what we eat; we're what we can digest. Specifically, and poignantly, we are also what we do *not* manage to digest (see chapter 3). Undigested or inadequately processed food creates aama. As the unwanted by-product of digestion, aama stays in the body and circulates through the entire physical system. It is this toxin that adheres to our teeth.

This sticky, soft, and often grimy substance builds up along the gum line. When this plaque hardens, which it does over time, it is called tartar.

Daily brushing and flossing and even regular dental visits for deep cleaning do not resolve the problem of plaque. Until the root problem—a compromised digestion and the toxins it creates—is corrected, plaque will continue to form.

Unlike conventional dentistry, which treats the teeth as sovereign structures quite independent of the rest of the body and its processes, Ayurveda views the body as an organic and unabridged whole in which everything is connected to everything else. When aama levels increase throughout the body, over time, one or

more of the srotas (the bio-channels throughout the body; see chapter 3) can become blocked. If nutrition cannot reach our teeth and bones, tooth decay will eventually result. This is one of the reasons it is important to keep our bodies toxin-free.

Additionally, without toxins compromising your system, the local immunity in your mouth is enough to ward off microorganisms. At any given moment, there are millions of bacteria in the oral cavity. According to one estimate, an average mouth contains 20 billion oral microbes. You can use the science of Ayurveda to fear these bacteria less and actually eat in such a way that your immunity to bacterial attacks increases. Ayurveda tells us that these bacteria become activated only when a buildup of toxins lowers immunity, and not otherwise. So, instead of being preoccupied with destroying bacteria, you can mindfully put your attention on eating healthy foods. Ayurveda's stance that you should improve your digestion in order to have healthy teeth is a revolutionary concept.

The one nutritional remedy for maintaining oral health that is encouraged by Western dentists is to stop eating sugar. Sugar, these dentists declare, is what attracts bacteria to our teeth. There are many people I know who have given up all sugars, following this modern instruction in an attempt to have healthier teeth. Yet even they develop cavities.

They may be avoiding sugars, but this isn't enough to prevent toxin production—and it's not just sugar, it's the toxins that promote the growth of bacteria in the mouth. Even if you give up sugar, if you continue to eat foods that are heavy and hard to digest, eat at irregular hours, or eat the wrong combinations of foods, your gastric cycle will be compromised, and—even without sugar in your diet—your body will still produce toxins.

Thankfully, Ayurveda unfolds a vision of life and health that is unabbreviated, comprehensive, and interconnected. Ayurveda always reaches for the whole, the indispensable big picture that surrounds and encompasses all of the particular and seemingly isolated facts. When any field is studied as whole, it becomes apparent that everything interlinks, interconnects. This is why Ayurveda's full-spectrum dental hygiene, established thousands of years ago, remains pertinent, ahead of its time, and of benefit to anyone who cares to employ it.

Ayurveda teaches us an amazing forward-thinking, deeply positive science of tartar prevention that encourages healing teeth in conjunction with rejuvenating the health of the entire body. Ayurveda's approach is subtle because it addresses not the tartar itself or the mouth in which the tartar appears but the root of tartar formation: our compromised digestion.

If we are to have perfect oral health, Ayurveda advises us to establish the healthy eating habits that will give us healthy digestion. If we do this, then the aama that is the precursor to plaque and tartar will never form.

Ayurvedic Diet for Healthy Teeth and Gums

It is important to choose foods carefully, not only from the point of nutritional content but also from the perspective of how easy they are to digest. Cooking with spices to make foods more easily digested, combining foods in the right ways, and choosing foods correctly for the season are all topics addressed in chapter 6.

There are, however, also certain foods that specifically support strong, healthy teeth and gums, and it's a good idea to include some of these foods in your diet on at least a weekly basis. Without this nutrition, no matter how "pure" your oral cavity is with brushing, scraping, and gargling, your teeth and gums—which are living, growing, self-sustaining structures—will not have the building materials they need to be strong. Here are the lists of recommended foods for healthy gums and teeth.

Foods Useful for Healthy Gums

- **Cereals:** Whole wheat and basmati rice

- **Pulses:** Lentils, *urad* (black gram or *Vigna mungo*) and mung (green gram or *Vigna radiata*)

- **Meats:** Well-cooked tender meat of deer, goat, and chicken

- **Dairy:** Ghee, or clarified butter made from cow's milk

- **Fruits:** Pomegranate, date, banana, fig (fresh or dried), and *amalaki* or *amla* (Indian gooseberry)

- **Nuts and seeds:** Almond, coconut, and black sesame

- **Vegetables:** Pumpkin, winter melon, and onion (cooked)

- **Sweeteners:** Pure sugarcane juice, jaggery, and honey

In short, a diet rich in goat meat, chicken, eggs, ghee, pulses, rice, wheat, and ghee (clarified butter) is beneficial for bleeding gums. If your gums bleed easily or are prone to disease, it's a good idea to avoid foods that are excessively pungent or salty. Other foods especially harmful to the gums are eggplant, any kind of fish (fresh- or saltwater), raw mango, and chickpeas, or garbanzo beans (known in India as *chana dal*).[30] If you have healthy gums, then you can always enjoy these foods.

Foods Beneficial for Teeth

- **Cereals:** Wheat and barley

- **Pulses:** Urad (black gram or *Vigna mungo*), chana dal (Bengal gram or *Cicer arietinum*), mung (green gram or *Vigna radiata*)

- **Meats:** Venison or goat meat (especially in a soup or a marrow broth), chicken, and crab meat

- **Dairy:** Fresh cow's milk, unsalted butter, and ghee

- **Fruits:** Ripe sweet mango, pomegranate, date, and amalaki or amla (Indian gooseberry)

- **Nuts and seeds:** Sesame seeds (tila)

- **Vegetables:** Winter melon, eggplant, and onion (cooked)

- **Sweeteners:** Sugarcane, jaggery, and honey

- **Spices** Garlic (fried in ghee)

If your teeth are susceptible to challenges, you should generally avoid sour foods such as yogurt, tamarind, lemon, oranges, and pineapple, or at the very least, eat them in moderation. You should also avoid eating hard or dry foods and drinking cold water and beverages—all of which will aggravate vata dosha.

A Radiant and Sparkling Smile

Ayurveda's approach to oral health calls on us to look at our total health. Partnering with Nature, we can employ Ayurveda's ancient wisdom as our daily guide to claim our health with a radiant and sparkling smile! And do not forget to look at appendix 3, "Oral Health Resource Guide," where I provide recipes that help keep our teeth and gums healthy and toxin-free. I invite you to enjoy whatever appeals to you from Ayurveda's expansive dental hygiene practices—you won't regret it, I promise.

CHAPTER 5

The Delight of Oiling, Bathing, Sense Care, and Beauty Rituals

 The flowing grandeur of the Sarayu, a holy river so ancient it is mentioned in the *Rig-Veda*, was a witness to so much that I learned in my childhood. And why not? She has been an eternal witness to my ancestors' journeys too—those who lived and taught the great knowledge of the Vedas, always near the river.

Almost every day I would make a pilgrimage to the river with my Baba. I prayed to the rising sun, listened to nearby temple bells, and learned pranayama and meditation on Sarayu's banks; I watched the sunrise across its placid surface and saw sacred lamps being lit and set afloat; and most of all, I bathed in its soothing, refreshing, and sacred waters.

I could hear the swish of the tossing waves, a sound that entirely matched my heartbeats. With all my senses alert, I would allow my gaze to span across the horizon. The rising sun would be spreading its auburn glory. I heard temple bells ringing with various frequencies, momentous temple gongs and sweet-sounding bells, amid rising chants that were thousands of years old. I could see lamps being lit and set afloat in the river atop tiny boats handmade from twisted and knotted dried tree leaves. I was so grateful to be awake and experiencing my essential oneness with natural and human-created splendor, wherein natural and divine artistry were intermingling and emerging in front of my child eyes.

Over the years, I noticed how River Sarayu's immense meandering and glittering body would change color based on the seasonal light she reflected back. However, her water, coming forth from a Himalayan glacier, and its sacred texture, velvety soft, always felt familiar, like my mother's lap. Since India is pretty hot nine months out of the year, it was a huge relief to dip my entire body on some days or parts of my body on most days into the cooling, soothing, and restful yet refreshing waters of River Sarayu.

The impact of those mornings with the Sarayu on my nascent consciousness was immense. The daily spiritual communion with a great holy river left an indelible impression on my being.

I believe the town of Ayodhya takes its character from its proximity to the Sarayu. The city is considered a *dhaam*, which means a "place of pilgrimage" and also a *tirtha*, which is the "ford" of a special river. Metaphysically speaking, by crossing the River Sarayu, which descends from the Himalayas (known as the lofty heavens), you are said to encounter your spirit ancestors. This is one of the reasons that every year Ayodhya attracts millions of pilgrims yearning to immerse their bodies in the Sarayu or, at the very least, to splash themselves with a few drops of its sacred water. They come, many of them, with hands folded in reverence to the divine presence of the Sarayu, and when they reach this holy river, the Sarayu absorbs the pilgrims' tears, right along with the exhaustion from their tired bodies and the malaise from their grief-stricken minds.

In the West today, many people spend a fortune to seek solace in health spas and retreats that offer water-based therapies. As a child, I witnessed the River Sarayu give gifts, day after day, free of charge. I saw people wade into the river, their bodies stooped, their spirits apparently broken, and then walk out of the river within minutes, taller versions of themselves, seemingly rejuvenated after being touched by the water. Today also, Sarayu is overflowing with love and receives over a million guests every year.

What Baba used to say to me is this: "Like the river, live the most authentic life you can. Make your own course. Never doubt how truly powerful you are. Do not stop until you encounter the ocean!"

Baba spoke these words, which were like commandments to my soul, in various conversations over the years as we stood gazing at the Sarayu, taking in her immensity with our human hearts. I would nod a silent yes, making my assent with heartfelt conviction. These were powerful, beyond-words moments of connection with the One, with all. ✒

Indeed, to this day, I hear the River Sarayu whisper this mantra of hope in my heart when I counsel people whose consciousness rises from the depths, moving between points of pain and relief, dismay and hope, disease and health. I remind them of the deepest healing yet to be achieved and the final and most significant journey yet to be undertaken—the journey of recognition that while this body is mortal, the true Self is immortal. A river does not perish or lose itself upon merging into the ocean. It finds the truth of its eternal existence, deep inside the ocean's depths.

This symbolic rite of purification of body, mind, and soul through contact with sacred water is a practice in many, perhaps most, cultures. Ancient Egyptians, Chinese, Native Americans, and countless other wisdom communities worldwide connected with sacred bodies of water in order to gain a greater spiritual communion. Be it the sacred Nile, the majestic Yangtze, or the branching Mississippi, each river has inspired humanity for thousands of years. Some of our deepest beliefs and highest aspirations find expression in these rivers, and keeping this in mind, to immerse ourselves in such a river is a potent ritual of worship.

Ayurveda shows us how to convert bathing in our own standard bathtub or shower stall into a divine ritual, a rite in which we connect with nothing less than the potent spiritual power of water. It's something we can do every day, if we wish, with every bath. And why wouldn't we?

Prayers for Bath Time

Perhaps that potent power is why India's Vedic tradition encourages us to make bathing a ritual by invoking the divine presence of holy rivers. Intention is the most important aspect of any rite, so I would like share some of the prayers my family recited during bathing. A chant I learned when I was little can be translated this way:

Ayodhya is my charming town.
River Sarayu is flowing in its northern direction.
Those who bathe in these waters
reside without effort near Lord Ram's[1] heart.[2]

Another prayer commonly recited throughout India is this:

In this water, I invoke the divine presence
of holy waters from the seven sacred rivers:
Ganges, Yamuna, Godavari, Saraswati,
Narmada, Sindhu, and Kaveri.[3]

Vedic bathing chants do not require the bathing water to actually come from a specific body of sacred water. Simply remembering the spiritual source is enough to transfuse our own tap water with spiritual effulgence. The Vedic sages were obviously employing the now-popular practice of creative visualization and positive affirmation. The popularity of these chants across India over the thousands of years of this ritual's uninterrupted practice is testament to its efficacy.

By the power of conscious thought, mantra repetition can convert the mundane into the sublime—turning the repetitive chore of bathing into a rite of spiritual purification.

I encourage you to compose your own bathtime chant. Repeat it aloud before bathing and often during the bath. Or if you don't like oral recitation, you can just think the chant, running the words silently through your mind. Perhaps something like this:

This water that falls on my body has
been kissed ever so gently by Mother
Moon and infused with fiery healing
light of Father Sun; it has flown through
the womb of Mother Earth, befriended
by herbs, to reach my being and purify
me. I receive you with love.

I'm sure you get the idea.

Care of Our Five Senses

Ayurveda lifestyle wisdom includes taking good care of our five senses, the powers of perception—seeing, hearing, smelling, tasting, and feeling—that operate through our eyes, ears, nose, tongue, and skin. Because the act of perception itself is a divine power, these organs of perception are literally doorways to our innermost being. The sense organs are subject to routine seasonal wear and tear as well as unwarranted use and abuse, especially if we live our lives unconsciously, taxing our senses and taking their strength for granted.

For this reason, it is vital in our modern lives that we mindfully incorporate five-sense rejuvenation and turn ourselves back toward health and well-being. The landscape of Ayurveda is dotted with flower-like rituals of five-sense care and love that are simple to perform and that bring us long-term benefits. Most important, these rituals awaken us from habits born of negativity and lethargy. The practices I highlight below are the ones I recommend to propel you into a constructive daily self-care routine.

Each time a sweet flower is smelled, bliss is a real-time experience. In the same way, each and every time you choose to participate in an Ayurvedic self-care and self-love ritual, your body and mind will take a leap forward and, in one way or another, you will experience real-time well-being.

Most of these rituals involve the sense of touch and care of the skin, the seat of vata dosha. By applying warm oil (*abhayanga*) or dried herb powders (*udgharshanam*) to your entire body and by following the Ayurvedic rules for bathing (*snanam*), you protect your skin, the largest sense organ, from disease and general wear and tear. Ayurveda also prescribes bath scrubs (*udvartna*) and herbal facial skin-care packs (*anulepana*) for full-spectrum skin care. I explore each of these practices below.

Ayurveda Self-Massage (Abhayanga)

Ayurveda recommends warming oils to a pleasant temperature and massaging them into the body with light, firm strokes. When the body is gently anointed with warm oils, the body's dryness is counteracted, the joints are lubricated, and the skin is sloughed and cleansed to shine and glow

with inner health. The medicated Ayurvedic oils strengthen the muscles, reduce pain and inflammation, and nourish the nerves. And besides all this, a warm oil massage is relaxing. What a beautiful way to begin our mornings!

It was perhaps the wisdom of Ayurveda that influenced Indians to incorporate oil massage as part of an everyday home culture. Self-massage with oil is practiced in almost every home. Massage professionals are a very recent phenomenon in India and are still restricted to select metropolitan areas. Most Indians apply oil to their own bodies—every part they can reach, including the head—and gently massage the oil in before bathing or showering. This happens daily or weekly and most certainly in preparation for holidays and festivals.

Massage also happens within a family. Mothers massage babies from the seventh day of birth onward with homemade butter or cream fresh from the cow. (Usually a pinch of turmeric is added to the cream.) Brides are massaged up to the day of their wedding, and so are their bridegrooms. Mothers-to-be are massaged, often by their own mothers, their aunties, or their sisters, and the elderly are massaged by their caregivers, who are often their grown children. Even livestock and pets—cows and horses, dogs and cats—are massaged when they begin showing signs of aging, and also to keep them in top form.

In India, oil massage is as much part of daily physical hygiene as bathing, shaving, and shampooing are in Western culture.

Even in the West, massage has become accepted as a complementary and alternative healing modality. We all know the power of massage to reduce stress and release the happiness hormones in the body and brain. I must commend the Ayurvedic sages, who incorporated this relaxing, rejuvenating, antiaging practice as part and parcel of daily hygiene.

There are, no doubt, benefits to our taking the time—an hour or an hour and a half—for the occasional professional massage, but it is much more beneficial to us to make massage a daily practice. Those precious ten minutes that we spend each day on self-massage will deliver regular sustenance to our skin, the organ that envelops our entire body.

The Sanskrit word for oil application, or massage, is *abhayanga*, whose syllables specifically refer to the movement of sustenance toward all the body tissues so that they glow with health. This sustenance comes through therapeutic oils, our healing touch, our intention, and our own energy.

This points to an important distinction between the way massage is viewed by Ayurveda as opposed to the West and even other Asian cultures. According to Ayurveda, the benefits of massage do not accrue only from skillful manipulation of the muscles but come as well from the application of the oil. The medicinal oil addresses the root of the problem by correcting the dosha imbalance and also by bestowing nourishment to the entire body through the skin.

For these reasons, only natural oils such as sesame, castor, and mustard are used in massage. The oils might be altered, but if so, they are infused by herbs and fragrant flowers—never by chemical perfumes. Ayurveda never recommends massage with commercial skin lotions or other synthetically derived compounds.

Oil versus Pressure

Applying warm sesame oil will correct vata or pitta dosha imbalance in the skin and muscles—which is what Ayurveda identifies as the underlying cause of pain, inflammation, stiffness, or dryness. Kapha-pacifying oils such as castor or mustard can also be used to counteract toxicity, cellulite, and obesity.

It's because of these balancing oils that we can experience all the benefits of a deep tissue massage in ten short minutes: improved blood flow, greater oxygenation, a release of any stress knots, a feeling of lightness, reduced pain and stiffness, deep relaxation in the body and mind, and heightened spiritual awareness.

So, in daily abhayanga, the strokes are deliberately kept light, and the hand pressure is almost imperceptible. However, great attention is paid to the temperature and type of oil. The massage oil must be warm even if you are pitta dominant, and the type of oil must be chosen for its impact on the doshas and body tissues.

The Five Pranas

In popular modern massage modalities, the focus is on addressing stiff or inflamed muscles. Students learning massage therapy in these traditions study the various types of muscles and muscle groups; how these connect, intersect, and overlay; and all of their names. Ayurveda massage, however, addresses prana, the invisible energies that underlie the muscles, fascia, joints, and bones, that move blood through the body and thoughts through the mind.

Prana is the essence of vata dosha. In one sense, prana can be compared to a mother energy that is flowing throughout the universe, much like the parallel concept of an all-encompassing chi in Chinese philosophy. Vata dosha is closely related to prana; in fact, vata is a subset of the greater concept of prana. And from this sense, vata and prana are synonyms, pointing to the same divine energy that connects and drives the mind and body of living creatures.

By tradition, prana has different names according to its function. There are five: the life-sustaining prana (*prana*), the downward-moving prana (*apana*), the upward-moving prana (*udana*), the circulating prana (*vyana*), and the prana that moves at the core, around the umbilicus (*samana*). Each of these pranas is influenced by the application of oils and light touch.

Through massage and slow, synchronized, mindful breathing, all five pranas spontaneously begin to come into harmony, into rhythm. All that is needed to communicate with the pranic system is our mindfully directed gentle touch and the application of warm, prana-balancing oils. This communication happens through the organ of touch, the skin.

Once this communication begins, each organ and body part—from the brain, heart, and lungs to the muscles and bones, literally every cell of the body—begins to synchronize automatically. This is what happens when the five pranas become more stable. So Ayurveda's targeting of the subtle often ends up being more powerful than the massage modalities that focus on muscles and bones, which are the gross manifestation of matter.

There are some modern authors who speak about how Ayurvedic massage works at the lymphatic level. There is some truth to this perspective, and I will not deny it. My own view, however, is the classic perspective that Ayurvedic massage works, first and foremost, at the energetic level, the prana. I believe that its initial impact is on the nervous system and mind, and that this, of course, then plays out in all of the other systems of the body.

This is why daily Ayurvedic massage seems to effectively release emotional tension,

discharge pent-up memories, and leave you feeling cheerful, optimistic, and deeply relaxed. The calm you experience after an Ayurvedic massage stays with you throughout the day, and when you do it over the long term, it can even lead to an enduring change in disposition. Even outsiders may begin to observe that you have become more trusting, optimistic, and able to endure the ups and downs of life with more ease and grace.

A self-massage that, by virtue of its oil usage, can make your body and mind more balanced is indeed a gift to you from Ayurveda. I urge you to unwrap this gift daily and embrace a deep restfulness, morning after morning.

The Miracle of Daily Ayurvedic Massage

Let me demonstrate how powerful this daily practice is by sharing my student Leeann Brady's story of how abhayanga turned around her health. When I first met Leeann, she was in her late thirties, juggling marriage and a demanding corporate medical job with the needs of her ailing mother. She had a beautiful face and a quiet dignity about her. Her pleasant demeanor left an impression on my heart, and I felt connected to her, wanting to look after her and protect her. It was dismaying to hear that she had been diagnosed with a grave illness, multiple sclerosis (MS).

On deeper investigation, I found that vata and pitta doshas, the energies of dryness and heat, were causing havoc inside Leeann's body. She was losing weight and becoming easily fatigued, and often when she woke up, her muscles were stiff and her eyes were inflamed and burning.

I prescribed sesame oil abhayanga daily, knowing that this would pacify vata and pitta doshas and also nourish her tissues. Leeann took on this one critical practice and virtually nothing else—and within six months she was doing much, much better. This inspired Leeann to move from being a clinic patient to an Ayurveda student, and in time, she graduated from my school Vedika Global's five-year Ayurvedic physician training program, the first of its kind in the West. Now, many years later, Leeann is healthy in spite of having MS, and she supports the health of countless others as director of Vedika Global's multiple wellness operations. Abhayanga made her a believer. Here is Leeann Brady's first-person account.

ONE WOMAN'S ACCOUNT OF ABHAYANGA

More than ten years ago, before I was introduced to Ayurveda, I watched a friend give her one-year-old baby an Ayurvedic oil massage. I was fascinated to see that the baby, usually so active, lay quiet and still. She was so relaxed that her plump little limbs, firmly rubbed and massaged, were like rubber appendages. I would venture to call it something more than relaxation, for as an adult, I feel it is difficult to attain such a state of both body and mind. Perhaps this is what I consider bliss to be—a rare moment when the outer world falls away from our adult consciousness and we truly *experience*.

Our eyes—the baby's and mine—met for a moment, and then hers moved on, back to her mom and to wandering around the room. I felt such intimacy with this child in that brief gaze. Recalling this later, I wondered why we share such moments of deep relaxation with another so infrequently. Perhaps because we seldom even experience them for ourselves. And when we do, to share such a moment would require

putting aside any fears or vulnerability. What I didn't realize at the time is that even just the warm oil itself would have been enormously helpful to me.

As an adult I always had dry skin. Every day after showering in hot water, I would slather gobs of white creamy lotion on my legs, arms, and midsection, hoping to stave off the horrible itchiness that would come later in the day, once my skin had absorbed all the lotion. This was a sure sign of my vata imbalance yet to come. But I had no knowledge of Ayurveda, so I slathered away daily with no hope of the skin condition ever subsiding. Those days are over now.

Daily abhayanga relieves my dry skin and so much more. This oil massage is an extremely important start to my day. It provides nourishment on many levels: skin, nerve tissue, muscles, joints, and more. It's the one thing I can always do to take care of myself, even when I am traveling, not able to eat a proper diet, or feeling stress or anxiety.

Let me say that my body does not always start the day feeling refreshed, light, and moving freely. Living with multiple sclerosis means waking most days with heavy limbs and stiff muscles. Rising early would help offset these discomforts. Given, however, that I may also wake with another common MS symptom, fatigue, I don't always manage to get out of bed before the sun. Most days upon awakening, my immediate goal is to care for myself in a way that allows me to move more easily through the day. After morning rituals of hot water, herbs, meditation, and some pranayama and stretching, I reward myself with abhayanga. Nothing soothes like a warm oil massage.

I consider my oiling ritual the most important thing I can do for my body to make it feel better immediately. And if my body feels more comfortable, then it will distract me less and serve me better through the rest of the day, so I can live my life more fully. No medication, herb, food, or exercise provides this kind of relief and nourishment. No matter how I felt before oiling, afterward I always feel deeply refreshed and nourished.

And when evening comes and I am ready for bed, sometimes my nerves are overactive from my full day—as if someone has plugged my nervous system into a wall socket. I might feel restless or have a jittery sensation in my legs and feet. Again, I reach for that warm oil to soothe myself. Abhayanga on my feet, ankles, and calves allows the hyperstimulated receptors to retreat, so I can get to sleep.

I am so grateful to Ayurveda and to my teacher Acharya Shunya, who changed my entire life when she initiated me into this one simple lifestyle practice, fifteen minutes of self-care that can lead to miracles. It is medicine to my body and mind.

Recently my neurologist commented that my MS was at the best possible level. She asked what I was doing to manifest this degree of health. Hearing about Ayurveda, she was curious to know more and even invited me to share Ayurveda's wisdom with other patients. Now, it seems that I am like the baby who amazed me with her ability to accept love and trust with all her being.

The Many Benefits of Ayurvedic Massage

As Leeann's story indicates, there are many benefits to daily self-massage. The ancient texts of Ayurveda say that daily self-oiling has ample antiaging befits. It improves bodily strength by directly nourishing the skin, muscles, joints, and tendons with nutritious oils, and it enhances physical stamina by removing tiredness or exhaustion. From an Ayurvedic perspective, oil massage effectively counteracts vata dosha aggravation. Further, application of specialized oils on the head and scalp can benefit vision, sleep, and complexion and increase your longevity. Self-oiling is seen to be a practice that can make you live longer.

According to a pilot study published in 2011 in *The Journal of Alternative and Complementary Medicine*, classic Ayurvedic oil massage significantly reduced stress levels in twenty subjects, leading the authors to suggest that abhayanga might also be beneficial in lowering high blood pressure.[4]

Because I feel that we benefit even more from lifestyle practices when we know what results to look for, I have listed below the benefits of daily abhayanga from four major classical texts.[5]

Slows aging: Increases in vata dosha in the body, which naturally happen over time, expedite the aging process. We are able to slow aging by balancing vata dosha, which is effectively done through regular oil massage. Oil massage also slows signs of aging on the skin. As irrigating a tree's roots will encourage the growth of new leaves, healthy tissues are promoted by oil massage.

Counteracts fatigue: Oil massaging relieves vata dosha buildup in the muscles, thereby normalizing and relaxing them. Pain in the calf muscles, neck, and shoulders, and a sense of overall heaviness—all signs of exhaustion—are reduced dramatically after even one self-massage session.

Balances vata: Massage with sesame oil—or a base of sesame oil that has been cooked with additional vata-balancing herbs, such as *ashwagandha*—not only reduces vata buildup in the skin and muscles, but in addition, through the absorption of this oil, vata is pacified systemically, imparting balance to body and mind.

Improves eyesight: The Ayurvedic sages say that massage of the feet and toes can, because of the movement of prana through the body's invisible channels (srota), have beneficial impacts on our vision, too.

Increases strength: Long before the era of dermal patches and supplying internal medicine by applying it externally to the skin, Ayurveda has delivered nutrition to the body via massage. The select oils that are applied act like nutrition to the body. Food-grade oils, often cooked along with strength-imparting (*balya*) herbs improve our biological strength.

Lengthens life-span: When prana, or bioenergy, is balanced, we are healthy. When it is corrupted, we are diseased. A massage that balances prana, nourishes tissues and sense organs, and makes the mind calm becomes our best strategy in preventing premature death or the onset of a deathlike disease.

Supports sleep: Any kind of massage can improve the quality of your sleep. The application of warm, vata-calming oils, such as sesame, to your feet and head calms the sense organs and mind, and this, most especially, induces deep sleep.

Nourishes skin: Skin is known as mirror (*darpani*). If we are happy, the skin shines; if we are sad or anxious, the skin is dull and dry. This is one way we age prematurely. Ayurvedic oils,

like sesame, are specifically chosen to nourish the skin and normalize all three doshas in the skin and, thereby, impart strength to withstand the seasons of life.

Increases resistance to disease: Oil application nourishes our tissues. These revitalized tissues can better withstand the natural wear and tear of life and aging without succumbing to microbes or disease.

Helps prevent injuries: Ayurveda texts contrast a well-nourished, sap-filled, green stem of a plant and how it resists bending to external pressure versus a dry, brittle stem that not only bends on lesser pressure, but also breaks off easily. When our tissues are oiled, they more easily withstand falls and other physical injuries with minimal impact.

Enhances beauty: The skin color and complexion improve with daily oiling. The texture of our skin becomes smooth and soft to the touch. Oil massage also has a beneficial impact on vata and kapha doshas, which are at the root of obesity. With daily massage, we lose unneeded weight and develop a more sculpted body.

How to Perform Self-Massage

Ayurvedic texts leave it to the oral tradition, master to disciple, to convey the method of self-massage. In my experience, there are no hard-and-fast rules for abhayanga as long as you lavishly apply warm oil to all parts of your body and do so in a gentle, loving, and mindful manner. Tradition recommends closing your eyes, slowing your breathing, and being aware of each incoming and outgoing breath as you massage your body. The effects are transformational.

To be a bit more specific, you apply up to a cup of warm oil to all parts of your body with your own hand. Don't stand for your massage—sit on a stool or the floor. With gentle rubbing and stroking movements of your hand, make sure that the oil is fully absorbed in an area where it has been applied. Then move on to the next area and repeat the process.

The best time for this massage is in the early morning, after eliminating and before bathing. Massage can also be done in the afternoon or evening, followed by a warm bath.

It is important that your stomach is empty whenever you perform self-massage. You can, as I've said, drink water right before a massage, but you should wait at least two hours after eating.

A daily oil massage practice of ten to fifteen minutes is great. If it is a weekly practice, then spend at least twenty-five to thirty minutes, dedicating more time to each area.

It is recommended to wait a few minutes right after the massage so that the oil has a chance to soak in before you bathe. This is, however, not mandatory. If you are self-massaging daily or almost daily, you can bathe right after completing your massage.

Choosing and Preparing Oils for Massage

Use table 18 to choose your preferred massage oil. You can also blend two or more oils in any proportions, depending on what effect you want.

Seasonal Recommendations

While massage with warm oil is recommended year-round, you can fine-tune your morning massage practice based on the following seasonal recommendations:

- **Winter:** Sesame oil is recommended.

- **Spring:** Mix 1 part mustard oil with 1 part sesame oil or dry massage with herbal powders.

- **Summer:** Mix 3 parts sesame oil with 1 part coconut oil.

- **Fall:** Mix 3 parts coconut oil with 1 part sesame oil.

Heating the Oil

You can reuse empty bottles—plastic squeeze bottles or glass—filling them with your chosen oil. To heat the oil, set the oil bottle in a pool of hot water in your sink. In a few minutes, the oil will be warm enough to use. Squirt a little oil on your arm to test temperature. Alternatively, you can invest in electric massage oil warmer or (my choice) a small electric crockpot. I also dedicate special towels and a bathrobe for this purpose.

Adding Essential Oils

You may wish to add essential oils to your warm massage oil for aroma and for the additional dosha-balancing benefits imparted by essential oils.

- **Vata balancing:** Use warming oils like cardamom, orange, lemon, or jasmine.

- **Pitta balancing:** Use cooling oils like rose, lotus, sandalwood, fennel, or coriander.

- **Kapha balancing:** Use warming and also penetrating oils like clove, holy basil, ginger, camphor, cinnamon, bay leaf, eucalyptus, and frankincense.

TABLE 18   Oils and Their Characteristics

TYPE	EFFECT ON DOSHAS	APPLICATION
Sesame oil	Three-dosha balancing Pure, cold-pressed oil from black seeds is best. Gray and white seed oils are of medium quality.	Useful in back pain, arthritis, sciatica, and muscle pain; best for hair disorders like premature hair loss and greying; has antiaging, anti-inflammatory, antimicrobial, and antioxidant properties.
Coconut oil	Mainly pitta pacifying Mix with sesame for more effectiveness.	Nourishes hair and skin; cools and lubricates skin; reduces heat and rashes. (It is not, however, as effective in pain management as sesame oil.)
Almond oil	Mainly vata pacifying A bit expensive. Mix with sesame for economy if required.	Revitalizes senses and nervous system; great antiaging, strength-imparting oil.
Castor oil	Mainly vata and kapha pacifying Mix with sesame oil for easier usage.	Antiaging and rejuvenating; helps counteract low back pain and stiffness; reduces abdominal distention upon massaging, improves skin glow; recommended for gout, rheumatoid arthritis, and general swelling; helps overcome inflammation of muscles.
Mustard oil	Mainly kapha pacifying (strong smell) Mix with sesame for easier usage.	Antitoxic, anticellulite, antiobesity; counteracts skin itchiness and fungal infections; relieves pain; warms the body. (Keep away from eyes.)
Butter	Homemade butter Made from cow's milk; use fresh.	Effective antiwrinkle therapy; quite cooling, soft in texture, and emollient, but gentle enough to nourish an infant's skin from seventh day onward.
Ghee	Vata and pitta pacifying Ghee provides an immunity-promoting ingredient.	Not typically used by itself but can be added as an extra ingredient to any oil, especially to counteract heavy-duty dryness, stiff muscles, or burning sensations on the skin.

The Strokes: Applying the Oil

You should follow your intuition in applying and massaging in the oil, but following are some suggestions you may wish to consider:

- Apply oil on your scalp and rub it in using your finger pads. Breathe deeply. You want to oil the scalp and not the hair in daily self-massage.

- Apply oil to your face gently in upward directions, pulling away from the center of the face. Also massage your ears (inside and out). Keep away from your eyes.

- Make upward strokes on your neck while gently cupping the neck with both hands.

- Use cupping, circular strokes on your shoulders.

- Use cupping, upward strokes on your chest.

- Massaging your heart chakra area is a matter of intuitive touch, so feel your way. You may feel like laughing or crying while touching heart chakra area with oil. If so, do let yourself do this. It is a release.

- Use clockwise strokes and breathe deeply a few times while oiling your abdomen. Let your belly swell up with the inhalation and collapse with the exhalation.

- For your limbs, use gentle strokes pulling downward and out (rather than up, toward the heart).

- Touch every finger and toe and rub oil between the digits also. Palm and foot massage are crucial.

- Extend your hands and apply oil on buttocks, lower back, and upper back—as much as you can without straining.

Three Areas of Special Focus

Ayurveda texts stress the oiling of the head, ears, and feet, so be sure to do this much, even if you cannot target the entire body daily.[6]

Head massage (*shirobhayanga*): Head massage includes both the face and the scalp—it not only prevents premature graying and hair loss but also nourishes all the sense organs, prevents headaches, improves sleep quality, and makes the facial skin beautiful and lustrous.[7]

Foot massage (*padabhayanga*): is the best remedy for overcoming fatigue. Several texts mention that it directly improves vision, and it stabilizes vata dosha in a major way. Massaging the feet is of great benefit when vata imbalance has caused pain and stiffness in lower limbs, especially sciatica or foot pain.[8]

Ear massage (*karnabhyanga*): is also vata pacifying, given that the ears are one of the seats of vata dosha. Massaging the ears is soothing to the senses. From personal experience, I can say that this is the best part of the entire massage. I look forward to it. I find that it calms my mind almost immediately and induces a meditative state of awareness. Texts declare that ear massage and drops of oil in the ear counteract the stiffness or pain in jaw or neck. It also prevents earaches, sensitivity to sound, and deafness.[9]

Oiling the Scalp

While the tradition of Ayurvedic massage recommends oiling the scalp with a full scalp massage daily, many people who lead busy lives in the modern world may find that this isn't feasible. If this is the case for you, I recommend applying the oil only briefly to your scalp before shampooing every day. This will ensure that your scalp gets a daily dose of health-promoting oil. Be sure to give yourself time to dry your hair before you leave for school, work, or wherever. If you suffer from dry scalp and dandruff, you can choose to wear a thin layer of oil on your scalp (not on the hair itself, which can remain relatively oil-free) and shampoo only every other day or every few days. You can do this by applying oil to your fingertips and inserting them carefully through your hair so as to only touch the scalp, as much as is possible. Then gently massage the oil in. This will recondition your scalp and reduce symptoms of dryness.

My recommendation is to oil your scalp lavishly on weekends, or whenever you have extra time. Massage oil into your hair also, including the ends. Each time you do this, you will be glad you did. This practice will wonderfully condition your hair, nourish your hair roots, and reduce the problem of frizzy hair and split ends.

Post-Massage Bathing

It is vital to complete the self-massage with hot or warm water bathing. The warmth of the water ensures that the oil penetrates even deeper to nourish the underlying tissues. To bathe, you can use any natural soap. Ayurveda recommends, however, using all-natural bath scrubs such as chickpea flour or green gram lentil flour on the body after an oil massage. This practice is known as *udvartanam*. Find recipes and step-by-step instructions on how to make your own bath scrubs known as *ubtan* later in this chapter.

When Not to Use Oil Massage

For years, I have been suggesting the oil application ritual to students and members of my extended family. My graduates are teaching the same art of self-massage to hundreds of clients via our clinics. As long as some simple rules of what to watch out for are respected, each and every person who embraces Ayurveda's self-massage ritual reaps the fruits of health, as promised by the sages.[10]

Of course, there are times when self-massage with oil is not recommended. If you have any of the symptoms or conditions described below, do not practice self-massage until the symptoms are gone or the weather has changed.

Excess kapha: The symptoms of increased kapha dosha include an active cold, cough, runny nose, sinusitis, or bronchitis as well as water retention (edema) and even obstinate obesity.

Indigestion and diarrhea: Indigestion and loose movements indicate compromised agni and presence of aama or food-based toxins in the gastrointestinal tract. The stickiness of the massage oil will increase aama, so it's important to wait until natural hunger returns (in case of indigestion) or your bowels normalize.

Fever and infections: Aggravated doshas combined with aama, or autotoxins, create fever and infections. So skip your massage until your fever fully subsides or your infection is cleared up.

Rainy weather: Avoid oil application on days when it's rainy or even looks like it may rain. At these times, agni is diminished, and consequently, autotoxins in the body are increased. Avoiding massage at these times is a precautionary measure.

Important Times to Receive Massage

As I've said, with the exceptions listed above, self-massage should be practiced daily. There are, however, times when we especially benefit from receiving massage. These include the following:

After childbirth: The Ayurveda system of health and healing prescribes forty days of full-body massage, with gentle but firm pressure on the lower back and lower abdomen of women who have delivered a baby. The massages should ideally begin on the day of delivery or the very next day. While childbirth is a natural phenomenon, vata dosha is invariably aggravated. The forty-day massage ritual ensures the pacification of the excited vata, without which there can be pain and aching in the lower back. Also, the attention a new mother receives through massage lends her emotional support, circumventing possible postpartum depression. This massage is usually offered by the new mother's female relatives, life partner, or a massage professional.

In infancy and childhood: Infants are massaged every day from the seventh day after birth until their third birthday. Preferably this early massage is done by the mother or caregiver. It promotes circulation, regulation of prana, and bonding. Most children love receiving massage, and since sesame oil is three-dosha balancing, any skin-based diseases and most other childhood diseases are inhibited. Of course, butter is also used for infants and children with sensitive skin, but sesame is a great economical and less greasy option. I was three or four when I learned how to apply oil to my body, and with a little help from my mother, I massaged myself quite well by age five. Children learn fast and love to self-massage—it empowers them to

learn a health-protecting, proactive ritual of self-care from an early age. Of course, I would not allow a child to heat the oil. I would give the child a preheated, lukewarm oil in an easy-to-handle squeeze bottle. I would also teach the basic steps several times and be nearby to prevent any accidents.

Other Types of Daily Massage

While an oil massage is the most optimum daily practice, Ayurveda tradition also specifies other varieties of massage, including dry powder massage and an extra-gentle massage.

Dry Powder Massage

A massage without oil is done with powdered lentils and herbs; this is known as *udgharshana*. This dry powder massage is especially useful for anyone trying to lose weight or having a tendency toward colds, coughs, or allergies, when an oil massage would be contraindicated.

Dry massage successfully reduces cellulite and fat deposits and overcomes a tendency toward water retention and itchiness of skin. This massage involves brisk rubbing, so it generates heat because of the friction. This heat opens the biochannels, liquefies subcutaneous fat, helps in easy absorption of the herbs, imparts a lightness to the body, counteracts itchiness, and makes even a drowsy or dull person wake up invigorated.

Further, the intense rubbing dilates the blood vessels and stimulates the agni in the skin (*bhrajak pitta*). Hence, the cellulite, water, and fat deposits in the skin get efficiently metabolized. [11]

For a dry massage scrub, you can use herb powders either singly or in combination. These include ground chickpea flour (*besan*), ground horse gram (*chana*), *Acorus calamus* (*vacha*) powder, *Pluchea lanceolata* (*rasna*), ginger powder (shunthi), *Santalum album* (*chandana*), *Crocus sativus* (*kesar*), and *Aquilaria agallocha* (*agaru*).

You can add water to the same herbal powder to make a paste and use this in massage, a practice known as *utsaadana*. Women often prefer this paste massage to a dry scrub, as women's skin is often softer and more sensitive. The paste-based massage has similar benefits to the dry massage powder, but the impact is a bit more tempered.

Extra-Gentle Massage

The special extra-gentle massage (*samvahana*) was first put forward by Ayurveda surgeon Sage Sushruta in the first-second century CE.[12] Samvahana consists of gentle and extra-tender thumping action and light and nonstimulating pressing strokes, ideally used on the crown of newborns, on infants, on young children, and on the abdomen of a pregnant woman. It is a massage that is done with little or no pressure. The medium of lubrication is often a form of dairy: either cream, ghee (clarified butter), or freshly churned butter. Any of these mediums can be used by itself or in combination with warm sesame oil.

The massage medium must be warmed before using. It could be warmed in the palm of the hand and should be at least room temperature. Never simply keep a massage lubricant—even dairy—in the refrigerator until massage time and then put it on the skin without warming it first. Be sure to let it sit out for several hours until it reaches room temperature.

I like to do samvahana massage when I want to give myself extra loving attention. I have suggested it for people who are too hard on themselves. In fact, the text by Sage Sushruta clearly states that this massage increases affection, and as he puts it poetically in Sanskrit, it increases *preeti*, or feelings of love.[13]

This massage is also great for increasing sexual interest as well as sexual pleasure. The gentle strokes and pleasing substances can act as aphrodisiacs if you undertake the massage with this intention.

Since this very gentle massage is also an effective sleep-inducer and pacifies vata dosha, which can be specifically aggravated from hard work or physical labor, I like to suggest it to those who hold physically demanding jobs or have suffered injury or emotional trauma. It is particularly well suited for anyone who has skin that is too sensitive to bear pressure, who is aging, or who does not have the stamina needed to keep strokes vigorous enough on a daily basis. In all such instances, the extra-gentle massage with gentle lubricants is the way to go.

The Ayurvedic Bathing Ritual (Snanam)

The Sanskrit word for bathing, *snanam*, means more than just bathing to remove physical dirt; it also has connotations of spiritual purification or ceremonial cleansing done for spiritual purposes. I find this enormously significant. The Ayurvedic bath is an elaborate ritual that invites you to connect with the purifying waters and healing herbs that are cleansing for your body, the receptacle of your divine spirit.

The spirit is always pure, taintless; yet the body benefits from regular cleansing. So why not make cleansing the body a ritual worthy of the majestic spirit that you are?

Sections below contain suggestions for adding specific flowers and herbs to your bath. These will impart immense healing properties to the water. My Baba used to say, "*Do not use anything for bathing that you cannot eat.*" And I convey this injunction to my students all the time. My family always made its own body care preparations—lotions, shampoos, and soaps that you can actually eat, using perishable ingredients that are completely biodegradable.

Growing Healing Herbs for Your Bath

Of course, it goes without saying that you can order the dried botanicals, either whole or ground, from trusted online sources. But if weather and space permit, you could also consider growing your own flowers and herbs. It's a good way to know for sure that what you're putting on your body is indeed pesticide-free. It is also gratifying to meet your own health requirements instead of expecting Mother Earth to deliver your order, without taking the responsibility to plant and nurture a few seeds.

I do purchase botanicals, but I grow those few that I can. There is something special about the healing you can experience from a plant you have grown yourself. You have put healing care into growing the plant; you and the plant have a relationship.

If you do not live in a situation that allows you to grow your own herbs and flowers, then think of these as ideas that may take root in the garden of your beautiful mind so that in the future, if you ever do have the privilege of possessing a garden or a sunny terrace, you will consider growing your own flowers, herbs, and medicinal trees.

Specifics about Bathing

The Ayurvedic bath traditionally follows the application of warm oil, abhayanga, described earlier in this chapter.

In regard to timing, traditional people like my Baba would always bathe pretty early in the day, and always before embarking on spiritual activities, worship rituals, yoga, and even meditation. But the timing of the bath does not seem to be a strict rule. Minor adjustments to your morning bath time are fine.

I do feel it's important that you bathe before eating breakfast, that you eat breakfast at the recommended time—before 8:00 a.m. and no later—and that you maintain consistency in your routine. You may want to review Ayurveda's guidelines for beginning your day, which are given in the introduction and chapter 1.

When bathing at other times of day, wait at least two hours after eating. In other words, bathing should always be done with an empty stomach. The process of digestion requires the flow of doshas and blood toward the stomach and organs of digestion. However, if we indulge in actions like bathing, heavy exercise, or sexual intercourse right after eating, the flow of doshas goes toward the muscles (periphery). This will potentially compromise digestion or definitely retard it, and the possibility of toxins (inadequately digested food) also cannot be ruled out. Hence, it is best to bathe before sitting down to a meal.

Various cultures encourage different bathing styles. Any of these would work as long as the water is clean and inviting. In the Ayurvedic tradition, bathing (snanam) includes any of these customs:

- Immersion in a bathtub (*avagaaha*)

- Showering with an overhead faucet or shower spigot

- Pouring water with a mug from a bucket while standing or sitting down

- Bathing in clean rivers, ponds, and lakes

Water Temperature

Ayurveda texts clarify the impact of various water temperatures on bathing. Obviously, if you're bathing in a natural body of water, you have no control over the water temperature, and it will likely be cool at least and possibly cold. That can be bracing, of course, and it's very good for some conditions. A cold-water bath pacifies aggravation of pitta dosha and is also beneficial in case of blood disorders. It can aggravate vata and kapha doshas.

A hot-water bath pacifies vata and kapha doshas but can aggravate pitta dosha. Ayurveda says that if hot water is used for washing the head, it almost always disturbs the vision because the eyes are the seat of pitta dosha. So even if you bathe the rest of your body with warm water, ideally you should wash your head and hair with lukewarm or even cool water. Warm water is used only in rare conditions to wash the head and hair.

Benefits of Regular Bathing

Ayurvedic texts beautifully summarize the benefits of bathing.[14] Regular bathing in the morning and with an empty stomach effectively counteracts fatigue or a sense of torpor, a tendency to sweat, and itching or sensations of heat in the body. In addition, bathing has the following benefits:

- Bathing enhances our life essence (*ayushyam*), removing disease-causing dirt, bacteria, and parasites from the skin.

- It enkindles our digestive fire (*deepanam*), often making us feel ravenous after bathing!

- Bathing can, in certain situations, act as an aphrodisiac (*vrshyam*).

- It improves our physical strength (*bala*) and immunity (*oja*).

- It increases our mental strength (*dhairyam*).

- It imparts an antidepressant effect by increasing the quality of sattva, which nicely jumpstarts the mind in its balanced mode (*sattva*).

- And it adds to our courage (*virya*) to deal with whatever lies ahead in our day.

This list is verified in the Ayurvedic scriptures, and I feel that anyone who bathes regularly can attest to each of these benefits as a matter of personal experience.

When Not to Bathe

Ayurveda suggests not bathing under the following conditions:

- When experiencing diarrhea or loose movements (because bathing will further compromise the digestive fire)

- When experiencing flatulence, especially when the smell is bad and you have acute indigestion (indicating poor agni and toxins)

- When you have a fever (indicating toxins)

- When you have recently eaten (wait until at least two hours after a meal)

In some of these situations, you may choose to bathe, but if you do, I suggest avoiding an extended session, whether it's a tub bath or shower. Keep the time to a minimum and, if possible, bathe simply with a wet sponge or cloth.

Crafting a Healing Tub Bath (Avagaaha)

When the body, having been gently anointed with warm oil, is immersed in a tub full of water in which tender leaves and flowers of healing botanicals have been added, it is called avagaaha, or Ayurvedic tub bath.

This kind of herb-infused tub bath is especially recommended to tranquilize the nervous system. It also benefits the circulatory system, nourishes the skin's hair follicles, and lubricates and rejuvenates the skin, muscles, and joints.[15]

Many of us can vouch for the exponential increase in well-being we experience when we make the extra effort to dissolve mineral salts, aromatic herbs, infused oils, or special soaps in our bathwater. The addition of lit candles, music, flowers, and incense can further transform an ordinary bath into an extraordinary and relaxing ritual of beauty, splendor, and rejuvenation. I encourage you to explore various ways to make your bath time special, and if you cannot do this daily, then try it at least once or twice weekly.

Adding Botanicals to Your Bath

Your time in the bathtub can be made all the more special by infusing your bathwater with healing botanicals. Botanicals are fresh or dried flower petals, leaves, roots, or fruits. Any of the botanicals mentioned in succeeding sections can be ordered online, purchased locally (at a grocery store or nursery), or grown in your own backyard.

When adding a botanical to an average-sized bathtub, be generous. Add one to two full eight-ounce cups of dry or fresh botanicals for each bath.

I like to have the bathwater on the warmer side in winter and room temperature or on the cooler side (but not chilled) in summer. In general, in warmer water, the medicinal quality of the botanicals will impact your skin and senses in greater capacity.

Add botanicals to the bathwater directly, or for greater medicinal benefit, boil 1 part botanical (fresh or dry, 8 ounces, for example) in 8 parts water (64 ounces). Bring to a boil and then reduce heat. Simmer until you are left with only 4 parts water (32 ounces). Add this reduced liquid (decoction) minus the cooked herbs (strain through a fine cloth) to the bathwater.

Bathe for a minimum of twenty to forty minutes. You will benefit from this healing bathwater only if you allow yourself time to soak in it. You may want to make some special time for this bathing ritual. When you are in a hurry, you will have to settle for a shorter bath or a shower.

If you wish, you can use an Ayurvedic soap in a healing botanical bath, but bring out the soap only toward the end of your bath time, after you have soaked for a while in the medicinal bathwater.

Even better than soap, however, is the ground powder of green mung lentils (green gram). Green gram flour can be purchased at Indian grocery stores (if you live near one, ask for *hari mung atta*) or ground into a fine powder yourself using a common coffee grinder. I tend to make my own more often than not. Make a wet paste by adding water to half a cup of the powder. After you have soaked for some time, rub this paste all over your body, even on your face, for exfoliating action. You can also refer to the section on crafting your own bath scrubs later in this chapter for additional ideas.

Following are some of the specific botanical tub baths recommended by Ayurveda.

Lotus Bath

For a lotus bath, add fresh or dried lotus petals to your bathwater. The lotus flower, known as *padma* and *kamala* in Sanskrit, is renowned for its beauty. It is India's national flower and is considered by Hindus and Buddhists to be the most sacred flower. The lotus is closely aligned with Shri Lakshmi, the goddess of beauty, abundance, and good fortune.

Lotus petals are mildly fragrant, cooling in their effect, and thus, pacifying for pitta and kapha doshas. Therefore, a lotus bath is especially recommended if you are recovering from any skin condition that involves itchy, blotchy, or red skin—chicken pox or herpes, for instance. The lotus has blood-purifying properties, and lotus petals refine complexion—a property known as *varnya* in Sanskrit.

The white lotus is most efficacious, but blooms of other colors will also work. I grow my own lotuses in large pots in my own backyard in California. Anyone who lives where there is a reasonably warm summer can do the same. Lotus responds well to direct sunlight.

White-colored water lilies (*Nymphaea alba*), sometimes known as pond lilies and called *kumuda* in Ayurveda, also possess similar qualities and can be substituted in a lotus bath with good effect.

Rose Bath

Rose, the most beloved flower of many, is a timeless symbol of beauty, love, and joy. In Ayurveda, rose is known as *shatapatri*, *taruni*, and *karnika*. Rose petals of any color can be used to make a tri-dosha-balancing bath. The impact of rose on the skin is clarifying and soothing and reduces redness. Rose bestows a healthy, glowing complexion every time since it is a complexion enhancer (*varnya*).

Rose also has a special potency to enhance well-being. In addition to its heady aroma, the rose has qualities that impact our hearts and emotions most positively. This is why rose is classified in the Ayurveda tradition as a *hrdya*, which translates as "heart-friendly." The rose makes the heart—whether it's the organ, the chakra, or just our emotions—stronger, happier, and more stable.

So add fresh or dried rose petals to your bathwater on any day when your mood needs a boost or your feelings need a peaceful release. Rose is also an effective remedy for anger and irritability, whether caused by overwork, heat exhaustion, or overstimulation.

Roses can be grown successfully in pots or home gardens as long as they get enough sunshine and water. Be sure to save those petals!

Jasmine Bath

The intensely perfumed jasmine flower has many varieties. For the purpose of a bath, I prefer using *Jasminum arborescens* (known as *chameli* or *saptala*) or *Jasminum sambac* (known as *mogra* or *varshiki*). This jasmine flower is cold in potency, yet it balances all three doshas, and jasmine leaves can be also added to the bathwater with similar benefits. You can add fresh or dried jasmine flowers and leaves to the bathwater.

Jasmine has a special healing impact on the eyes, ears, and mouth, and acts as an agent to protect and detoxify the skin. The aroma of jasmine is heady. It can soothe headaches induced by mental tension and can rejuvenate the body after heat exposure and heat exhaustion.

The jasmine plant can grow in both shade and indirect sunlight, so it flourishes as an indoor plant as long as it has access to some light. Jasmine is extremely easy to care for—I consider it a plant of very easy access—and I recommend that you invest in a jasmine plant today. It will give you aromatic gifts and countless healing bath times year-round!

Marigold Bath

The marigold, known as *zendu* in Sanskrit, is cooling. It balances pitta and kapha and has a special property of purifying blood. It is antibacterial, antiseptic, and antifungal. Because of these properties, the marigold has been used as a skin salve and medicinal oil for thousands of years. It has been used as a remedy for candida, athlete's foot, and ringworm.

Marigold benefits both oily and dry skin. It normalizes skin tone and complexion, imparts a glow to the skin, reduces redness, and acts as a natural moisturizer to keep wrinkles at bay. It also clears blemishes. Marigold soothes skin and prevents further dryness and, at the same time, keeps excessive oiliness in check. The juice of this useful flower is a traditional Ayurvedic remedy to eliminate ear pain, reduce eye inflammation, and (as a gargle) to cure mouth sores or stomatitis. Marigold is even effective in healing vaginal and bladder infections, hemorrhoids, and post-childbirth sutures.

With all of this, you can just imagine how healing a marigold bath is, not only for your skin, but for all of your other sense organs as well.

Add fresh or dried petals and leaves of marigold blossoms to the bathwater.

Marigolds almost seem to grow themselves once you drop the seeds in the ground or plant the saplings. They are low maintenance, but they love full sun and grow in well-drained soils and also in pots. You will love them, I promise you!

Musk Rose Bath

Musk rose is an intensely sweet-smelling flower with a cooling potency and a balancing effect on all three doshas. Musk rose or *Rosa morchata* is known as *kubjaka* or *surabhi* in Sanskrit. This remarkable flower is classified by both the Ayurvedic texts and oral tradition as an aphrodisiac (vrshyam). It is said that bathwater fragrant with the petals of musk rose naturally and pleasantly stokes sexual desire. The musk rose is safely used for this purpose, and the list of its positive benefits does not end there. The potency of the musk rose, which is slightly warming, can help ward off colds.

Add fresh or dried musk rose petals to your bathwater.

Musk roses will grow even in shade or indirect light, otherwise requiring very much the same care of any other rosebush.

Turmeric Bath

Turmeric (*haridra*) is an ancient herbal remedy that purifies the skin, brings it beauty, and gives it a glow. Since turmeric also acts as a potent antibacterial, antifungal, and antiseptic, it is clearly an Ayurvedic bath ingredient of choice. The only downside is that turmeric's deep-yellow color tends to stain the bathtub and towels as well. Fortunately, this is not a permanent stain; it goes away in time, effortlessly without bleach.

After a turmeric bath, it may also be important to bathe or shower with plain warm water and to clean the body well with a body scrub consisting of finely ground mung lentil (green gram) to ensure that the turmeric residue has been fully removed. It is well worth undertaking this effort because turmeric is a renowned anti-inflammatory and analgesic. So if you have muscle aches, back pain, or joint pain, then a warm bath soaking in the healing goodness of turmeric will go a long way. Additionally, a turmeric bath will also soothe and begin the healing of many troublesome skin conditions—acne, boils, blemishes, itching, excessive redness, eczema, or allergic rashes.

To use turmeric, you can either add the powder directly into warm water (it does not mix as well with cooler water) or make a decoction from its fresh rhizome (rootstalk) and then add this to the bathwater.

I have begun to grow turmeric recently in my backyard, in a large pot, and am finding this easy to do, so I recommend that you do the same. Turmeric also grows very nicely indoors, as long as you have a sunny room. It is a low-maintenance plant.

Amalaki Bath

Amalaki refers to the fruit of *Emblica officinalis* or *Phyllanthus emblica*, or malacca tree. It is a deciduous tree known for its edible fruit, called amla, or Indian gooseberry. Amalaki has such an impact on the skin and hair that an Ayurvedic text proclaims, "One who bathes with water in which fruits of amalaki has been soaked will surely get rid of wrinkled skin and gray hair and will live for a hundred years."[16] That is a weighty claim to make; it almost sounds magical. But given the potent antiaging and antioxidant qualities of amalaki, I can understand why the sages were so enthusiastic about an amalaki bath. Amalaki is considered foremost among the antiaging drugs and best among the rejuvenating herbs, *and* it improves complexion.[17]

In bathwater, you can use amalaki by adding its dried fruit powder to the water directly, or if you live in a place where its fresh fruit is available, you can make a decoction from its fresh fruit and add this to your bath. In the bath, amalaki imparts its potent and scientifically validated antimicrobial and antiviral properties.

Ayurvedic Bath Scrubs (Udvartana)

I recommend replacing ordinary soaps for your bath routine with more natural preparations. Most commercial soaps contain artificial fragrances, petroleum derivatives, and other chemicals that damage the skin. In Ayurveda, body scrubs are part of the daily cleansing regimen and are often used in place of soap. These body scrubs, called udvartana or ubtan, can be modified based on your skin type.

If you would like to craft your own scrubs, you can begin with the recipes below, which are ones my family has used for generations. Scrubs are to be used daily as a soap substitute and after oiling as a cleanser. Simply scrub the powder gently over the body and rinse off. The scrub recipes here are nondrying and do not contain any harsh chemicals.

It's best to grind all ingredients to a fine, powder-like consistency or to purchase them preground. The base of these scrubs is often made of one or a combination of these three natural ingredients:

Green gram flour (hari mung): Whole green gram strikes a balance between oiliness and dryness and ensures that the natural moisture of the skin is maintained. Mung is cooling, clarifies complexion, gently exfoliates, gets rid of unwanted facial hair, and overcomes whiteheads. This base can be used safely by all.

Chickpea flour (besan): Chickpea flour lightens complexion and removes tan. It imparts instant glow and can also be used as a quick pick-me-up before a special event when you want to look your best. Its impact is cooling, and it absorbs excessive sebum, so it is helpful with oily skin.

Red lentil flour (masoor): This is best used as a base to counteract oily, blemish-prone skin. It effectively controls sebum production and counteracts acne. Red lentil is cooling and soothing and is useful by itself or in conjunction with green gram lentil for any skin that tends to break out easily.

The following recipes are for a one-time use after you add the liquids, or you can store the dry ingredients for future use.

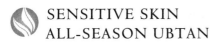 SENSITIVE SKIN
ALL-SEASON UBTAN

Sensitive skin needs extra care, and medicated products are often suggested for such skin types by "experts." Make your own medicated ubtan at home with this recipe.

INGREDIENTS

- ½ cup green gram flour
- 1 teaspoon turmeric
- 1 teaspoon milk or water, or enough to make a paste
- 1 teaspoon coconut oil or sesame oil

Note on ingredients: Milk and coconut oil are preferred in summer and fall, especially if your skin is oily. Use both ingredients throughout the year if your skin is on the dry and hot side. Sesame is a tri-dosha-balancing oil; however, it is especially helpful for dry skin, premature aging, or wrinkles.

METHOD

1. Mix the dry ingredients. Add the oil and milk or water.
2. Stir lightly, though thoroughly, to make a paste.
3. Apply on your body and gently rub. Rinse with water.

 SPRING SEASON
PRE-SHOWER UBTAN

This ubtan provides exfoliating action and helps balance natural skin oils. It removes dead skin and leaves skin looking tremendously fresh.

INGREDIENTS

- ½ cup green gram flour
- 1 tablespoon minced fresh fenugreek leaves or 1 teaspoon ground fenugreek seeds
- 1 tablespoon water, or enough to make paste

METHOD

1. Mix all ingredients until dry ingredients are incorporated. If using fresh fenugreek leaves, mix until they are coated with the powder and liquid.
2. Apply this paste on your face, neck, and arms. It starts drying as you apply.
3. Once you have completed the application, start rubbing off the paste with fresh water. The removal of the paste through rubbing, versus simply spraying water on yourself, is the exfoliating action.

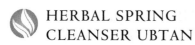

HERBAL SPRING CLEANSER UBTAN

This ubtan is great for balancing aggravated kapha dosha in spring. Use as a bathing scrub in lieu of drying soaps.

INGREDIENTS

- 1 **cup barley flour**
- 1 **tablespoon Indian gooseberry (amalaki) powder**
- 1 **tablespoon ground coriander**
- 1 **teaspoon neem powder**

METHOD

1. Mix all ingredients.
2. Rub gently all over the body. Rinse with water. (Try to not introduce any water into the stored dry mixture.)

SAFFRON SKIN GLOW-ENHANCING UBTAN

Saffron is the best antiblemish and complexion-enhancing agent. Oats are highly absorptive and soften the skin. Red lentil has excellent skin-cleansing properties. It can be used on the face as well as all over the body. Milk has a nourishing quality. All of these wonderful ingredients, when mixed and applied on the face, clean it as well as soften it and add a glowing quality.

INGREDIENTS

- ½ **cup red lentil flour (masoor)**
- ¼ **cup ground oats**
- ¼ **teaspoon saffron strands**
- 1 **tablespoon cool milk, or enough to make a paste**

METHOD

1. Mix all ingredients into a paste.
2. Apply a thin layer on face and body. Wash off with cool water after ten minutes.

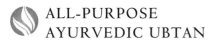

ALL-PURPOSE AYURVEDIC UBTAN

Use this scrub once or twice a week.

INGREDIENTS

- ½   cup rice flour
- 1   tablespoon green gram flour
- 1   tablespoon milk, rose water, or plain water, or enough to make a paste

METHOD

1. Mix all ingredients into a soft scrub.
2. Apply the scrub with your fingertips. Massage your skin gently with the facial scrub for one minute with gentle, circular movements of your fingers. Be extra gentle on the skin around the eyes.
3. Rinse the scrub off your face with water.

Ayurvedic Face Packs
(Anulepana)

Naturally, Ayurveda has some wonderful suggestions for homemade preparations to use for facials and as masks for various other parts of the body. You can apply Ayurveda face packs daily, weekly, bi-weekly, or once a month, based on your personal preference. Wash them off after they dry (but do not allow to dry so much that they crack), and then apply your preferred day moisturizer, if you need one.

From the time I turned thirteen until I was almost twenty-two, I treated my face and neck with one or another homemade facial pack recipe nearly every day. It was part of my daily routine. Even today (and I have crossed the half-century mark), I get compliments for my skin. It is blemish free, and I am told I look younger than I am. With my busy schedule these days, I have little time to apply facial packs, but it looks like my early concentrated investment into my skin is still paying off.

I do still like to pamper myself with a facial pack every three months or so, on those rare weekends when I am not teaching. The aromas bring back such lovely memories from a beauty-filled life growing up in India. And even now, the transformation in my skin is dramatic! Try for yourself. Each time, you will be glad you indulged your skin with a luxurious, all-natural face pack treatment. It is never too late to begin, and there is no day like today to love yourself a little more!

The face pack recipes that follow are all lovely, traditional in origin, and easy to prepare. For the most part, I have grouped them by their major ingredients.

- **Cucumber:** Cooling, soothing, and oil-balancing

- **Rose:** Medicinal for skin that is aging, sensitive, red, or inflamed

- **Cow's milk:** Soothing for skin that is mature or sensitive (Use organic, whole raw milk if available.)

- **Turmeric:** Purifying for the blood and a miraculous nourishment for the skin that leaves it glowing and radiant

There are also masks using sandalwood, marigold, chickpea flour, and coconut milk. Following are several recipes for every skin type!

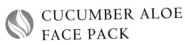 ## CUCUMBER ALOE FACE PACK

This pack is beneficial for oily T-zone skin (forehead, nose, chin, and area around your mouth).

INGREDIENTS

- 1 tablespoon grated cucumber
- 1 tablespoon *Aloe vera* gel (squeezed from a leaf from of a homegrown plant, if possible)

METHOD

1. Mix ingredients together. Apply to face and neck.
2. Wait 15 minutes. Rinse with lukewarm water. Pat dry.

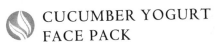 ## CUCUMBER YOGURT FACE PACK

This pack is also beneficial for oily T-zone skin.

INGREDIENTS

- 1 tablespoon grated cucumber
- 1 teaspoon whole-milk yogurt

METHOD

1. Mix ingredients together. Apply to face and neck.
2. Wait 15 minutes. Rinse with lukewarm water. Pat dry.

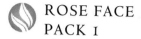 ROSE FACE
PACK 1

This pack is good for dry, red, inflamed skin and is great in fall. This is a nonhomogeneous mask; in other words, it will not be uniform and will contain bits of organic matter.

INGREDIENTS

- ½ cup fresh crushed rose petals (aromatic, no pesticides)
- 1 teaspoon whole milk
- ½ teaspoon coconut oil

METHOD

1. Mix all ingredients. Apply to face.
2. Lie down and leave on for 5 to 10 minutes.
3. Rinse with cool milk or water and pat dry.

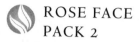 ROSE FACE
PACK 2

This pack is especially useful for dry, sensitive skin year-round and is great in the summer for normal skin.

INGREDIENTS

- ½ cup crushed rose petals (fresh, aromatic, no pesticides)
- 1–2 tablespoons raw honey (enough to coat the rose petals)
  A few drops rose oil, optional

METHOD

1. Mix ingredients together. Apply to face.
2. Cover eyes with whole rose petals and lie down or recline. Let mask sit for 10 minutes or until it starts to feel tight.
3. Rinse with cool milk or water. If the honey is sticky, use a gentle cleanser after rinsing with milk and then follow your normal face care routine.

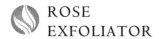 ROSE
EXFOLIATOR

This recipe is for good for all skin types
including extremely sensitive skin.

INGREDIENTS

1   teaspoon rock candy, ground into
    a fine powder
1   teaspoon whole milk
1   teaspoon rose water
½   teaspoon honey (for oily/hot skin)
    or ghee (for dry skin)

METHOD

1. Mix all ingredients to make a paste.
2. Use both hands to exfoliate the face by
   rubbing the mixture gently on the skin.
3. Rinse with warm water after a few
   minutes. Moisturize if desired with a
   light moisturizer.

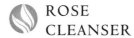 ROSE
CLEANSER

This is a simple but excellent cleanser for all
skin types.

INGREDIENTS

½   tablespoon rose water
½   tablespoon whole milk

METHOD

1. Gently splash on face or dip cotton in
   the cleanser and apply to face. Use your
   fingertips to gently scrub your face.
2. Rinse with lukewarm water and pat dry
   with a clean towel.

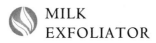 ## MILK EXFOLIATOR

This exfoliator is good for all skin types for use once a week.

INGREDIENTS

- ½ teaspoon rice powder
- ½ teaspoon almond power
- 1 tablespoon whole milk, or enough to make a paste that's not too runny or gritty

METHOD

1. Mix all ingredients together.
2. Gently rub in a circular motion over face (don't scrub too hard).
3. Rinse with lukewarm water and pat dry with a clean towel; follow with moisturizer if desired.

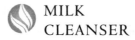 ## MILK CLEANSER

Use for dry skin, wrinkles, red bumps, and inflamed skin.

INGREDIENTS

- 1 teaspoon whole-milk cream (top of milk/ skin that forms on milk when boiled)
- ½ teaspoon ground green mung dal

METHOD

1. Mix whole-milk cream and lentil powder to make a gentle cleansing scrub (mix ingredients together so it is not too gritty or runny).
2. Rinse with warm water. Pat dry and moisturize if desired.

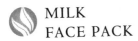 MILK
FACE PACK

This is a nice pack for all skin types. It is a very thin mask that is quite luxurious on application.

INGREDIENTS

1 tablespoon whole milk
1–2 threads saffron, crushed
¼ teaspoon or a small pinch of turmeric

METHOD

1. Mix all ingredients together and apply to skin with clean fingers or a specialized mask brush (with natural fibers).
2. It will dry very quickly and once it does, rinse with lukewarm water and pat dry with a clean towel; follow with moisturizer if desired.

Note: Turmeric and saffron may temporarily color the skin.

 COCONUT AND TURMERIC
FACE PACK FOR FALL

INGREDIENTS

2 tablespoons chickpea flour (besan)
2 tablespoons raw organic honey
¼ teaspoon ground turmeric
1 tablespoon whole-milk yogurt
1 tablespoon coconut milk, or enough
   to make a smooth paste

METHOD

1. Mix all ingredients. Apply to clean, dry skin, and leave on for 15 to 20 minutes.
2. Rinse thoroughly and tone and moisturize your skin as desired.

ANTIAGING TURMERIC FACE PACK

INGREDIENTS

- 1   tablespoon chickpea flour (besan)
- 1   teaspoon turmeric
- 1   tablespoon whole milk or whole-milk yogurt

METHOD

1. Mix all ingredients. Apply paste evenly on your face and let it dry.
2. Wash off with lukewarm water while scrubbing your face gently in a circular motion. Pat dry.

 ## ANTIPIGMENTATION TURMERIC FACE PACK

INGREDIENTS

- 1   teaspoon ground turmeric
- 1   tablespoon mashed papaya
- 1   teaspoon whole milk

METHOD

1. Mix all ingredients. Apply to face and wait 20 minutes.
2. Wash off with warm water and pat dry.

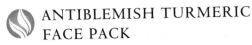

ANTIBLEMISH TURMERIC FACE PACK

This mask is for daily use. This mixture can also be applied on burns, acne, and wounds for faster healing.

INGREDIENTS

- 1 teaspoon ground turmeric
- 1 tablespoon *Aloe vera* gel

METHOD

1. Mix ingredients together and apply to face.
2. Leave mask on for 20 minutes. Wash off with warm water and pat dry.

TURMERIC STRETCH-MARK PACK

This pack can be used daily until stretch marks fade.

INGREDIENTS

- 4 tablespoons black gram (urad dal) flour
- 4 teaspoons turmeric
- ½ cup whole milk

METHOD

1. Mix all ingredients. Apply pack on designated area.
2. Allow to dry and then rub and peel off. Wash with warm water.

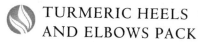 ## TURMERIC HEELS AND ELBOWS PACK

Use this pack daily for cracked heels or elbows. Continue until the issue is resolved.

INGREDIENTS

1   tablespoon castor oil
1   teaspoon turmeric

METHOD

1. Mix ingredients together and apply to desired areas. Rub in and leave on for a minimum of 30 minutes or keep on feet overnight by wearing socks.
2. Wash off with warm water.

Note: Turmeric does not stain your skin or sink permanently, but it does stain temporarily. A mild yellow staining of your facial skin will go away after several washes, or more quickly by gently scrubbing the affected area with a few drops of a mild facial toner on a cotton ball. Yellow staining of ceramic sinks can be removed with any bathroom cleaner or even simply soap and water. However, watch out for artificially colored, extra-bright turmeric—use only the organic kind.

 ## SANDALWOOD RADIANCE FACE PACK

The benefits of this mask are innumerable. First, sandalwood purifies blood, and hence it reduces rashes, blotches, and pimples. Also, since rose water and sandalwood are both varnya (good for complexion), this mask enhances the glow and makes the skin soft and naturally radiant. Sandalwood powder is a rare herb; it is seriously endangered. Hence, use this pack only if you already have an old stock of sandalwood powder.

INGREDIENTS

1   tablespoon sandalwood powder
1   tablespoon water or rose water, or enough to make a paste

METHOD

1. Mix sandalwood with water or rose water and apply it to the face.
2. Allow it to rest for 15 minutes and then wash it off. Use it every day for best results.

GLOWING SKIN MARIGOLD/ ROSE FACE PACK

Have you ever tried face masks with flowers? Marigolds have antibacterial and antiseptic properties that heal acne. Honey works in the same way. Milk softens the skin. Doing this at least one or two times a week helps tighten the pores and leads to glowing skin. This is a perfect Ayurvedic face pack for oily skin. Alternatively, you can use petals of roses in the same manner.

INGREDIENTS

   5   fresh marigolds or roses
1–2 tablesoons whole milk, or enough
      to make a paste
   1   tablespoon honey

METHOD

1. Using a mortar and pestle, pound flowers with milk to make a fresh, flowery paste.
2. Mix in honey.
3. Apply this paste to your face and leave it on for 10 to 15 minutes before washing it off with lukewarm water.

 CHICKPEA FLOUR FACE PACK FOR DULL SKIN

This is one of the most effective and efficient face packs for dull skin. Its exfoliating action takes away the dead cells, and it is a famous Ayurvedic remedy for blemishes too. Regular usage will result in soft, smooth, and glowing skin, and slowly, blemishes will start fading too. There is no other face pack that takes sun tan away like this one does. It clears the skin of tan and gives it an added glow.

INGREDIENTS

   1   tablespoon chickpea flour (besan)
      Few drops fresh-squeezed lemon juice
      Pinch of turmeric powder
1–2 tablespoons rose water (for aged skin) or
      milk (for dry skin) or yogurt (for acne
      or oily skin), or enough to make a paste

METHOD

1. Mix all ingredients to make a paste.
2. Apply the mask to cleansed face and leave on for 10 minutes. Rinse with warm water.

SUMMER SKIN CARE FACE PACK

This pack is my favorite for summertime use because it hydrates the skin.

INGREDIENTS

⅛ cup coconut milk (grate coconut and squeeze out the milk)

1 teaspoon castor oil

Pulp from one medium-size avocado or ½ large avocado

METHOD

1. Mix all ingredients. Spread over face and leave on for 15 minutes.
2. Dip a clean, soft cloth in cool water and wring out so that it is not dripping. Wipe mask off gently.
3. Rinse with cool water and finish with a rose water spritz and light moisturizer if desired.

Wash Your Hair with Botanicals

The lather that emerges from commercial soaps, shampoos, and bubble baths is from sodium lauryl sulfate (see the box, "Why You Should Stop Using Commercial Shampoos"), a common surfactant that traps oily residues and creates foam. This and other surfactants have been proven to irritate the skin, compromise the immune system, and in some cases, increase the chance of cancer. The ingredients in natural Ayurvedic shampoos will not create this kind of lather—but they don't have these side effects either.

Personally, I prefer the goodness of herbs that nourish and protect my body from disease rather than leaving a chemical footprint on it.

There are a number of botanicals that you can dry and prepare as powders, which can then be made into a paste for a natural shampoo. Store these botanical powders in a glass or ceramic jar with a tight lid, keeping the jar away from sunlight. Herbs are usually fine for up to six months from day of purchase. If, however, you notice a significant change of color, an unpleasant smell, or the presence of a fungus, discard immediately, even if it hasn't yet been six months.

Begin preparations for your Ayurvedic shampoo the night before you wish to wash your hair. Measure some of the botanical powder (four ounces of powder for short to medium hair or eight ounces for long hair) into a glass bowl and mix it with enough hot water to form a watery paste. Allow it to rest overnight. The next morning, check the consistency. It should be runny. If needed, add more water. While it is preferred to soak the herbs overnight, if you forget to do this, you can simply add lukewarm water in the morning to make a paste before use. It's not ideal, but it will suffice.

Why You Should Stop Using Commercial Shampoos

One of the ingredients in commercial shampoo is sodium lauryl sulfate (SLS), which is also used as a detergent to clean floors. That's right, floors! SLS creates those beloved bubbles. Unfortunately, SLS builds up in the heart, liver, and lungs. SLS also causes the skin to flake, destroys hair follicles, and impairs the follicle's ability to grow hair.[18] SLS is banned in Europe and Central America—but it is still used in other countries openly!

An ingredient in dandruff-control shampoos is coal tar. Coal tar is a recognized carcinogen by the Environmental Protection Agency (EPA), the National Institutes of Health, the Agency for Toxic Substances and Disease Registry, the International Agency for Research on Cancer, and others. According to the World Health Organization's International Agency for Research on Cancer, there is evidence that coal tar is mutagenic (changes the DNA), phototoxic (chemically irritates the skin), and carcinogenic in animals.[19]

Another ingredient, formaldehyde, which appears in many shampoos as a preservative, may be carcinogenic. On the National Cancer Institute website, formaldehyde is linked with a variety of cancers.[20] Shampoo manufacturers, however, are not even required to list formaldehyde as an ingredient; and they label it instead as "Quaternium-15."

And this is just the beginning. Commercial shampoos are rife with artificial fragrances, undeclared chemical contaminants, and other petroleum by-products that can harm you.

To shampoo, apply the botanical paste lavishly to your scalp and rub vigorously. Then apply the remaining paste to the hair itself, massaging it gently from roots to tips. Massage your scalp and hair for a minimum of three to five minutes and for up to as long as you wish. This allows the herbs to impart their benefits. Then rinse with tap water. There is no need to repeat steps. The herbs are potent, and once is enough for them to do their job well.

To make your own shampoo, choose from the ingredients described in the following sections: shikakai, soap nut, amalaki, and hibiscus flowers and leaves. You can stick to one botanical or mix them in equal quantities.

Shikakai

Shikakai is a shrub that grows wild in the hot and humid parts of India and other parts of Southeast Asia. Its fruit pod, bark, and leaves are collected, dried, and ground to make shikakai powder, which is renowned for its benefits to the hair. Thanks to a growing worldwide popularity of shikakai, it is being commercially planted now and is easily found online. The benefits are as follows:

Controls dandruff: Dandruff is a common scalp disorder that has not, unfortunately, been arrested by commercial antidandruff shampoos (that use zinc pyrithione, selenium sulfide, salicylic acid, imidazole derivatives, sulfur, coal tar, and whatever else). Daily use of these commercial shampoos can lead to brittle hair and dry the scalp, and they can even cause allergic reactions. Shikakai, a natural astringent, protects the scalp from dandruff and soothes the scalp's itchiness and flaking.

Antipruritic (anti-itching): Shikakai gives almost overnight results on patches of seborrheic dermatitis (on the brows and forehead) and psoriasis patches, and even on acne due to excess sebum production.

Cools brain: My teacher once said that after a head wash with shikakai, you can expect sound sleep that night since its cooling potency pacifies pitta in the brain, inducing sweet sleep.

Nourishes hair roots: Shikakai contains vitamins C and D as well as other essential phytonutrients to nourish the hair follicles and promote hair growth.

Soap Nut

Sapindus mukorossi, known in India as *reetha*, is a flowering tree that flourishes in India and Nepal. Its round, nutlike fruits ripen in winter months (after November). These dried fruits are called soap nuts in English, and they contain a natural surfactant called saponin. Thankfully, this natural surfactant is friendly to both the body and the environment.

I grew up recognizing this tree and watching for its ripened fruit. We would bring home the nuts, separate the seeds, and use the soft pulp as a soap. Today, both reetha powder and the soap nut are available online.

For thousands of years in the Ayurveda tradition, soap nut powder has been used for washing hair, clothes, utensils, ornaments, and even hands and bodies during bath time. After all, it is Nature's own detergent, so it is the natural soap substitute of choice for washing practically anything and everything. It is free of side effects and has these benefits:

Three-dosha balancing: This in itself spells health and a beautiful head of strong and luxurious hair![21] Reetha powder is also a natural hair conditioner, hair softener, and detangler. I love this quality, since I have long hair, and all women who possess long hair know how easily it can get tangled.

Natural antibacterial and antiparasitic: Ayurveda texts clarify that reetha is a natural antibacterial. Modern research and clinical studies also support the fact. In a study published in the International Journal of Pharmacy and Pharmaceutical Sciences, aqueous biosurfactant extracts prepared from fruits of *S. mukorossi* were found to be effective against *Micrococcus luteus*, *Brevibacterium linens*, *Bacillus subtilis*, *Staphylococcus epidermidis*, *Escherichia coli*, and *Pseudomonas fluorescens*. The authors conclude that "biosurfactant (saponin) extracts from *S. mukorossi* can be included in herbal care products not only for their emulsifying properties, but also for their antimicrobial effect."[22]

Similarly, in another study, reetha demonstrated significant antimicrobial activity against twenty phyto-pathogenic microbial strains and showed to be a potential biofungicide. Further, soap nut powder was not found toxic, even at high doses.[23]

Hence, reetha is very effective against lice and other parasites that may consider our scalp their home, and it is also an effective antifungal, antipruritic, and anti-infective agent. That is good to know, especially if we have schoolchildren, who sometimes come home with lice!

Amalaki

I have spoken quite a bit about amalaki—the Indian gooseberry, also known as amla—as it is a prestigious herb in Ayurveda. It is classified as an immunity-enhancing, disease-preventing, anti-aging, longevity-promoting agent. Ayurveda also classifies amalaki as a top hair-health-promoting ingredient, known as *keshya* in Sanskrit. To make a powder from this fruit, first remove the seeds. Washing your hair with this finely ground powder will support a healthy growth of hair, prevent hair loss, and also arrest premature graying of the hair.

When I was growing up, we would collect the fresh fruit in the fall, and cut them into pieces, and dry them for several days in indirect sunlight, or preferably, in the shade. These dried pieces were later boiled in coconut oil until the solid matter became charred. The oil was filtered, and this clean oil was used to condition the scalp and hair before and after a shampoo. Also, dried amalaki fruit pieces (which will keep for an entire year) were soaked overnight and the soaking water used after a shampoo for the last rinse. This amalaki water would leave a lasting sheen, similar to a modern leave-in conditioner.

You could try this amalaki rinse by soaking 1 tablespoon of amalaki powder in 24 ounces of water. This amalaki rinse may enhance your sense of well-being and peace. Students have reported feeling almost as if a new happiness had descended on them after washing their hair, and I believe it is due to the amalaki in the shampoo. Those who had burning eyes or even a headache from heat or sun exposure have reported a definite, even dramatic, decline in these symptoms after their shampoo.

Hibiscus Flowers and Leaves

Hibiscus flowers and leaves nourish your hair with natural moisturizer and prevent hair loss. They add a beautiful luster to the hair, prevent split ends, and remove dandruff from the scalp, normalizing the pH.

You can grow and collect your own flowers, dry them in the shade, and then grind the dried flowers into a fine powder. Or you can easily order the dried powder online.

And if on the day you plan to shampoo your hair, you have only fresh flowers and leaves, then you can use those instead. Simply wash the fresh flowers and leaves well in tap water and mash them into a paste with a mortar and pestle. If you're in a hurry, add water and use a blender for this step. You can also combine this paste with the other possible shampoo ingredients mentioned above before finally adding water to make a wet paste.

Hibiscus has a natural reddish pigment in it. But the color from Hibiscus washes off completely, leaving the hair strong, soft, and shiny and the scalp clean and refreshed.

Ayurvedic Hair Conditioner

The shampoo ingredients provided above are perfectly balanced, neither drying the hair nor leaving it sticky or oily. If, however, you feel that you would like to add extra conditioning and shine to your hair, then I have a three-step suggestion for you:

1. First, after shampooing, towel dry your hair. Please avoid or minimize electric blow-drying as it can potentially overheat your scalp (which aggravates pitta dosha) and dry out your hair (especially the ends).

2. Next, when your hair is almost dry but still somewhat damp, mix together a pea-sized dollop of pure coconut oil with an equal quantity of pure *Aloe vera* gel, and massage this into your hair. Pay special attention to the ends.

3. Leave in this conditioner. If required, you can reapply each day until you shampoo again.

This mixture of coconut oil and fresh *Aloe vera* gel immediately counteracts frizz. Each of these ingredients is, in itself, celebrated by Ayurveda for its benefits to hair. With this combination, your hair will shine with a beautiful glow, and it will never be sticky.

Having spent so much time on the skin and hair, let us now move to caring for our other sense organs.

Care of Ears

Filling the ear cavity with warmed medicated oils is known as *karna purnam*. This practice is recommended to those who have healthy functioning of ears (to keep them healthy) as well as to those who have ear issues, either occasional or frequent. These issues might be such problems as frequent wax buildup, ringing in the ears, or loss of hearing. While this therapy works directly on the ear canal to improve the sense of hearing, it works indirectly on the entire body to address the prana or systemic vata dosha. Remember, the ears are one of the important seats of vata dosha.

You can perform karna purnam during your daily oil massage. Here's how:

1. First, during your daily massage, pay extra attention to your outer ear.

2. With a dropper, pour a few drops of warmed sesame oil into one ear. This should be 2 to 6 drops per ear—enough to fill your ear cavity with the warm oil.

3. Keep your head bent slightly for 30 to 90 seconds to allow deeper penetration of the oil.

4. Now, turn your head over to the other side, and repeat the ear-filling process in other ear.

5. Once your bathing is complete, you can wipe any remaining oil from the ear cavity with cotton balls.

This practice is wonderful for all-round prevention of the ear conditions mentioned above as well as itching and a tendency toward ear infections. Further, it works brilliantly for neck and jaw pain (TMJ) and can even calm vertigo.

Try to do this for your ears every day, even if you do not give yourself a massage every day. On such days, simply do a very short local massage of your outer ears and then fill each cavity with oil.

After treating your ears, it is important that for the next several hours you avoid exposing your ears to heavy wind. Light, normal breeze is okay. If needed, wear a head scarf or a hat that covers your ears.

You should not put oil into your ear cavity if you experience any of the following:

- Middle ear or inner ear damage or a perforated eardrum

- An active ear infection

- Cold symptoms (fever, runny nose, sneezing, coughing)

- The feeling that a cold is coming on

- Allergic rhinitis, sinusitis, or tonsillitis

- Living in a country or state where the law prohibits it

Care of Eyes

Our eyes are one of the seats of pitta dosha, and so they must be protected at all times from excess heat. It is true that this instinct exists in most of us. We squint spontaneously if we stare too long at sources of heat or bright light. If we feel our eyes are overheated—perhaps we've been staring too long at a computer screen—we close our eyes briefly or put our cooling palms on them.

Ayurveda tradition is all too aware that with advancing age, many of us will be subject to the discomfort of dry eyes, burning or hot eyes, red eyes, and even pain in the eyes. With this in mind, the following self-care practices for our eyes are recommended:

- Hot water showers and steam baths do not help our eyes. Hence, Ayurveda recommends that we never wash our eyes with hot water. Wash your head and eyes with cool water only.

- Avoid gazing directly into heat and bright light sources, and wear sunglasses on bright days.

- Avoid eating overly spicy foods (the heat escalates pitta dosha) and include ghee or clarified butter in your diet. Ghee is a substance that is known to pacify pitta.

- Massage your feet with sesame and other warm oils. According to Ayurveda, there is an energetic and invisible connection between the soles of our feet and our eyes. Hence, massaging the feet with oil directly benefits our eyes and even improves vision.

You can also give yourself an eye wash, put on a medicinal eye salve, or immerse your eyes in a bath—all of which I describe below.

Eye Wash (Netra Prakshalan)

A special eye care practice involves washing the eyes with cool water. Do this upon waking up and splash the cool water directly into your eyes. This not only wakes you up, it also provides your eyes with the coolness they need.

A special eye wash can be made by soaking *triphala* powder in water. This powder, which is available online, is a mixture of powders made from the dried fruits of *Terminalia chebula*, *Terminalia bellerica*, and *Emblica officinalis*. Triphala is renowned in Ayurveda for its ophthalmic benefits.

To make the eye wash, soak 1 teaspoon of powder in a glass of hot water. Let it stand overnight. The next morning, filter this room-temperature solution through a fine cloth to remove the triphala particles. Wash your eyes with the clean, filtered water. Then wash your eyes with plain tap water. You will find that any redness in your eyes is diminished or gone entirely and that your eyes are revitalized. If you are a computer user, this is a vital practice to adopt in the mornings before you begin work or at least on weekends.

Eye Salve (Anjana)

The practice called anjana involves applying salve made from healing herbs to the inner eyelid after bathing. The salve, often called a collyrium, is cooked to a thick honey-like consistency. The benefit of all types of Ayurvedic eye salves is that they specifically soothe the eyes and prevent eyestrain and sun sensitivity. You should widen your eye with one hand and apply the salve using an applicator or wand with the other hand. Always apply the salve moving from the inner to outer corners of the eye.

Though this practice is greatly beneficial, it can also be potentially a bit uncomfortable to some, since it can make the eyes tear up a bit. But the eyes tear up only for a minute or so, so once you get used to it, it does not feel uncomfortable. Try it the very first time, perhaps, over a weekend when you are staying in, not wearing eye makeup, and can take the time to clear any tears from your face. Remember that the tears (if any actually show up) are pretty clarifying and ultimately end up refreshing the eyes. Or simply search online for "Ayurvedic kajal" or "Ayurvedic anjana," which give a similar eye-purifying benefit.

An alternative is to apply one drop of pure honey in the lower eyelids at night. This may sting a little, and your eyes may also water some, but not much. Soon, however, all redness and burning will subside, and if there are any impurities on the surface of the eye, they will be eliminated. You will experience a cleaner and fresher eye. This also promotes sound sleep.

It is important not to apply this honey anjana any more often than three nights per month. You can repeat it each month. Also, after the honey-based anjana, avoid reading or watching television that night. Simply meditate or go to bed.

Eye Saturation (Netra Tarpanam)

This unique eye care practice, netra tarpanam, is to be done only by those who experience intense dry eyes. *Netra* means "eyes," and *tarpanam* means "nourishment." In this practice, you will nourish your eyes by applying cooling ghee.

This is a simple do-it-yourself procedure that can be done at bedtime. Benefits that you can expect include the balancing of pitta as well as vata dosha in the organ of the eye, moisturizing of dry eyes, cooling the burning sensation in eyes, a decreased sensitivity to light, improvement of any blurred vision, and the prevention of conjunctivitis and cataract.

This is a three-step process:

1. First, you will need a dropper, a hand towel, and a small vessel in which you have about a teaspoon of melted ghee. The ghee should be room temperature, not warm.

2. Now, lie down. Gently put a drop of ghee inside one eye. Open and shut your eyelids so that the ghee spreads across the eye surface.

3. Now repeat this with the second eye. Flutter your eyelids open and shut a couple of times. If any tears or ghee come out of the eyes, you can use the hand towel to wipe the moisture away.

The eye surface may feel negligibly irritated, but it will not burn. Once you become used to the sensation of ghee in your eyes, you will not notice it at all. Of course, you cannot read, text, or use the computer after this. You can only meditate or go to sleep.

The next morning, you will wake up with refreshed, cooled, and well-nourished eyes. You will find that the sclera of your eyes is whiter, and gradually with daily use, you can say good-bye to dry eyes.

Care of Nose

The benefits of the daily oil cleansing of the nostrils (*pratimarsha nasya*) is not only for the nose, but also prevents diseases of the eyes and ears. Oil in the nose is even a beauty treatment of sorts. The sages of Ayurveda discovered that it prevents or arrests premature graying of hair and hair loss. It also nourishes the facial skin and deepens the voice. So it is a great practice for singers and public speakers. It also works to offset minor stiffness in the neck, headaches, and stiffness of the jaw. Nasya also works great for insomnia.

The practice of cleaning the nose involves instilling two drops of sesame oil or liquid ghee into each nostril daily. Tilt your head backward, either while sitting or lying down. Then instill two drops in a nostril, one at a time, through a dropper. Inhale the oil deeply by closing the second nostril and breathing in with the open nostril until the oil reaches all the way to the throat. You will be able to taste it. You should then spit this oil out through the mouth. It's best not to swallow it, though don't panic if you do. The oil has been through your nasal system, but it's edible.

Nasya practice can be done either before or after bathing or showering. Time it so that it's either thirty minutes before showering or thirty minutes after showering. Do not do it immediately before or after. In any case, complete it before you have breakfast. I prefer doing nasya after showering because the oil massage (abhayanga) and the shower with warm water, and the steam generated, open up my nasal channels to receive the oil.

Of course, do not perform nasya if your state laws prohibit putting oil drops in your nose or if you have fever, active cold or cough, or it is raining or about to rain.

Neti Cleanse

Irrigation of the nasal passages using pleasantly warm saline water is a yoga-based technique used in Ayurveda for several centuries. The neti cleanse is especially beneficial if you have a chronic tendency toward colds, sinus blockages, rhinitis, sneezing attacks, or headaches. However, to follow up a neti cleanse with oil in the nostrils (nasya) has double benefits.

Below are instructions for getting started with a neti cleanse:

Neti pot: It is important to source the right equipment. Fortunately, neti pots are now sold in mainstream drug stores and, of course, online.

Saline solution: Prepare a saline solution by mixing lukewarm water from the tap (or even better, distilled water) with rock salt (not ordinary table salt; see appendix 4). Add $1/16$ teaspoon rock salt to every 8 ounces of water. The temperature of water should be comfortable to inhale, never hot. Be careful.

Time of practice: Neti cleansing is best undertaken in the morning, ideally after elimination of bowels but before bathing. A neti flush can, however, be done any time before sunset, as long as it is not right after eating a meal.

Frequency: Neti cleanse is typically done once daily. From a seasonal perspective, it is of greatest benefit during spring.

Method: Tilt your head sideways, trickle a fine stream of water through the upper nostril, and let it come out through the lower nostril. The water will be dropping below you, so naturally, you will do this activity over a sink. Simply use half of the water in the pot in the first nostril; save the remainder for the second. In between nostrils, you can take a break, stand erect, and blow your nose (very gently) if required (you will want to).

Post-flush: You can again gently blow your nose to clear all solution. Rinse out your neti pot and put it away until next time.

Neti is contraindicated if you experience occasional bleeding from your nose, or you have a deviated septum.

A World of Sensual Delights

Ayurveda lifestyle wisdom unfolds a variety of ways in which you can care for your skin, hair, and senses. Each practice opens a door into a whole new world of healing botanicals and timeless ingredients that promise rejuvenation and well-being. While it is not necessary that you start doing every practice today, you should find it reassuring to know that when you are called to do so, the knowledge awaits you in this book. At any time, you can come back to this chapter, thumb through its pages, and begin experimenting with some of the practices elucidated here.

CHAPTER 6

Crafting Sacred and Seasonal Meals

When I met Beverly Herrera nine years ago, I saw her as an inherently powerful woman who was demoralized by an ongoing health issue. Beverly was a successful Realtor, life coach, and women's leader in the San Francisco community, but crippling stomach pains were holding her back. This stomach condition had resisted all treatment modalities—conventional and alternative—for thirty years and was worsening year by year. The pain, which Beverly said felt like "a hole in my stomach," was holding her back from living with real joy.

I won't give a detailed description of the remedies Beverly tried. They involved multiple cycles of antibiotics (which gave temporary relief), a medication to address bile accumulation (which had intense nausea as a side effect), and a diet of mostly raw, organic fruits and vegetables with yogurt (which caused more problems than it resolved). Here's Beverly's experience with an Ayurvedic diet.

BEVERLY HERRERA'S JOURNEY OF CONVICTION

Nine years ago, Beverly Herrera adopted an Ayurvedic diet, and what happened then is nothing short of a miracle. That's the way she describes it. Within one month of beginning to eat foods that were attuned to the season and that provided balance for her aggravated doshas,

Beverly felt noticeably better, and half of her stomach pain was gone. Within three months of following the Ayurvedic approach to eating, Beverly felt almost completely cured—she put it at 90 percent. For many years now, she has had no stomach pains.

Some of the foods Beverly let go of to follow an Ayurvedic eating plan had been, as she put it, "staples" in her diet—yogurt and cheese, for instance, which are difficult to digest. She simply had to make new eating habits, find new staples, adopt a new rhythm for her meals, and be careful about food combinations

Inspired and excited by the age-old food wisdom that allowed her to recover from a three-decade food problem in just three months, Beverly and her two grown daughters enrolled in a beginner's course at Vedika Global. Beverly continued on through five years of dedicated study to graduate as a doctor of Ayurvedic medicine, and Beverly now makes a difference in the lives of many people who suffer from their own digestive problems. She has become an inspiration to others in the way she looks (much younger than her years!), in the way she eats (what she wants—without breaking Ayurveda's food rules, of course), and in the way she works (professionally, she is stronger than ever). What is even more inspiring than all of this, however, is the compassion that regaining her health brought about in her soul.

Learning recently that the nineteen-year-old daughter of one of her neighbors was diagnosed with Hodgkin's lymphoma and concurrent thyroid problems, Beverly phoned the girl's mother and said, "Your daughter has to change her diet right away, and I will cook for her."

Beverly did cook for this ailing young woman, not for a few days or weeks but for four full months. (Some of the recipes she used are in appendix 4, "The Ayurvedic Diet Resource Guide.") In time, others in their community joined a meal train, cooking organic and fresh food and delivering it to their young neighbor.

I cannot say how much this food, prepared by Beverly and others with full conviction in the science of Ayurveda dietetics and offered as an act of selfless service, helped support this young woman's recovery from cancer, but the upshot is that she no longer has Hodgkin's lymphoma. She is in complete remission and in excellent spirits.

Beverly was inspired to this act of neighborliness by both her compassion and her deep belief in Ayurveda. She explained to me, "I had information about food choices that other people didn't have, and I wanted to be able to provide that information to them."

In the following pages, I give that information about healing food to you.

Food, Mind, and a Sacred Life

Ayurveda tells us that food provides much more than physical sustenance for the body. Food shapes and shifts the mind, influencing our ability to think and to conceptualize. Food affects our deepest emotions. When we consume food with reverence and loving meditative awareness, our bodies become filled with radiant health and divine well-being. And when we eat with

a toxic attitude, the very act of eating otherwise healthy food can disturb the quality of our consciousness and disconnect us from our own source. Pure foods, carefully cooked and eaten mindfully with prayer and connection to the Universal Truth that manifests within and through the food, can lead us back to this source. We experience spiritual serenity, physical vitality, and psychological hope and joy.

Thus, a paramount concept in Ayurveda, one that sets it apart from all other dietary systems and world cuisines, is its focus on spiritually charged foods. These are called sattvic foods. Sattvic foods are not only pleasing to the senses and nutritious, but they also have a calming and pleasing effect on the mind.

The Vedic concepts of sattva (purity and balance), rajas (agitation), and tamas (inertia) are seen as the three modes of mind-based consciousness. These are the inherent vibrations, or qualities, of all material objects, including food. Ayurveda emphasizes the importance of eating sattvic food to support both physical health and a peaceful, elevated state of mind. For food to be sattvic, it must be eaten in right measure, be balanced in its qualities, and always eaten fresh, which means that it must be recently harvested and recently cooked.

Let me describe more fully these three types of food.[1]

Sattvic foods: These foods make the mind relaxed and serene, are full of life force (prana), are cooked in ghee, and are light and easy to digest, yet they impart stability and strength to the body. Organic vegetables and ripe fruits are never eaten out of season, so seasonal awareness is important in constructing a sattvic diet. All foods are lightly cooked in ghee (clarified butter), which is preferred over all other cooking mediums, with enough fragrant spices added to make the recipe optimum for digestion (however, spices must not cause burning sensation or heartburn, so moderation is advised). Among salts, only rock salt, or what is also known as Himalayan pink salt, is considered sattvic. Rock salt should be used with care, since sattvic foods are generally on the low spectrum of saltiness, rather than the high end. Nuts and seeds also impart sattva and work as great sattvic snacks. Raw honey, sweet fruits, and all-natural (non-fermented) grains are also important ingredients of a sattvic meal plan. Cow's milk is considered the most sattvic milk in Ayurveda (versus goat, sheep, or buffalo), especially if taken from cows raised in a peaceful environment. Cow milk–derived natural butter, cottage cheese, and yogurt (sweetened with natural sugar) are also considered sattvic.

Food can take on a sattvic energy when it is mindfully sourced and cooked peacefully with attention to freshness, hygiene, and personal spiritual vibration and consumed with gratitude and spiritual awareness, without speed or greed (and without waste). Since plant-based foods digest easily and do not clog the body's bio-channels, they are considered more sattvic than eggs, meat, and fish. Naturally, simply cooked foods will be more sattvic than overly processed foods. Fruits and raw vegetables possess maximum sattva; however, digestibility is an issue, so light cooking (such as steaming or sautéing in ghee) makes food sparkle with sattva. This is why Ayurveda recommends cooked foods over an exclusively raw diet.

Rajasic foods: Rajasic foods overstimulate and irritate the body and mind because of inherent or added properties such as excessive pungency, sourness, or saltiness along with undue hotness, sharpness, and roughness (dryness), often overly stimulating the gastric enzymes. From this logic, garlic is a naturally occurring rajasic food, and adding chili sauce or wine to any recipe will add rajasic qualities. These spicy, alkaline, and salty foods include what we call processed foods, junk food, and fast food, as well as alcohol or caffeine, and even small amounts of marijuana or other drugs. A diet that is largely vegetarian, but nevertheless cooked with excessive salt and burning spices and consumed along with caffeine, alcohol, or soda, or in hurried manner, will be rajasic.

Tamasic foods: These are foods that lack prana and are harmful to mind and body. They include foods that are stale (lacking freshness), putrid (foul smelling), or excessively heavy due to being overly fatty. Eating meat is recommended in Ayurveda to improve physical strength, but a diet that is dominated by meat will increase tamasic qualities—this is especially true of old, canned, or frozen meats, versus organic meats that are cooked fresh and consumed in moderate or low quantity. All meat and egg recipes do impart some heaviness and even dullness in body and mind, especially when eaten in excess. Sometimes that can be a good thing, such as when we want the mind to slow down or we want to sleep.

Classifying all vegetarian foods as "sattvic" (and by that logic, all vegetarians as sattvic beings) and all spice and garlic eaters as rajasic, and all meats and meat eaters as tamasic is an extreme generalization, and Ayurveda has never made this crude mistake. People eat the foods they eat due to geographical-cultural reasons, and above all, based on what foods (plant or animal) were historically available in plenty.

Hence, Ayurveda makes no moral assumptions about vegetarianism being somehow superior. Rather, it is the manner in which food (plant- or animal-based) is procured (ethically or not), cooked and consumed (mindfully or not) with other ingredients (old or fresh, and calming, exciting, or dulling), that has the most impact.

I like this approach; it elevates this concept beyond the meat-versus-vegetable debate (since the Vedas say that both are sentient anyway). This is a mature ideology, in my opinion.[2]

By this logic, a person who follows a sattvic diet will develop a sattvic frame of mind, and a person with a sattvic frame of mind will prefer the sattvic food that increases their vital force, energy, strength, appetite, and health. This is true of rajas also: rajasic people prefer foods that are sour, salty, hot, and pungent and foods that cause pain, bitterness, ill health, and a temperamental mind. Tamasic people are naturally drawn to food that is old, stale, canned, dirty, or very heavy. It may be surprising to learn that foods have this kind of influence over your thoughts and state of mind, but it is true. It's a fact. And I am witness to this fact day after day in my work.

My Baba's Healing Kitchen

 My earliest memories of Ayurveda are visceral, not intellectual. My grandfather was a humble householder and teacher of the spiritual wisdom from Upanishads and other Hindu texts to the people of our small town Ayodhya.

Baba was born in the year 1900 in the changing landscape of India's social-political destiny. This means that my grandfather was educated in Vedic texts and yogic practices by his own father, who was a Hindu saint, and by study in the Indian school system. As an adult, he even took a government job to support his family, and he imparted Vedic wisdom on his own time.

But a light that would serve the world, and change it for the better, cannot remain hidden forever. Long before I came into the world, my grandfather became a full-time spiritual teacher, surrendering his livelihood to God and dedicating his life to the upliftment of his community. Without fee, Baba shared his knowledge and blessings to whomever showed up at our door. When a higher power beckons and a calling is answered, sincerely and from the heart, it all works out in the grand scheme of things.

I never took a count, but every day there was a long line of visitors at our door. Between his packed sermons held in the inner courtyard of our ancestral home, Baba sat in the outer courtyard to meet with these people, who came with their suffering bodies and minds. Baba met with as many souls as he could in a given day, addressing their physical distress and mental anguish. Nine times out of ten, he would suggest changes in their food and lifestyle, along with giving spiritual advice. That was enough. Only rarely would Baba suggest someone take an herb. His prescription worked each time. The crowds continued to grow in numbers, and the healed would return to express their gratitude.

So our home was always filled with people who sought Baba for a variety of reasons. There were the pilgrims and spiritual devotees who came not only from Ayodhya but from far and wide. They sat in equanimity, many with monastic shaven heads or traditional Brahmanic tufts of hair, dressed in white or in saffron shawls and robes, awaiting Baba's exposition of Vedanta, the knowledge of the spiritual Self that transcends birth and death. These people were mostly introspective, silently performing tasks that supported Baba to carry out his spiritual work.

And then there were the lost and broken ones, the suffering ones, who often had potent symptoms of disease. Some would be shedding tears of pain or be lying on the floor from weakness, waiting for Baba's attention.

A number of the people who came to see Baba were well-off or middle class, but the majority were extraordinarily poor and often needed mats and blankets from us just so they could be comfortable during their wait. Invariably, all of the souls who came to Baba's home, be they enlightened or lost, healthy or sick, were given nourishing food.

The hearth in my Baba's home was always lit; his family members and our kitchen helpers were always cooking meals—all of which happened under my grandmother's dedicated and amazing stewardship. Her kitchen was so inviting that visitors would often step forward to cut vegetables, churn buttermilk, wash the pots and pans, or any of the other myriad tasks my grandma required to be done before a meal was served. Each meal was sattvic and was an Ayurveda delight: seasonally attuned, medically potent with healing spices, and tasting absolutely delicious!

Many people stayed in and around our home waiting for Baba's attention, and they would eat several meals at our home during their wait—sometimes for days or even weeks at a time. Something I cannot forget is the transformation around the food that I repeatedly witnessed with my own eyes. While people waited for an audience with Baba, their heartburn or gas and stomach pains would recede, their fevers would subside, their skin conditions and rashes would spontaneously begin to clear, and their anxieties would lessen. A man whose knees were locked and stiff began walking again, one step at a time. A widow who could not cry after her husband's death, finally wept, releasing the pent-up grief that had been poisoning her entire being. A schizophrenic man who was violent and restless when his parents first brought him to our home, calmed and settled down like a happy and contented baby does after a satisfying meal. People wondered about this and would speak among themselves about it: was it the blessings and energy of Baba that were curing people, or was it the sattvic food his wife and family cooked? ✐

A Teaching and Healing Kitchen in America—Continuation of a Legacy

Food eaten in the right season, with the right spices, and served with a blessing or mantra—Ayurvedic food!—makes all the difference. Today, I have come to realize that any cuisine can be transformed from a mundane meal to a sublime and healing experience if Ayurveda's universal rules are used in its preparation.

As you know by now, I have been deeply inspired by my teacher's life and the living lessons he imparted to me. When I set the foundation for my school of Ayurveda, not surprisingly, I modeled it after the traditional gurukulam of my Baba. That meant that Vedika Global had to have a kitchen. In the first two years, our rented facility did *not* have a kitchen, so we improvised. My husband, who is a passionate and creative self-trained chef, and I would cook Ayurvedic meals on a camping stove, feeding and teaching our students core self-care recipes.

The students loved this, but Chef Sanjai (as students call him) and I were both thrilled when, in 2010, the school moved into its current facility with its beautiful, sunny, fully equipped kitchen. Once we had a kitchen, everyone who came to my gurukulam could be fed an Ayurvedic meal before class.

This meant that after working all day as a finance professional in the corporate sector, Chef Sanjai would often drive an hour in traffic

in order to prepare a fresh meal for students. Sanjai would painstakingly research recipes in Ayurveda's ancient texts and draw from its rich tradition of healing foods. He also recreated recipes of Baba's that I shared with him.

The cooking in the gurukulam kitchen has always been a delight. We laugh a lot, taste batches, debate the science behind the recipes, adjust the food, and then share with all our students the exact recipes. It is a wonderful tradition for us to cook together in this way, feeding the school's students and those who attend the clinic and community events that Vedika Global sponsors.

It wasn't very long before I started hearing new stories of transformation through food. The characters had changed over time, and a fancy modern stove had replaced my Baba's traditional hearth, but the knowledge about healthy foods in Ayurveda is *sanatana* (eternal), and it was once again delivering the same results.

Sanjai and I are no longer doing all of the cooking. A team of dedicated volunteer students came together under my teaching and my husband's cooking directions, and they form the heart of our kitchen crew. We all chant together while we cut the vegetables and grind the spices—working as one body and one heart to feed our community. What we are cooking is not just food but Ayurvedic elixirs—and these create medical miracles.

Agni: The Inner Altar of Divine Fire

The Vedic sages saw this entire world as a field of sacred experiences, an expression of infinite consciousness. The sun in the universe is also situated inside our bodies, where it is known as agni. If the sun were to disappear, all life as we know it would come to an end. In the same way, if our inner flame, agni, were to be extinguished, we would die. Whenever this flame of agni flickers, our health vacillates. When the flame is steady, we too become stable in body and mind.

Agni comprehends the body's various biophysical and biochemical processes by which ingested food is converted into vitality *(tejas)*, immunity *(oja)*, and energy *(prana* or *urjah)*. Metaphorically, agni is like the hearth of the body. This is where the body "cooks" our food to become our cells and tissues *(dhatu)*. In fact, even our minds are fed by the subtle essence of food that has been processed by agni. Our physical and mental strength, our enthusiasm and courage, our beauty and complexion, and most especially our longevity and ability to resist disease are directly related to the health of our agni.

By choosing to eat certain foods rather than others and to employ rules of cooking processes and mealtimes, we can proactively keep our personal agni in balance. We need to protect our agni by the proper intake of food and drinks.[3] For this reason, the rest of this chapter discusses the specific rules that serve agni.

Ayurveda recognizes that maintaining an optimum digestion capacity is even more important than the properties and nutritive value of the foods we eat. Without agni, our body cannot assimilate a food's nutritive value.

Four Physiological States of Agni

Genetics determine our dominant dosha at birth, and this dominant dosha influences which of the four types of agni we inherit—balanced, slow, sharp, or changeable. The difference between the types of agni is mainly the time it takes the body to digest food, as shown in table 19.

The balanced agni state is coveted and ideal, but it's also rare. This agni endows natural health. The other three types of agni do not create disease, as such, as long as their variability from the balanced state remains within certain limits. Following Ayurvedic food rules restores agni to a balanced state and prevents it from becoming pathological. According to Ayurveda, even if an imbalanced agni has caused illness, it is never too late to address the problem.

Normal Variability in Agni

Agni is never fixed. Throughout the day, throughout the year, and throughout our lives, our agni is continually undergoing changes in its intensity or the level of efficiency with which it digests foods. There are the three normal kinds of variability that affect agni: the season, the time of day, and our biological age. Let's explore each of these.

Variation in the Seasons

Variations in agni induced by the changing seasons are physiological changes, and we can adjust for them easily, returning to a balanced state of agni by eating a seasonally prescribed diet. Table 20 explains the basic principles of this.

See appendix 4, "The Ayurvedic Diet Resource Guide" for seasonal diet recommendations that ensure that your agni never becomes taxed in a given season.

TABLE 19   Agni Characteristics

	BALANCED AGNI	DULL/SLOW AGNI	SHARP AGNI	CHANGEABLE AGNI
Dosha	All doshas balanced	Kapha dominant	Pitta dominant	Vata dominant
Digestion Time	Optimum time	More time	Less time	Variable time
Normal Response to Meals	Enthusiasm and alertness after meals	Some fullness sensation in belly; some sleepiness or loss of energy after meals	Hunger returns soon after meals	Variable responses to meals

Variation in the Time of Day

The variation of agni induced by the movement of the Earth around the sun is also not a cause for concern. Simply follow instructions on mealtimes given in table 21.

Variation in Biological Age

These variations are also considered normal. The young, middle-aged, and elderly cannot eat in the same way because agni varies based on age.

Pathological Imbalance of Agni

When we overtax our system with the wrong diets or lifestyle choices, first the doshas become imbalanced, and thereafter, we manifest pathological states of agni, which cause symptoms and diseases. Therefore, imbalanced agni is directly related to aggravated states of doshas:

- When vata becomes aggravated due to chronic lifestyle and food errors, agni too

becomes highly unpredictable or erratic, giving rise to flatulence, burping, and stomach pain. In Ayurveda, we refer to this state as *vishama*, which means "variable" or "changeable." This word pretty much sums up what to expect when vata dosha is afflicting the fire in our bellies. Imagine a fire exposed to harsh winds—what happens to the flames? The flames will flicker; they can become either excessively enraged or subdued and even extinguished. Likewise, digestion is unpredictable at best. On some days, large amounts of food will digest well, and on other days, even small amounts of food will simply not digest, giving rise to uncomfortable symptoms of gas, bloating, heaviness, and even belly cramps.

- When pitta becomes aggravated, agni becomes hyperactive, giving rise to acid, heat, and exhaustive hunger along with potential weight loss. In Ayurveda, we

TABLE 20   Agni Variation by Season

Season	Dosha in Macrocosm	Agni State	Recommendations
Spring	Kapha peaking	Somewhat challenged because the peaking kapha in macrocosm also induces slowness in the agni process in the microcosm (body).	Eat light.
Summer	Vata accumulating	More challenged because vata induces variability in the microcosm, making the digestion process somewhat unpredictable.	Eat lighter.
Late summer/ rainy	Vata peaking and pitta accumulating	Maximally challenged because when vata peaks in macrocosm, it naturally causes disturbances in microcosm, and agni can quickly become erratic, and indigestion or other gastric disturbances are more commonly seen.	Food choices should be the lightest possible at this time.
Fall	Pitta peaking	Improved because the increased pitta in macrocosm helps pick up agni in the microcosm.	Food choices should be balanced between light and heavy.
Early winter	All doshas balanced	Optimum because all doshas are naturally balanced in the macrocosm).	Choices can safely include heavy foods.
Late winter	Kapha accumulating	Good because accumulating kapha in macrocosm begins to induce some fullness but not a lot, and previous months' improvement is still supporting digestion in general.	Choices can safely include heavy foods.

TABLE 21 Agni Variation by Time

Time of Day	Dosha	Agni State	Recommendations
6:00 a.m. to 10:00 a.m.	Kapha time	Dull/slow	Eat breakfast as early as possible to give it time to digest since agni is not at its optimum strength. Keep breakfast light.
10:00 a.m. to 2:00 p.m.	Pitta time	Sharp	Eat your heaviest meal of the day, ideally at noon or close to noon.
2:00 p.m. to 6:00 p.m.	Vata time	Variable	Do not snack; simply sip warm water or tea instead or eat a very light snack (if really needed).
6:00 p.m. to 10:00 p.m.	Kapha time	Dull/slow	Eat dinner as early as possible to give it time to digest since agni is not at its optimum strength. Keep dinner light.
10:00 p.m. to 2:00 a.m.	Pitta time	Sharp	No meals. Sleep.
2:00 a.m. to 6:00 a.m.	Vata time	Variable	No meals. Sleep. Can begin waking up one and a half hours before sunrise (based on where you live and what time the sun rises in a given season).

use the word *tikshana* for this state, which means "sharp," or "quality of sharpness," as if the fire inside the belly has become so heightened (sharpened) that we feel hungry again soon after eating, almost as if we are starving. Naturally, food is digested quickly in this state, sometimes even twice as fast as what is otherwise normal, and even large amounts are digested expediently. In absence of timely ingestion of food, sharp hunger pangs, dizzy spells, and heartburn may arise, and even ulcers and rapid weight loss can occur in extreme cases.

- When kapha becomes aggravated pathologically, agni also drops critically in its function, and you may have a hard time digesting even a small meal. This state is called *manda*, which means "a state of dullness or slowness," wherein the fire in the belly is inadequate (due to increased water and earth elements from the escalating kapha dosha). A dull agni will not be able to digest even small amounts of food in a reasonable time, and ingestion of large quantities of food or fluids with heavy qualities can all but wipe out this flame. Naturally, digestion time is maximally extended in this state of agni, and what is not digested frequently deposits as fat tissue (and also toxins).

Table 23 summarizes the process of dull, erratic, and sharp types of agni. A quick glance at the pathological features and effect on bowels will help you determine what type of agni you possess generally.

The Six Flavors in Food

One of the keys to finding what kind of effect a food will have on your system is its flavor, its taste. Everything that we eat, whether plant, animal, or mineral, possesses a specific taste. This taste, referred to as *rasa* in Sanskrit, impacts the body and mind in specific ways. Ayurveda identifies six tastes,[4] which are composed of an eclectic combination of the five elements. Most foods are a blend of these tastes, or are dominant in one with a secondary or latent taste.

Sweet = Water + Earth
Sour = Fire + Earth
Salty = Fire + Water
Pungent = Fire + Air
Bitter = Air + Space
Astringent = Air + Earth

Each taste has corresponding therapeutic value:

- Sweet taste promotes growth (example: milk).

- Sour taste increases agni (example: lemon).

- Salty taste enhances the taste of the food (example: salt).

- Pungent taste helps open the bio-channels (example: black pepper).

- Bitter taste destroys toxins (example: turmeric).

- Astringent taste ceases the flow of fluids by constriction (example: tea).

Based on the principle of "like increases like," when tastes are ingested, the five elements that make them up either aggravate or pacify the corresponding doshas.

In the following sections, I explore the impact of these six fundamental tastes on the doshas, states of agni, and the body, along with listing their general properties. You may want to review this section often so that the concepts of the six tastes gradually become internalized. When I am biting into an apple, for example, and based on the taste my tongue first perceives, sweet or sour, I know what the corresponding impact on my doshas will be. I find this knowledge truly exciting and empowering!

Sweet Taste (Madhur Rasa)

The first taste that we "receive" in that first moment of life is none other than the sweet taste itself. After all, mother's milk is sweet. For those of us who got the canned stuff instead for whatever reason, well, even that is sweet! How punishing can the sweet taste be when Nature herself poured her nurturing, loving, pleasing, and pampering intentions into it?

Is it any wonder that half the world dreams of sweet foods after wishing each other sweet dreams, and in those dreams we long for our sweethearts in sweet embraces, whispering into their ears sweet nothings? Oh, the unspoken desires for a life sweetened by the magic of sweet smiles, sweet babies, and sweet homes! The sweet taste has entered our ethos, it has

TABLE 22 Agni Variation by Age

Age	Dosha	Agni State	Recommendations
Birth to 18 years	Kapha dominant	Dull/slow	Eat nourishing but very digestible food, with added spices to counteract the dull agni; otherwise, allergies and fever can manifest.
18 years to 45 years	Pitta dominant	Sharp	Eat nourishing foods with added coolness from cooling spices like coriander and fennel to counteract sharp agni; otherwise hyperacidity and other heat conditions can manifest.
45 years to death	Vata dominant	Variable	Eat small and nourishing meals that are light and easily digestible; keep fixed mealtimes and maintain warming, vata-balancing strategies; otherwise, flatulence, chronic constipation, hemorrhoids, and IBS can manifest.

TABLE 23 Pathological States of Agni with Symptoms

	PATHOLOGICAL DULL AGNI	PATHOLOGICAL SHARP AGNI	PATHOLOGICAL ERRATIC AGNI
Digestion Time	Excessively extended, or slowed down	Excessively shortened, or speeded up	Excessively erratic and unpredictable
Pathological Features	Loss of appetite, nausea, stasis of food, flatulence, malaise, generation of toxins	Intense and excessive appetite, no satiety, loss of body strength and tissues, exhaustion	Changing appetite, variable time to digest same quantity of food, flatulence, pains that come and go during digestion
Effect on Bowels	Possible constipation	Possible diarrhea	Constipation alters with diarrhea, along with flatulence, bloating, or hemorrhoids

determined our culture, it has juiced our desires, and it has nourished our suckling infants since the beginning of time.

When the sweet taste is banned from our lives due to a fad diet, an inconclusive scientific theory, a sort of self-punishment, or any other reason, we are as if deprived of the very essence of life that nurtures and soothes us.

Insatiability is what the sweet taste forces us to contemplate. No matter how much of the sweet we get, by mouthful, armful, and wallet full, we are left wanting more and more. One who masters the sweet taste and is not mastered by the sweet taste has in essence understood what life is all about. Our relationship with the sweet taste is really symbolic of our ability to enjoy and engage without the pathological attachment and entrapment. We must moderate our consumption or else negative consequences follow in the fields of body, mind, and life. And finally, know that naturally occurring sweet tastes such as in fruits and dairy are here to support us and sweeten our journeys!

Examples: Sweet taste is dominant in breads, pastas, sweet fruits, starchy vegetables, dairy products, fats, green gram, wheat, rice, coconut, meats, and all types of natural sweeteners.

Properties: Oily, cooling, heavy, pleasant, soothing.

Action on doshas: Pitta ↓ Vata ↓ Kapha ↑

Action on agni: Induces fullness and dullness (in excess). Sweet taste is recommended in order to slow and control a pathologically sharp agni.

Action in body: Sweet taste is the dominant taste in most carbohydrates, proteins, and fats. It is considered wholesome since it promotes bulk, prolongs life-span, increases the body's strength and the skin's luster, and promotes expulsion of urine and feces. Eating sweet-flavored food is useful to counteract a burning sensation, thirst, a feeling of weakness, exhaustion, or if you need to gain weight.

Who can benefit? Those who wish to balance vata or pitta doshas; those who feel hungry quickly and urgently and need to calm this pitta-influenced, sharp state of metabolism (*tikshana agni*); those who require general strength (*bala*) or need filling out of their body tissues; and those who have an instant need for energy and stamina, such as athletes during competition, can benefit from consuming sweet foods.

Who must use caution? Those who have excessive kapha and, therefore, pathologically dull agni; those with excess body fat; those experiencing active phlegm, cough, or asthma; those who have parasites or fungal infections; those who have diabetes or other medical disorders requiring abstinence from sweets, and those who typically feel heavy and sleepy (due to the presence of kapha dosha or due to habits) should limit or avoid sweet foods.

Sour Taste (Amla Rasa)

According to Ayurveda, sour taste is required by our agni, but only in measured quantities. This precious amount serves to stimulate, reawaken, refresh, and energize us. It helps us break down our food and also destroy gas.

It is when we get addicted to this taste (and believe me, this can happen), all hell breaks loose. What do you expect will happen if you choose to coat your insides with a mild acid daily? It can lead to burns, suppuration, ulcers, bleeding, and other heat-related explosions, eruptions, flare-ups, and discharges.

The body, in its supreme intelligence, produces its own acid, the mighty hydrochloric acid, and this acid is an intrinsic aspect of agni. When Nature's other freely occurring food-based acids, such as ascorbic acid (vitamin C) found in sour fruits, citric acid found in oranges and lemons, acetic acid in vinegar, tannic acid in tea and wines, and tartaric acid in grapes, are consumed as Ayurveda's sour taste, naturally they aid agni and carry out their essential roles in the body according to a divinely programmed, preexisting intelligence.

If the sweet taste is like a mother, ever accommodating, then the sour taste is like that helpful friend who can turn vicious all of a sudden. Maintain your friendship judiciously and at a distance, and your agni and sour taste can have a lifelong relationship. Abuse it, and wonder what got into you! No wonder relationships go sour and at times—sour grapes may well be the reason we stay away, and stay safe as a result.

Envy is an emotion that is sometimes attributed to the overconsumption of sour taste. Perhaps the curdling, fermenting, putrefying, and stirring effect of sour taste manifests as the convulsion of desires and the mutiny of dissatisfaction with the current state of affairs. As sour as it gets, the stew of envy is fermented some more.

Examples: The sour taste naturally occurs in citrus fruits, such as lemons, limes, oranges, and grapefruit; as well as tomatoes, vinegar, and alcohol; and fermented foods like pickles, cheese, and yogurt.

Properties: Oily, liquid, light, hot (cold in mouth but hot in potency).

Action on doshas: Pitta ↑ Vata ↓ Kapha ↑

Action on agni: Picks up a dull state of agni due to inherent heat. Sour taste is classified as a first-class digestive stimulant, and its intake begins the salivation process.

Action in body: Promotes both appetite and digestion when consumed in moderation (as with sour buttermilk), but in excess it causes acidity and heat. Produces a cleansing of the mouth, refreshes taste buds and senses.

Who can benefit? Those who need to improve appetite can consume sour foods (lemon in hot drinking water, for example). Those who need help with digestion can also benefit (for example, dried mango seed powder aids digestion). Vata dosha also comes into balance with a few special sour foods such as Ayurvedic buttermilk (takra) or wine in moderation.

Who must use caution? Excessive consumption of sour taste increases pitta. Various types of burning sensations, excessive thirst, and diseases of pitta (such as heartburn and skin rashes) can become aggravated.

Salty Taste (Lavan Rasa)

The main attributes of salty taste are hotness and sharpness. It is not as heavy nor as oily as the sweet taste. If used in moderation, a salty taste promotes the deliciousness of our food (which is important for digestion too!) and has a moistening effect on body tissues along with a mild laxative impact on the bowels. But in excess, salt literally burns through the tissues and loosens them, causing premature wrinkling, blood disorders, and so forth.

CRAFTING SACRED AND SEASONAL MEALS

Ancient Ayurvedic texts comment that city dwellers who get addicted to salty foods are developing "malaise, laxity, and debility in the body."[5] Moreover, the texts remind us of the fate of shrubs, herbs, and trees that try to grow in areas where soil is excessively salty. Damage, stunted growth, and dead plants are what we witness on a large scale.

Sometimes, an excess consumption of salty taste is said to stir emotion of greed in the mind. What is the imparting quality of salty taste that attracts us to it in the first place? And once attracted, are we hooked for life? Is that why the hand does not stop until it has put every last overly salty potato chip in the mouth? What if a wholesome experience becomes a need, what if a need becomes a want, and what if a want becomes an obsession? And then, what is to stop our minds from spilling over and spreading this pattern to every area of our lives? Greed is to salt as unchecked wants are to life.

Examples: The salty taste is present in things that are naturally salty, such as seaweed, soy sauce, fish, mineral salts, and certain vegetables (such as celery).

Properties: Oily, hot, and heavy. Salty taste also makes food tasty.

Action on doshas: Pitta ↑ Vata ↓ Kapha ↑

Action on agni: Due to its heating property, salt is naturally both an appetizer and a digestive. It directly imparts its heat to the process of agni and hence food is digested more expediently.

Action in body: In the right dosage, salt promotes appetite and digestion and acts as a mild laxative. Its searing and heating qualities help break down food (splitting action) and aid in absorption of food. It removes stiffness and coldness in muscles.

Who can benefit? Those who wish to pacify vata dosha will benefit from more salty foods.

Who must use caution? In excess, pitta and kapha will become aggravated. A burning sensation in the mouth or throat, giddiness, heartburn, hot rashes, and high blood pressure are also signs of overconsumption. Due to the heat it creates, overconsumption of salty taste can cause graying of hair and even premature hair loss. Salt in excess will worsen skin conditions.

Pungent Taste (Katu Rasa)

The pungent taste reminds me of the fine line between being assertive and being aggressive. While salty and sour tastes assert their influence on agni, pungent taste is aggressive, assailing, attacking, combative, and at times even quarrelsome.

Like a militant fireball, the pungent taste enters our bodies via the mouth and gets to work with speed and energy, inflaming the agni first and then riding through the various bio-channels, mercilessly scorching obstructions such as parasites, tissue cells, excessive fluid, and lumps. You can imagine how necessary this divine but obsessive cleaner is for the body's daily cleanup.

As a housekeeper, this taste gets full marks for leaving nothing unattended. As a homemaker, the pungent taste is a bit of a perfectionist who sometimes tosses out the wanted stuff with the unwanted stuff (such is the compulsion to clean up!). Thus, the ruin of healthy body tissues, the impairment of oja or immune factor, and the destruction of sexual potency and fertility are all thanks to the overly efficient pungent taste!

But cleaning is necessary, so if the pungent taste is well guided, allowed in only for short and supervised visits, and accompanied with sweet taste, if necessary, as a moderator and soother, we can get our house cleaned and keep it that way. If pittas and vatas exercise extreme caution, and always use the sweet taste in association, and kaphas use the pungent taste happily every day (in moderation, of course), maybe we all can benefit from this hot and dry fire, in our own unique manner, as appropriate for our doshas.

Often anger as an emotion is associated with the intake of pungent taste. Anger, when appropriately felt and used (when required), serves as a tool of conscious living. The fire within is sometimes accessed through the emotion of anger. Pungent taste feeds this fire.

The ferocious ginger, the spitfire chili, the fierce garlic, and the angry human have one thing in common: the fire that burns, the fire that purifies, the fire that says no, the fire that sets limits, the fire that overrides boundaries, the fire that compels, the fire that enlivens, the fire that consumes, the fire that begins life (or anything) as a first spark, and the fire that ends life (or anything) as the last, extinguishing, devouring flame.

Examples: The pungent taste naturally occurs in vegetables such as garlic, ginger, radish, mustard, and the pepper family. Most Ayurvedic spices such as asafoetida, cumin, and mustard seeds are pungent.

Properties: Hot, dry, and light. It also causes salivation.

Action on doshas: Pitta ↑ Vata ↑ Kapha ↓

Action on agni: Agni flares up most quickly with pungent intake (even more so than sour and salty).

Action in body: In moderation, the pungent taste promotes agni and unblocks the stagnant secretions (phlegm) and hence counteracts colds, cough, and congestion. It also improves absorption and assimilation. It makes the body an inhospitable environment for worms and other parasites (such as yeast), and to an extent, it acts as an antitoxin, aiding breakdown, circulation, and elimination of wastes. It is antiobesity and anticholesterol (for example garlic).

Who can benefit? If kapha is aggravated, then judicious use of pungent spices such as ginger and cloves will be of great benefit. Pungent taste also helps ignite a dull agni.

Who must use caution? Excessive intake of pungent taste can cause serious imbalances manifesting in a dry, scorching, and burning heat in the body. First pitta and then vata dosha get aggravated, resulting in the following conditions: constipation, dizziness, giddiness, exhaustion, fainting, tremors, cramps, pain, burning sensation, dryness of mouth, heartburn, nausea, muscle fatigue, excessive weight loss, impaired fertility, skin rashes, hair loss, premature graying, and a host of other conditions.

Bitter Taste (Tikta Rasa)

To my taste buds, the bitter taste feels like a strict teacher. Here I was, having a party with sweet, salty, and sour tastes with a dab of passionate, pugnacious pungent, you know, to heat things up, and then came along bitter to remind me of my homework.

All this mindless partying has caused my body to accumulate food toxins, perhaps a parasite or two (also having a party!), along with congested body fluids and lots and lots of obstructions in my bio-channels. I need to clear out, lighten up, and start again. Well, the bitter taste will see to that all right.

Bitter is cold and indifferent, and does not bother to beguile us with its taste. Rather, it almost punishes us with its taste. Yet we need it to do what it does: reduce fevers, remove poisons, dispel infections, clear out parasites, and heal skin diseases. Without the bitter taste, we would never learn our lesson, get a fresh start, and begin with a blank gastrointestinal canvas.

When desire has taken birth, it first manifests as a state of dissatisfaction with what is and externally manifests as envy, and then it advances itself as absolute greed. When the greed is not met (can greed ever be satiated?), anger manifests. And when anger has wrung us inside out, what is left but grief? It is said that an excess of bitter taste induces grief.

I now am left picking some bitter memories from my otherwise sweet, sour, salty, and pungent past; all excitement and anger have been washed away by striking grief with a bitter aftertaste. How did this taste and all its stark aloneness enter into my psyche? Bitter enemies, bitter friends, bitter relationships, bitter thoughts, and bitter desolation loom large. Is the grief induced by bitter taste indicative of remorse? Is it a reflection on how too much of anything hurts? Is it a protest against the nonfulfillment of desire? Is it that basic resistance we all offer when life forces on us a spiritual lesson? The bitter taste is my teacher after all.

Examples: The bitter taste is naturally found in most green and yellow vegetables, including kale, brussels sprouts, dandelion greens, spinach, endives, broccoli, cauliflower, and asparagus. It is also found in bitter melon.

Properties: Dry, cooling, and light. This taste overpowers all other tastes.

Action on doshas: Pitta ↓ Vata ↑ Kapha ↓

Action on agni: When consumed in moderation, bitter taste supports the agni by imparting the quality of dryness.

Action in body: It cleanses the taste buds, allowing for receptivity of fresh tastes. It specifically aids the metabolism of food toxins and unblocks bio-channels (for example, the bitter spice turmeric is effective in relieving arterial blockages). Foods with a bitter taste are generally antiphlegm, antiparasitic, antipyretic, antitoxic, and antiobesity (but can reduce muscle bulk, too). Due to its cooling and cleansing qualities, bitter taste helps offset blood toxins causing obstinate skin conditions. Bitters such as neem, turmeric, and fenugreek are used topically to control itching and treat infection. In extreme moderation, the bitter taste is a great digestive tonic, keeping the body clean and unburdened by parasites and food toxins alike.

Who can benefit? Bitter vegetables and spices are a great asset in pacifying aggravated kapha. Incorporate some bitter in your diet (such as leafy greens or the naturally bitter spices turmeric and fenugreek) on a daily basis, especially in spring, which is the season of kapha aggravation. Or add bitter to your diet to pacify kapha that is currently expressing itself in heaviness in body and mind, extra fat deposits, or dullness in mind. Since bitter is a cooling and dry taste, it also helps balance pitta dosha's heat and oily quality. In summary, bitter taste works best to balance overexpressed kapha and pitta doshas.

Who must use caution? In excess, the dry and cold qualities of bitter taste tremendously increase vata dosha and associated conditions, such as emaciation (reduces tissue bulk), weakness, sexual dysfunction, dizziness, dryness of mouth and skin, abdominal distention, abdominal pain and spasms, and pain in heart and other muscles, and it can even lead to aggravation of mental disorders.

Astringent Taste (Kashaya Rasa)

The astringent taste imparts a puckering effect on all the bio-channels of the body. At times this works great, especially if the bio-channels should be constricted to prevent excessive leakage of fluids such as blood, urine, or water via bleeding, diarrhea, or vomiting. At other times, however, an unnecessary contraction of bio-channels, as in constriction of the bronchi, results in breathlessness.

Anytime the channels close more than normal, or close prematurely, the substances flowing inside the channels are impeded. Since vata is the force that is transporting all substances inside every channel, an increase and disturbance in vata dosha is immediate and imminent.

Nature in her supreme intelligence has sparsely distributed this astringent taste in her edibles. The modest astringent taste helps keep a lid on our bio-channels and prevents us from spilling over and coming apart at our seams, so to say.

Some say the intake of astringent taste induces fear. If closure and restriction are symptoms of resistance, then what is it that is resisted? And more important, I ask, why did I resist in the first place?

Is it the fear of sweet taste stirring from our subconscious—deeply embedded, voluptuous desires that stare us in the face and demand to be fulfilled? The fear of sour taste's hidden urgency playing out as chronic dissatisfaction? Or is the fear a fear of salty taste's pushy greediness? Is it the fear of pungent taste's angry explosion, inside and outside—how would that make us look? Or is it the fear of bitter loss, too wretched to be mentioned?

Let's look first at this fear that prevents desires to take root and manifest. This fear itself is astringent—a restriction of flow, a caustic compression, a shrinking of desire, an impediment of wants, a restriction of needs, and a curtailment of our very self.

Perhaps losing nutrition during uncontrollable episodes of diarrhea or bleeding drums up the fear of death itself, the ultimate fear lodged inside all of us? Perhaps fear, then, is a safety device, and the desire is really the desire to be healthy and to stay alive at any cost. So we close up, shut down, zip up, tighten, withdraw, compress, and restrict our self, all thanks to the cautious and ever mindful astringent taste. I bow to this fear that is more like caution and that makes me want to be healthy at any cost.

Examples: This is not a taste that can be identified easily but observed through its actions of imparting a drying and puckering effect on the tongue. It is most noticeable in unripe bananas, lentils, dried beans, peas, pomegranate, green tea, cranberries, and tart apples.

Properties: Dry, cold, heavy, nonslimy, light, compressing, moisture-absorbing. This taste checks discharges, restrains, compresses, and creates roughness and compactness.

Action on doshas: Pitta ↓ Vata ↑ Kapha ↓

Action on agni: In low amounts, the astringent taste prevents or counteracts excessive salivation as well as water in the stomach, both of which can make agni dull.

Action in body: Taken in moderation, it brings about necessary drying and helps in the healing of wounds and ulcers by the action of constriction of skin and vessels. Astringent taste helps tone the bio-channels and provides benefits by slowing or stopping the flow of various substances, which can be seen in cases of bleeding and diarrhea.

Who can benefit? All doshas can benefit when consumed in very small doses.

Who must use caution? This taste can aggravate vata quickly, hence it must be taken with caution if vata is already aggravated. Drying of mouth; chest pain; flatulence; bloating of abdomen; obstruction in passages of circulation (srotas); obstruction of feces, urine, flatus, and semen; spasms; convulsions; and other diseases of vata can occur due to its overuse.

How to Work with the Six Tastes

If your agni has only the normal variants and is not pathological with adverse dosha symptoms, then simply consume all six tastes. You would modify your taste selection by choosing some tastes over others because of the fluctuating seasons but for no other reason. And this injunction applies to all creatures that live with the seasons, not just you.

Appendix 4, "The Ayurvedic Diet Resource Guide," provides food recommendations for the seasons. As long as you pay attention and make these necessary seasonal modifications, you will be fine. Eating for the season will keep your doshas in balance, and the doshas will in turn keep your agni at its maximum physiological strength. Thus, eating for the season is Ayurveda's primary preventive health principle.

The corrective recommendation—the rule you must follow if your agni has become pathologically variant, due to previous lifestyle and diet errors, with adverse dosha-related gastric symptoms (refer back to table 23 on page 186)—is to eat according to the season and balance the doshas. In other words, beyond addressing the macroenvironment, the seasons, you also need to adhere to the needs of the microenvironment if you have imbalances in your body. Dosha-based diets are corrective prescriptions and not universal diets to be followed by all pittas, all vatas, or all kaphas under the sun.

This is important to understand, and so I will say it again. Throughout your life, you should follow a diet appropriate to the current season. This is the universal prescription. Only in periods of specific imbalance should you embark on a dosha-balancing diet, which is always a personalized prescription.

Doshas are balanced primarily by tastes or flavors. See table 24 to choose the tastes that must be consumed to balance a given dosha. More details on a dosha-balancing meal regimen are provided in appendix 4. To find out if you have a dosha imbalance, you do not need to know your dosha constitution, called your *prakriti* in Ayurveda. (It is interesting that the Sanskrit word *prakriti* also connotes "Mother Nature.") You can simply see if your agni has dosha-related

TABLE 24   Dosha and Taste Potency

	INCREASING IMPACT			DECREASING IMPACT		
	Maximum	Medium	Minimum	Maximum	Medium	Minimum
Vata	Bitter	Pungent	Astringent	Sweet	Sour	Salty
Pitta	Pungent	Salty	Sour	Bitter	Sweet	Astringent
Kapha	Sweet	Salty	Sour	Pungent	Bitter	Astringent

symptoms. (See pages 40–43 in chapter 1 for a list of the symptoms of aggravated doshas.)

Additionally, to restore balance, you may want to increase a certain quality, such as dryness or lightness. In this case, you would select some tastes over others. See table 25.

Think of the six flavors as paints in six colors—and use these colors daily to make a new portrait of your health. The canvas is ready. When you make a wise color selection, the radiance of health comes through!

I have yet to encounter another system of mind-body-soul medicine with more comprehensive dietary recommendations than Ayurveda. Food is the best way to prevent disease and optimize health. Food guidelines and recommendations in Ayurveda have been well researched, tried and tested, and validated in the living laboratory of humanity. Let's look at one instance of this.

ONE WOMAN'S RECOVERY THROUGH AYURVEDIC FOODS

Tracy Cunningham, an award-winning art director, illustrator, and graphic designer from the San Francisco Bay Area, lost forty pounds and eliminated severe hives, high cholesterol, and symptoms that presaged diabetes within one year of adopting Ayurvedic eating habits. The main thing she did, though, was pull herself back from the dark and frightening experience of being trapped in a very sick body and regain a happy and serene mind.

Tracy had begun suffering from debilitating bouts of hives about five years earlier, when she was in her early thirties. She had no idea what caused these outbreaks. She frequented the emergency room, and she regularly took over-the-counter anti-inflammatory medication so she could tolerate the inflammation and itching. Her constant scratching of her flaking and cracking skin created huge abscesses on her face. Tracy moved through life like a zombie, under the influence of allergy medication. Over time, her hives became systemic, and the outbreaks spread to every part of her body.

Tracy's job was a series of daily stress-laden deadlines, twelve-hour workdays with rare lunch breaks. Taking a vacation was frowned upon. Not only did all of this stress keep her body poised for hives, but it also triggered emotional eating. She began to pack on weight.

TABLE 25   Quality and Taste Selection

| Quality | INCREASING IMPACT | | |
	Maximum	Medium	Minimum
Dryness	Astringent	Pungent	Bitter
Oiliness	Sweet	Salty	Sour
Heaviness	Sweet	Astringent	Sour
Lightness	Bitter	Pungent	Sour
Hotness	Pungent	Sour	Salty
Coldness	Sweet	Astringent	Bitter

"I'd always filled a void in my life with processed foods and sugar," Tracy said. "Now it was a way to deal with stress as well." On her five-foot-three frame, she was carrying two hundred pounds.

By the time Tracy signed up for the beginner's Awakening Health course in Ayurveda at my school, she was constantly exhausted and beginning to show signs of depression. She knew she had to do something.

Through Ayurveda, Tracy gained an understanding of what was happening to her body and the reasons for the hives and weight gain—and she found those answers, which had eluded her for years, within weeks of starting the course. Finally, she could relax. She had found a system of knowledge that would help make her whole again.

The first and most important skill Tracy learned in her first few classes was how to assess her digestion. Ayurveda says that digestion is a fire that should be neither blazing nor weak. Tracy realized that her digestive fire was naturally slow and that she had slowed it down even more through her nonstop emotional eating, her high sugar intake, and those long periods of hives. Instead of a warm brick fireplace, the metaphor I like to use, Tracy's digestion was like a drippy, leaky, barely warm potbelly stove. Tracy quickly saw that her slow digestion was the cause of her hives and weight gain.

By eating prescribed foods at the prescribed times, Tracy began to notice miraculous differences in her body. For one thing, her energy increased. For another, she began to feel hungry at the right times.

Within a few months, her hive outbreaks became rare, and within six months, the extra weight began to drop off, effortlessly and at a healthy pace. "I wasn't even following a strict exercise routine," she said. "The weight loss just happened naturally, through minding my digestion!"

This meant that the weight loss was sustainable—something she had never experienced with the diets she'd tried in the past. But it's been four and a half years since Tracy started eating an Ayurvedic diet, and her body has simply refused to gain that weight back. She has maintained her weight loss effortlessly!

By following a customized Ayurveda plan, Tracy's cholesterol dropped several points and her prediabetic readings also improved.

Here are a few of the foods and dietary habits that Tracy tossed out of her kitchen to make this amazing change in her health and body.

Seafood: Fish is considered light and healthy, and so it is freely recommended by medical professionals, nutritionists, and media. Ayurveda's perspective is that fish lives in water, embodying the quality of water, which makes it kapha increasing. Itching is one symptom of kapha aggravation. By this logic, fish—whether it's fresh- or saltwater—will never help you lose weight, because weight loss requires kapha reduction, not addition. And because of the salt, saltwater fish is additionally considered heating (pitta increasing). Heating foods would aggravate Tracy's red-hot hives, which were a result of increased pitta. For this reason, seafood is prohibited for people with hot and itchy skin conditions in Ayurveda. As a first move, Tracy stopped all seafood for a trial period of three months—and she saw that she was, indeed, recovering from hives and losing weight. Tracy could see she was on to something!

Frozen, microwaveable meals: Frozen and stale foods are difficult to digest. Tracy realized that, for the sake of convenience, she was wasting money on dosha-aggravating frozen dinners that made weight-loss companies richer and herself poorer in health.

Yogurt, juices, and smoothies: These are kapha-increasing and agni-dulling. "They may work for some people," Tracy said, "but certainly not for me." In America today, yogurt is touted as the ideal food for weight loss. In Ayurveda, it is considered the ideal food for weight gain—since even low fat increases kapha with each bite.

A meat-centric diet: Tracy was used to eating meat at every meal. She learned that she can cook the same meats with Ayurvedic spices (such as turmeric and cumin) to make this heavy food more digestible. She also learned to eat more lentils, beans, and vegetables at dinnertime—these foods are easier than meat to digest—and to restrict meat-eating to lunchtime, when her agni is naturally sharper.

In this way, Tracy weaned herself away from the generic wisdom spawned by modern, popular so-called diets that push the same strategy "to lose weight and be happy" to one and all, no matter what the age, constitution, or season. Instead, she turned to the sanity of individualized Ayurvedic diet recommendations based on the consideration of individual state of agni, the season, the time of the day, and doshas.

Now five years later, Tracy has graduated as an Ayurveda practitioner, and she has a less stressful day job as well: she coordinates all of Vedika Global's Ayurveda community programs with great success. Once she was healed and restored, Tracy asked me for a spiritual name, and I gave her the name Lakshmi, the goddess of perfect health, abundance, and beauty, who dwells in the lotus of the heart. She smiled, her being radiating with health and eyes content with the recognition of her inner Lakshmi.

Three Approaches to Ayurvedic Eating

We've been over a lot of territory so far in this chapter, and I want to summarize what I feel are the most important points. There are three approaches to Ayurvedic eating; two of them—eating for agni and eating for the season—are actually two sides of the same coin. When you're doing one, you're doing the other. It just depends on which you would prefer to hold paramount in your mind. Either way, this is how Ayurveda recommends eating pretty much all of the time.

The third approach—eating to balance a specific dosha—is more specialized. It's a style of eating you would embark on to correct an imbalance you perceive, to address troublesome symptoms—let's say intestinal gas or afternoon headaches. Think of it as a self-administered prescription and undertake such a diet for a specific length of time. You would eat to pacify a dosha only for a short time. Here are more details about each approach.

Eat for Your Agni

This is a cardinal rule in Ayurveda: you should eat according to the status of your agni. For one thing, if you're not hungry, don't eat. Also, you must modify your meals—the quality, quantity, and frequency—according to the physiological rhythms of your own metabolism. This is an intuitive matter. It's something we all do. When people experience heartburn, even if they've never heard of Ayurveda, they look for cooling foods, they avoid ginger and wasabi, they eat lighter foods, or they may skip a meal. They don't tell themselves that they're

igniting their agni, but that's what they're doing, and this helps them overcome indigestion. If eating certain foods results in intestinal gas, then after a while, we will avoid those foods. These healing insights do not require advanced knowledge. If we are attentive, such wisdom comes from within us. Ayurveda has honored people's intelligent responses to food and expressed them as principles of agni. So, in Ayurveda, we *always* eat according to agni. You could think of this rule as a gentle reminder of what you already know deep down. Without concern for doshas, think about whether your agni is normal or sharp, dull or variable—and eat accordingly. Here is a list to help with this:

- For sharp agni, eat heavy, cooling, dense, dulling foods. Do not miss meals, and know that you may require a larger meal and a snack.

- For dull agni, eat highly digestible, warming, nondense, sharp foods. You may require detoxing for few days. Of all your meals, dinner especially should be very easily digested and quite small.

- For variable agni, be open to making new choices, meal by meal, and counteract sharpness or dullness by the law of opposites. Also, make sure you eat by the clock and slowly regularize the digestive clock and process.

- For normal agni, simply continue following all the food rules provided in the rest of this chapter. You do this to keep your agni normal. Also, know that you do not require any specific food lists as long as you eat seasonally.

Eat for the Season

When people come to study at my school, even before I tell them about the doshas, I teach them how to eat seasonally. At the heart of it, this is so simple: warming foods in winter, cooling foods in summer and fall. (See appendix 4, "The Ayurvedic Diet Resource Guide" for some specific suggestions.) As students take in the concepts of seasonal eating, they always have several aha moments as they begin to recognize that Ayurvedic eating is simpler than they had thought—or had been told. Entire civilizations of human beings, past and present, and all animal species know how to eat according to the season. Ayurveda has studied this inborn intelligence and has expressed it as precepts that we can follow. These laws belong to Nature; Ayurveda has merely interpreted them and written them down for our convenience. And I want to point out that when my grandmother cooked for dozens, and sometimes hundreds, of people, she always cooked seasonally appropriate food. As I've said, those foods were healing—for everyone.

Eat to Balance a Specific Dosha

As I've mentioned, you would embark on a specific dosha-balancing diet for only short periods of time, never as a lifelong strategy. This prescription may be contrary to popular ideas of eating a one- or two-dosha-balancing diet, based on your dosha type (constitution), all your life. But I am merely stating what the sages have clarified in the core texts. So this is the fundamental approach, as opposed to the "dosha type" fad diets made popular in the West by modern interpretations of Ayurveda's science of nutrition. In general, by eating seasonal foods, you are already offsetting a potential dosha imbalance. That is why seasonal diets automatically focus more on kapha-balancing foods in spring, vata-balancing foods in summer and rainy seasons, and pitta-balancing in fall. In the winter, no single dosha can go out of balance—this is due to scientific principles too involved for me to explain here—and so the dietary recommendations for winter are based not on doshas but on nutrition for the season. Also, if a certain dosha is aggravated, and this is expressed through obvious symptoms—intestinal gurgling for a vata aggravation, heat in the belly for pitta, or phlegm in the lungs for kapha—then, for a specific period of time, you can select dosha-pacifying foods in your daily meal planning, until symptoms subside. (Refer back to tables 4, 5, and 6 on pages 38–39. Also, see the dosha-based diet tables and dos and don'ts on dosha management in appendix 4.)

Please note that anyone with a serious illness needs the assistance of a qualified vaidya, an Ayurvedic doctor, to find the right diet. Such a diet is a one-of-a-kind prescription—the specifics of it and the length of time it should be followed are individual. Setting such prescriptions is well beyond the scope of this book.

Another Consideration: Qualities

We have talked about the flavors of various foods, but there is more to a food than just its flavor. If you want to eat something that tastes sweet, you might have a handful of grapes, or then again, you might eat a banana. Grapes and bananas are both sweet, but they are very different foods—and they have different effects on your system. They have different *qualities*.

What Ayurveda calls qualities are the twenty physical attributes that determine the constitution (prakriti) of a food. Rather than just your sense of taste, you are calling into play your senses of touch and vision and, in some cases, even hearing to gauge a food's fluid content, density, or stickiness. What is most significant about the qualities, however, is not the physical properties of a particular food but the effect this food will have on your system once you have eaten it. You might not think of licorice as cooling or a tomato as warming, but these are, according to the Ayurvedic sages, the qualities that these two foods have based on the effects they have on your body.

Before I list the qualities, I want to acknowledge that it may seem daunting to some readers to receive yet another list, another new—new to you—perspective on foods. Yet using this tool, food qualities, is not rocket science. This is how native peoples in all world cultures have eaten over the centuries. In dry desert climates, they looked for oily, slimy foods (cactus, okra, fleshy fruits); in humid or wet climates, they went for more fiery foods (peppers and chilies). When they were aging, they ate light (easily digested) foods, and when they were growing or pregnant, they ate heavy foods. There was no food packaging then, no added vitamins or calcium, and people used the foods' qualities to judge what was best for them in their particular, individual circumstance.

Somehow, in the modern world, we seem to have forgotten this wisdom. Thankfully, the sages of Ayurveda observed Nature and gave us the list of twenty qualities to use as a tool in selecting foods (see table 26). Remember the principle of "like increases like; opposites decrease each other." This is the principle to apply when looking at the qualities of the foods you eat. It is in this way that the heavy can lose weight, the thin can gain weight, the unstable can become stable, and the stagnant can become mobile.

These twenty physical qualities represent a matrix of physical transformation. I suggest that you keep this list in mind when you're grocery shopping. Simply evaluate your food choices in light of their qualities, and you will know what these foods will do to your body. If you are thin and want to put on weight to fill out your curves, then choose foods that are dense rather than porous and heavy rather than light (pork or beef versus chicken) and oily instead of dry (dairy versus popcorn). This is easy, no? And it's intuitive, too! So give the knowledge of doshas a break and simply use your five senses plus your common sense when you go grocery shopping! Now you get to make your own diet that works for you.

Ayurveda Food Disciplines

The Sanskrit word for the disciplines we mindfully and voluntarily take on in order to reach a certain goal is *sadhana*. In Ayurveda, the goal of our sadhana is aiding the health of body, mind, and soul. In Ayurvedic food sadhana, we embrace certain rules that are inspired by the timeless wisdom of the sages of Ayurveda. There is a famous Ayurveda proverb: When diet is wrong, medicine is of no use. When diet is correct, medicine is of no need.

What follows is a discussion of the major food disciplines put forward by Ayurveda. Some may seem obvious, and some you may never have thought about.

Eat Fresh Foods, Not Stale

Stale foods have a mind-disturbing quality. They induce tamas. With tamas, the mind gets filled with negative vibrations. Heaviness, dullness, and even sadness and depression are found to

TABLE 26   Ayurveda's Twenty Qualities

QUALITY	EFFECTS ON BODY	EXAMPLES	DIGESTIBILITY INDEX
Cold	Contracts, halts, lowers body temperature	Grapes, milk, coconut water, aloe, licorice, cucumber, fennel, rose, coriander, cane sugar, milk, ghee (clarified butter), cold water	Slow
Hot	Causes perspiration, raises body temperature	Peppers, garlic, saffron, chilies, honey, mint, ginger, cumin, black pepper, wasabi, mustards, horseradish, daikon, tomato, hot water	Rapid
Heavy	Builds up, promotes bulk (weight gain)	Black gram, wheat, fish, yogurt, cold water, nuts, meats of large animals (like cows and pigs)	Low and slow
Light	Imparts lightness, reduces bulk (weight loss)	Mung bean; puffed rice; bottle gourd or opo squash; hot water (air and fire added by boiling); cumin, fenugreek, and other digestive seeds; dried rice flakes; millet; barley; meats of small, lightly moving birds and animals (like rabbit and deer)	High and rapid
Oily	Lubricates, smooths	All vegetable oils and lards; dairy fat, like butter; ghee; oil in nuts and seeds	High but slow
Dry	Dries, absorbs moisture	Millet, barley, popcorn, chickpeas, dry cereals, toast, dried fruits, salads, raw foods	Fast
Dull	Slows activities, dulls physical responses and the doshas	Whole grains, nuts, wheat, roots, brown rice, black gram	Slow
Sharp	Quickens activities, sharpens physical responses, excites, can irritate	Citrus, all peppers, wasabi, radish, horseradish, cloves, chilies, ginger, nutmeg, cinnamon, mustard, black pepper	Rapid

QUALITY	EFFECTS ON BODY	EXAMPLES	DIGESTIBILITY INDEX
Mobile	Stimulates movement, such as laxative action	Senna leaves, castor oil, milk	Rapid
Immobile	Prevents movement, makes firm (especially in regard to potential hair loss or bone dislocation), makes you fall asleep	Goat meat, nuts, wheat, ghee, black gram, nutmeg, poppy seed, opium (medicinal use only), slow-cooked food, fresh-cooked food, bone soup, most roots	Slow
Soft	Softens (especially in regard to a physical organ or body part)	Castor oil, licorice, wheat, ghee, butter, milk	Rapid
Hard	Makes hard or resilient (especially in regard to a physical organ or body part)	Nuts, meat, roots	Slow, resistant
Sticky	Softens, lubricates by introducing a coating or covering	Milk, milk cream, fish, okra, tapioca, sticky rice, chia seeds, aloe, edible gum, yogurt, psyllium husk	Slow
Clarifying	Eradicates or cleanses away irritants and pathogens	Turmeric, neem, castor oil	Rapid
Smooth	Can smooth and make uniform (especially in regard to bones)	Avocado, whipped cream, butter	Slow
Rough	Can increase skin dryness and sensitivity; can produce physical gas	Bitter melon, broccoli, popcorn, chips, rough crackers, cauliflower	Resistant
Bulky	Increases bulkiness, causes weight gain	Black gram, heavy, thick meat (buffalo, beef)	Slow

TABLE 26 Ayurveda's Twenty Qualities (cont.)

QUALITY	EFFECTS ON BODY	EXAMPLES	DIGESTIBILITY INDEX
Subtle	Penetrates through the minute channels of the body; can be mind-altering	Alcohol, salt, marijuana, caffeine, opium	Rapid
Dense	Provides density, bulk; leads to weight gain	Starchy foods, swollen tapioca (semisolid), jams and jellies, pastries, meats	Slow
Fluid	Causes fluidity in the body	Water, milk, coconut water, fruit juices	Rapid

manifest in the mind of a person who has eaten stale foods. In time, the immune system (oja) also becomes weakened. I have helped countless people battle depression simply by having them eat fresh food. "Fresh food" means, as I've said, food recently grown and recently cooked.

So make cooking fresh your daily sadhana. Minimize leftovers, and when food is left over, eat it quickly so that it doesn't sit in the refrigerator. Your own leftovers are better than those you bring home from restaurants and cafes because when you cook the food yourself, you know what has gone into it—both in terms of the ingredients and the emotions of the cook.

I suggest beginning a collection of simple-to-cook recipes like the ones I share in this book. Make them your staples. For your dinner, a cup of hot milk or cooked oatmeal is preferable to processed, packaged, frozen, or canned entrees—all of which are not only stale but have been manipulated by additives and processing that dampens your agni and seriously disturbs the doshas.

Take Your Time in Food Preparation

Ayurveda recommends preparing fresh foods in a slow and relaxed manner in a spirit of joy and with the keen anticipation that will make the salivary glands and other digestive juices flow. When we take the time to prepare our foods from natural ingredients available on our planet, these foods will, in turn, give us more time on this planet.

Food preparation begins with its purchase. I suggest that you buy your groceries from natural markets or vendors who offer pure, organic, seasonal, and fresh foods. The next step is food prep—mindfully cutting, chopping, and otherwise readying the food to be cooked. Then, there is the cooking itself, the final step in a process that should delight the soul. I suggest that you drop any habit you may have of rushing thorough your preparation. Instead, choose longer stretches of time for cooking. Then you can begin viewing food and its associate processes, equipment, tools, and gadgets as friends, not tasks.

In fact, watching food manifest from its initial raw stage to its final, ready-to-eat state is a meditation itself. Hold this thought: *The world stands waiting while I cook my food as an offering to myself.*

Make It Fine Dining Every Day

Based just on the length of its history, I think I can safely say that the art of fine dining was first given to the world by Ayurveda. The ancient texts of Ayurveda recognize the importance of eating in a beautiful place and of eating on appealing vessels and dishes (*ishta sarvopakarana*). It is clear that the sages of Ayurveda were aware of the role that psychological factors play in optimum digestion. Ayurveda fine dining includes, at the minimum, setting the stage with beautiful, clean, and inspirational crockery and eating utensils—whether flatware or chopsticks—with music in the background (wind chimes are great), perhaps a lit candle or two or oil lamps, and fresh flowers and fruits as an eye-catching centerpiece. Sage Charaka further recommends dressing up for meals, wearing fragrant flowers on the body or perfumes, and also chanting sacred mantras before eating to set the right vibration and prepare the body and mind to accept the food with ease and grace.[6] This is all pleasurable for our senses and plays a part in enhancing our anticipation of a meal, which in turn, stokes agni.

I suggest that when you eat, you press the pause button on your other activities, bring yourself to your usual dining spot, and sit comfortably at a table or mat to eat. The digestive juices will begin flowing instantly, in that very moment. Your outer clock and conscious choice have activated your inner clock and some inner choices. Ayurveda recommends eye-catching utensils, fragrant spices, beautiful garnishes, and tasteful presentations of food to evoke excitement and enthusiasm and enjoyment in our act of eating. Fold away those TV trays and bring out your "guest" dishes—you should be giving yourself the care and beauty that you deserve. To put yourself in the center of your own lotus is extremely good for your health.

Fix and Follow Regular Mealtimes

In general, the time between meals can vary from three to six hours, depending on your digestion. The evening meal should be taken before sunset or just after. You should retire two to three hours after the evening meal. Eating late at night, right before going to bed, produces indigestion, gaseous distention, hyperacidity, and disturbed sleep.

Follow these simple guidelines or, if you must, make up your own schedule. Whatever you decide on, stick to it. I suggest eating breakfast before 8:00 a.m., lunch between noon and 1:00 p.m., and dinner between 5:00 p.m. and 6:30 p.m. If you must eat later, then do, but pick a time and stick to it. Keep variations to your meal schedule to a minimum. Having a somewhat fixed timing for eating strengthens agni. Consuming food at random times confuses and derails agni. To a great extent, agni operates as an autonomous conditioned mechanism, with the digestive juices and processes activating according to a time-based rhythm. This is how, when it is lunchtime, we know it without even looking at a clock. But when food is thrown into the body indifferently at varying times each day, agni is unable to settle into a rhythm and will become activated at the wrong times. When we finally take the time to eat, our agni may not even be awake or not functioning at its full power.

Solitude or Company over Meals— Make It Count

If you are eating alone, then make the best use of this opportunity for spiritual solitude. Take your plate to a backyard or a lovely, quiet area of your home and seek your own sweet company over food. Your silence during eating can include a state of mind in which you practice thankfulness. You offer the food your own quiet focus, your serene mind, and your sense of respect and gratitude.

If you are going to have company while you eat, then it would be great to ensure that the mealtime is companionable. The dining table is definitely not a place to settle grievances and wage arguments. Leave the struggling world alone for at least the thirty minutes it takes you to eat.

Simply focus on the plate or bowl of food and the act of eating. With each bite, you are recreating your own body and mind, no less. You might post a sign in your home near the eating area: "Thank you for respecting my silence. I am practicing mindfulness."

Watch Your Emotions while Eating

Ayurveda was the first science to see the connection between our mental states and our metabolism. If you are feeling anything other than okay—anything other than what most of us would call "normal"—then walk away from food. Don't eat right now. You can eat a little later. This exception to the rule of having set times to eat points to the way Ayurveda sages appreciated the complex human psyche. After all, a disturbed mind will disturb all three doshas, and agni won't remain stable for long either. In fact, when we are emotionally upset, we often feel a sinking sensation in the pit of the stomach, and a mild to strong aversion to food is common enough (though transient). So it is best to take time out from eating in such situations and, instead, first center ourselves and regain a fresh perspective. A short meditation can restore agni and appetite quickly by restoring a more detached and observer state of consciousness toward the (unwanted or unpleasant) situation at hand.

I suppose this is why Ayurvedic texts underscore the importance of a calm mind and pleasant company during meals. When family dinners become a form of torture, and food is eaten in rage or self-pity, it is natural to associate our anger or grief with food. We end up disliking or fearing food, or—the opposite—we see food as replacement of what we think we are missing in life, and we eat for comfort.

Make it a practice to begin eating only after washing your hands—and face as well, if possible—and then close your eyes for a moment of meditation. Consciously attend to the food on your table. You can recite food mantras or prayers from your culture, and this will support you to manifest serene mindfulness as you eat.

Pace Your Eating— Not Too Fast, Not Too Slow

When you eat in a hurry, it is impossible to remain aware of whether you are still hungry or have become full and should stop eating. Eating at the right pace also facilitates the all-important (but often forgotten) act of chewing. Food that is inadequately masticated taxes our agni. Chewing sufficiently also directs our attention to what we are eating, to how it tastes, and to what we are experiencing from that flavor. Consequently, when we eat at the right pace and truly chew our food, we become in touch with our own needs and can know when we have had enough.

Then again, always seeking the happy balance, Ayurveda also advises against excessively slow eating because this does not give the agni enough stimulation. Also, when you eat very slowly, the temperature of food drops, and hot items may become cold by the time you finish eating them. This coldness further impedes the agni, and your meal will not be processed and assimilated suitably.

So, pace yourself with mindfulness. The food and the act of eating this food deserve your attention. Mindfulness can be achieved by preparing yourself to eat ritually; each meal, this is possible.

Mindfully Judge How Much Food to Eat

According to Ayurveda, the appropriate quantity of food is different for each person, each state of agni, the season, the time of day, and the dosha that we need to balance. There is no one recommendation for the amount of food to be eaten for all people at all times. When you eat the correct quantity, you will feel active, energetic, and happy. Undereating brings about a feeling of weakness and a loss of zeal and weight. Excessive eating, in turn, will cause heaviness, lethargy, sleepiness, and constriction in the chest and abdomen.

So here is what I have to say: eat until you feel pleasantly satiated. When you walk away from the table, you should not have any discomfort in your abdomen, your breathing should be comfortable, and your mind should feel content. Only you know where to draw the line. Get back in touch with your instinct and then follow its inner dictates. Reclaim your instinct. Don't give it away ever again. Ayurveda provides three commonsense tips for eating the right amount of food.

First, eat less than your maximum capacity. This suggests that you stop eating just before reaching satiety. If you walk away from your meal just a teeny bit hungry, you are doing great. Actually, this teeny bit of hunger doesn't exist in the belly; it exists in the mind. That hunger is the lust or greed factor we must choose to transcend if we are going to reap the benefits of abiding health.

Second, imagine your stomach is divided into four parts. Think that two parts are for solids, one part is for liquids, and keep the last part deliberately empty so that digestion can take place appropriately.

Third, eat according to the strength of your digestive fire. If you have sharp agni, you can eat a large quantity at each meal, and you may find that you have no problem digesting it. If you have dull agni, you should measure out food carefully on your plate and begin with smaller amounts at each meal, making sure you can digest what you are ingesting. Eat slowly, and go back for seconds only after evaluation of real hunger versus your mental hunger (often they don't match up). If your agni is variable, you will need to adjust the quantity you are consuming meal by meal. Don't simply follow fixed quantities day after day as agni will be variable at every meal. Feel your way and then feed yourself accordingly, with utmost respect of your agni.

One final factor in determining the right quantity to eat concerns the qualities of the foods. If the foods of a particular meal are oily, heavy, and dense, then you should consider eating less than you usually do. If the foods are light, airy, and dry, then you can eat a bit more. As we've discussed, these qualities have varying impacts on agni, so it's only common sense to make these adjustments in quantity.

Do Not Skip Meals

Eating less than the body requires can have adverse consequences. Eating nothing, excessive fasting or dieting, or simply forgetting to eat when we're busy—these are all serious factors that contribute toward a full-blown agni disturbance. To starve ourselves is to starve our agni. Lacking fuel, the agni dies on us just as a fire in our fireplace would die out if we forgot to feed it another log of wood.

A weak agni cannot digest even water or simple soups. Once you have weakened your agni by not eating, then eating anything can become a liability. A weak agni can create only toxins. In time, the agni we have underfed is suffocated by the increasing toxins, suffocated under the aggravated vata dosha, and lacks adequate fuel to regenerate itself. At this point, the agni is extinguished forever, taking the individual with it. No agni means no life.

For this reason, weight loss in Ayurveda is never accomplished by missing meals. Weight loss happens by your eating digestible foods, at regular mealtimes, and drinking warm water.

Eat Only If You Are Hungry

One strict rule of Ayurveda is to eat only if you feel the previous meal is completely digested. If you eat another meal when the earlier meal is not yet through your system, there is a danger that the newly ingested food will mix with the partially digested food, and this will disturb the agni and all three doshas. It will create toxins (aama).

The ideal time to eat is when significant hunger is present and your bowels and bladder have nothing pending. (While the ideal time to move the bowels is in the morning, if you feel you must do so later, then definitely do that, and do it before eating rather than after.) If there are any burps or belches coming up, then they should be pure air with no aftertaste or smell. Also, there should be no bloating in the stomach. You should feel light, not heavy, and you should keenly anticipate the next meal. This signifies that the ideal time to eat has arrived.

If we are not in touch with our own state of hunger or fullness or if we don't follow the above guidelines—if we eat whenever we come across tasty food or feel emotionally empty—then our agni will continue to be compromised and we will continue to generate toxins. This is also one reason snacking is cautioned against by Ayurveda.

In an ideal world, when we eat at set times, we feel hungry at those set times. However, Ayurveda never asks us to follow any rule blindly. It is also important to gauge whether you have real hunger—let's not stuff our faces just because the clock says it is our mealtime! Let's examine our lifestyle and train our agni first so that when the outer clock strikes a certain time, our belly clock (agni) also sends us the signal of hunger.

Snack Only When Agni Permits

Unfortunately, eating frequently, known as *adhyashana* in Ayurveda, seriously compromises agni and generates toxins. By constant snacking, even if we snack in very small quantities, we are overloading our agni, giving it more fuel than it can handle. Imagine a fire in your fireplace. If you load too many logs on a tentative flame, this flame will die out. For the fire to catch, you may have to remove a few of the heavy logs and feed it some light twigs. And if you fan a fire that has just enough wood and kindling, in time, it will pick up intensity. An intense fire that is fed additional wood will become even more intense. Use this image when you decide whether to have a snack. Snacking is permissible only if the agni is fairly sharp. That's when it needs more fuel. If you have a sharp agni, then be careful to set specific times for snacking and don't just eat all day at random times.

For most of us, however, and most of the time, we require more time between meals to build our agni to the point that it can take more food. This means that we need a prolonged gap between meals to allow for the full digestion of the previous meal, the cleansing of clogged bio-channels, and the release of urine and stool. All this stimulates hunger, hunger stimulates digestive juices, and when the next meal is also moderate in quantity, there is a good chance that your agni will shift into a higher gear and remain there.

Pick Up a Dull Agni with a Hot Drink

Instead of frequent small meals, Ayurveda suggests building up a weak agni by drinking hot water to which you have added lemon juice or salt or both. All of these—the heat, the sour, and the salt—will stimulate agni. Once you are clearly hungry, you can then eat a small, adequately spiced, well-cooked meal—the small amount, the spicing, and the cooking of the food will also serve to help revive agni. In this way, slowly and steadily, agni can be restored in strength. In short, spices, herbs, digestive gruels, and some careful fasting are the Ayurvedic methodology for aiding digestion. See appendix 4 for tips on Ayurvedic detox.

Eat When Hungry, Drink When Thirsty

With thirst, as well as with hunger, stay tuned in to your inner knowing. Don't believe anyone who tells you to drink water to satisfy your hunger! Ayurveda is very clear that we should not eat when we are thirsty nor drink when we are hungry. Hunger and thirst are symptoms of completely different inner processes. The new fad of drinking water to drown hunger is extremely disturbing to agni and to the doshas. Usually when agni sends out hunger signals, it is saying that the body requires more of the five elements—through the flavors—so that the task of building and maintaining the body can go on. So that life can go on. When we deprive ourselves of the all-important biological fuel of the five elements, we enter the danger zone. Water is neutral and, unless herbs, juice, or vegetable extract is added to it, carries none of the six tastes.

Warm Foods Are Preferable to Cold

Food tastes better when it's at a warm temperature, and the heat stimulates the digestive fire, pacifies excess vata in the digestive tract, and leads to elimination of flatulence and bowels with ease. Avoid excessively hot foods, however, since the disproportionate heat eats away at pitta dosha, leading to burning sensation, excessive thirst, a dry mouth, and the aggravation of any existing bleeding conditions from nose, anus, or skin.

Excessively cold foods aggravate both vata and kapha doshas and ultimately lead to the cooling down of the digestive fire, with consequent loss of appetite, metabolic deficiency, gas, and flatulence. The effect that cool food has on the agni depends on its degree of coolness. Food at room temperature is somewhat agni-upsetting, while chilled foods are agni-distressing. As I've said many times, warm foods support agni best.

Take Responsibility for What You Eat

The person who eats the food—that's you—is the very person who has the responsibility for making what you eat and the way you eat to support and nourish you. It is not enough to simply follow external rules, even those rules that come from Ayurveda. You must observe your own response to foods and come to understand your relationship with food. If you take into consideration your own digestive power, the season, the time of day, and whether the food you last ate has been digested, you will be way ahead of the game.

So even though the disciplines suggested are for universal benefit, you play the greatest role in your Ayurveda food sadhana. Ayurveda teaches many dos and don'ts regarding food, yet it also makes this bold declaration: Regardless of how healthy it may be, if the food you are eating does not delight your senses and please your mind, then it won't be of any help to you! Ultimately, the sages declare, that the food you do not enjoy eating will disturb your agni and shatter your strength.[7]

Now this is certainly food for thought. We must sit down to each delicious health-promoting, dosha-balancing meal with a sensitivity to what impact this food will have on the mind. It's a very good idea to make any efforts needed so that each meal is garnished and presented in such a way that the mind is pleased by the food.

Your Food Preferences Matter

Whenever you eat foods that you feel that you should eat but, for whatever reason, do not want to eat, then you end up creating food toxins. So think before you force-feed any food to yourself or anyone else—and I am definitely including your children here. Feeling that you must eat food you find distasteful can actually do more damage to your agni than it does good.

I recommend that you rack your brain to see how you can cook those healthy foods in a more delicious manner so that you and your family will want to eat them. Remember, mealtimes should never be wars, and meals are not merely a mix of vitamins, proteins, and minerals. Don't ever think that you can plug your nose while eating a food you don't like. Any meal you eat should look good, taste good, smell good; it should be served in an aesthetic manner; and it should be consumed with a sense that the food itself is sacred.

Avoid Processed (So-Called Miracle) Foods

A frozen smoothie may be jam-packed with wonderful vitamins and minerals, but it may very well freeze your agni while you drink it. A dehydrated, commercially prepared, brilliantly packaged powder may boast rare proteins and promise the world of health to you but be a challenge to your agni to break down (and your mind gags at the thought of it)! Raw vegetable juices may be full of live energy—vitamins and minerals—and may be low-calorie, too, but they might just drown the agni with all that fluid. A food bar may be low in calories and packed with all the latest nutritional must-haves, yet this "food" may have such a complex molecular structure that it's difficult to impossible for agni to break it down, and toxins are the inevitable result. Count your recommended fruit servings and eat them too (good for you!), but all those fruits may very well do in your already collapsing agni—and leave you feeling a little nauseated and gassy.

What is wrong with this picture? I'm not saying that the modern, commercial prescription is *always* wrong, but it is often not the absolute truth either. In a world of shifting scientific "facts" and conflicting theories, not only is it difficult to know which of these "miracle" foods is right for you—but so often your agni does not cooperate. The best thing you can do is to keep it simple. Have you ever wondered why your so-called miracle foods leave you even more tired or exhausted or why the latest nutritional supplement gives you stomach cramps or diarrhea?

Whatever the claim and whatever the content, if a food or food supplement is not amenable to digestion by your unique agni, it is as good as poison for you.

Avoid Mutually Incompatible Foods

Let me begin by saying this very clearly: do not combine foods in a meal that are mutually antagonistic or incompatible. Foods work in varying ways within the digestive system, and therefore, certain foods should not be eaten together. Food combining is a complex science, and the principles of why certain foods are incompatible are outside the scope of this book. Here is a list of common but infelicitous combinations that a wise person will choose to skip:

- Milk is incompatible with salty and sour tastes, meat, fish, all vegetables, fruits, lentils, beans, millet, honey, yogurt, oils, alcohol, anything with a salty or sour taste, and certain types of basil, especially the holy basil (tulsi).

- Melon is incompatible with grains, starch, fried food, and cheese.

- Honey is incompatible with ghee (at the very least, do not mix them in equal proportions).

- Radish is incompatible with milk, banana, raisin, potato, tomato, eggplant.

- Chili pepper is incompatible with yogurt, milk, melon, and cucumber.

- Yogurt is incompatible with milk, sour fruit, melon, meat, fish, mangoes, banana, and breadfruit.

- Egg is incompatible with milk, meat, yogurt, melons, cheese, fish, and bananas.

- Mango is incompatible with yogurt, cheese, and cucumber.

- Corn is incompatible with date, raisin, and banana.

- Banana is incompatible with buttermilk.

- Chicken is incompatible with honey, sesame, jaggery, milk, radish, and lotus stem.

- Lemon is incompatible with yogurt, milk, cucumbers, and tomato.

Avoid Frozen Foods

Frozen foods present a real dilemma for people beginning to embrace Ayurvedic wisdom. Frozen foods bring so much convenience into our modern lives, yet they can upset our agni, especially if we have a dull agni to begin with. Possibly this rule is different for those whose ancestors come from a polar region, but for the rest of us, eating food that has been frozen creates problems. This is one of the hardest modern habits for people to wean themselves from—but it's not impossible. All of the people whose success stories I have shared in this book have said a permanent good-bye to frozen foods. Yes, they even cook Ayurvedic recipes like lentil soup (dal) in smaller batches and let go of the convenience of frozen peas or corn, ubiquitously available in supermarkets. In the beginning, it feels like an impossible feat, since frozen vegetables are almost a fixture in every home today. However, once I explain the reasoning, I often find that frozen foods are easily minimized if not completely eliminated. Besides, the joy of shelling fresh peas or cobbing the corn in the right season is a great feeling!

Frozen foods are not only stale, but they are also cold, which makes them tremendously vata aggravating. Oh yes, I know that we can measure and calibrate the vitamin, protein, and mineral content in frozen foods, but the prana, the life force, is completely destroyed by freezing a food—and this makes it stale.

If you have no choice but to eat food that has been frozen, then try doctoring it. Before cooking, warm it up with hot water if you can. Make sure you use some ghee and warming spices like cumin to counteract vata-aggravating qualities enhanced through the process of freezing. And, gradually, eat less frozen food. Cultivate a preference for fresh-cooked meals. Slowly but steadily, move away from a choiceless, industry-determined existence to a personally determined universe, filled with individually crafted choices that work for you and your agni.

Limit Raw Foods

Here is a tip for salad lovers: I recommend getting off of exclusively raw diets and reevaluating frequent raw salads as a food choice. Raw foods do not satiate our sense of hunger and often leave us craving more food. Also, and even more important, most raw foods are inherently dry; they are not oily or moist; they do not add the lubricant quality that helps digestion. Raw foods actually slow down the digestion process and, over time, form hard stools and promote constipation. One way to ensure that a raw salad has that moist and lubricating quality is to include foods that are naturally oily such as avocado or nuts. You can also add oil as a dressing.

Because Ayurveda suggests that we consume food in its most pristine form, it would seem that raw foods would make great sense. But it takes a pretty sharp agni to digest raw foods. For many people, eating raw foods can actually contribute to the creation of toxins in the body. So before you eat raw foods, ensure that your agni is sharp enough to take them on. If so, then please enjoy those raw foods. But if not, then you should boil, bake, steam, char, or otherwise cook those foods—and don't forget to add a good-quality natural fat like ghee or at least olive oil. In the next section I speak about how important this natural fat is in our diet, but for now let me say that Ayurveda recommends that unless a food has its own fat (like a meat that releases fat when it cooks), we should add oil or ghee during cooking.

Please understand that I'm not saying that raw foods are bad or that Ayurveda has a fixed (and negative) opinion about them. Clearly, raw foods have more prana, more living energy, than cooked foods. There can be no doubt about this. Ayurveda's sister science, yoga, recommends raw foods for refinement of consciousness. But while our remote ancestors consumed a lot of raw vegetables and fresh fruits, they were much more physically active than we are. Many of us in the modern world are mostly sedentary, and as a result, our agni is duller and more erratic.

This means that raw foods have become a liability for the agni of many people and are no longer the asset they once were.

So unless you have a sharp agni, raw foods will create gas and bloating, will aggravate vata, and will disturb the agni, if not immediately, then over time. I have so many stories of recovering raw-food regulars and their out-of-control vata that I can't possibly tell them all here.

Of course, there is no one right way to approach food. Ayurveda does not put forward only one type of food ideology—either raw foods or cooked—for all people. As I've said, the most important consideration is the state of your own agni. You can't go wrong by tuning in to your own agni and its strengths and limitations. I promise.

Drink Water Consciously

I've already commented on the ridiculous "rule" that everyone should drink eight glasses of water each day. Ayurveda recommends that we drink only when we are thirsty. Drinking water is not fixed in the way mealtimes are fixed. Your thirst is bound to fluctuate based on your agni, the time of day, the season, the air temperature, and your level of activity. Respect your natural instinct, and drink water when you are thirsty. Here are some additional guidelines from Ayurveda:

- Drinking a full glass of water immediately before meals weakens your agni.

- Drinking water immediately after meals increases kapha.

- During meals, it's best to drink a small quantity of water (two to four ounces), sipping the water whenever you wish.

- Drinking water two to three hours before or after a meal is also fine.

According to Ayurveda, boiled water that becomes cool naturally, while the lid of the boiling vessel is still covered, is highly digestible and mitigates all three doshas and relieves thirst and fever. This water is additionally helpful in igniting agni since it has been processed by heat earlier. It is helpful in combating constipation, flatulence, abdominal bloating, and hiccups. When water is boiled down to half its original quantity, then it is said to be three-dosha balancing. This water is said to help with weight loss as well as counteract toxins (aama) within the body channels. It is especially recommended in spring and during the rains (regardless of where you live). The sages explain that water boiled down to three-quarters its original quantity has similar benefits and is even more suitable for consumption in summer and autumn.

Regular, unboiled, and naturally cooled water can also be used for pitta management. Water can be kept in a clay, stainless steel, glass, or silver jug and exposed to the cooling moon rays. Here are some additional suggestions regarding drinking water:

Herbal water: Add two teaspoons of coriander seeds to a gallon of unboiled water in a stainless steel or glass container and place it near an open window to catch the cooling rays of the moon in the night. This water is especially cooling and thirst quenching in summers.

Naturalized water: Expose unboiled pure water in a container to the rays of the sun during the day and the rays of the moon at night. Drink the water the following day. Because it is energized by two cosmic entities—the sun and the moon—this water is slightly balancing to all three doshas and rejuvenates body and mind.

Nighttime water: According to Ayurveda, we can drink warm (previously boiled) water at night, especially in place of dinner if we are experiencing indigestion. This nighttime water enkindles agni, dispels gas, and helps expedite digestion.

Just like food, water can become stale. Boiled and cooled water kept for more than a day is considered stale or old and loses all its benefits. Water for day use and night use should be boiled separately just a few hours before consumption.

Well, so much for purified bottled water, which is, at its best, sealed staleness!

Cook Right by Cooking with Ghee

Remembering that like increases like, consider that oiliness in your foods will impart a healthy oily sheen to your skin, a silky softness to your hair, kapha strength to your organs, and vata pacification in body and mind. And above all, it will ignite your agni. Know that a no-fat diet or ultra-low-fat diet is not considered ideal in Ayurveda. Additionally, I recommend that you use ghee (recipe in appendix 4, "The Ayurvedic Diet Resource Guide")—the clarified butter that is sold in almost all major grocery stores and also online—as your main cooking medium. Ghee is not the same as butter. Ghee is a special cooking medium and a favorite of the sages who were the original seers of Ayurveda.

Followers of Ayurveda have always eaten ghee. This is historical, and it has continued in modern times through the rise and fall of the various "fat is good" or "fat is bad" or "some fats are bad" theories. The Ayurveda followers continue to enjoy ghee in moderate quantities, and while they do, they often experience weight loss, lowered cholesterol, healthy digestion, lubricated skin and hair, lubricated joints, and soft, well-formed stools. In the meantime, the modern world has become seriously divided about fats—those who love them and those who hate them.

There are, of course, hydrogenated fats and polyunsaturated fats—and we know what they can do to us—but modern attitudes for and against pure fats have proven to be detrimental. The fat haters paid a stiff price with their physical and even mental ill health. The fat lovers, on the other hand, preached that you can eat all the fat you want with no price to pay. Well, they too were proven wrong because excess fat consumption can be harmful to health.

In the Ayurvedic world, fats were never crowned, nor were they dethroned. Fats have always been appreciated as an intrinsic component of our food, required if our agni is to function properly and required as well if our food is to be tasty and appreciated by our minds.

When fat is consumed regularly and in a moderate manner, it feeds the agni in the same way that fuel feeds a fire. Without fats, the agni becomes weak and erratic. Fat helps digest proteins, carbohydrates, minerals, and all other nutritional components of food.

According to Ayurveda, of all fats, ghee best contributes to the healthy functioning of agni, immunity (oja), strength (bala), the balance of our all-important kapha dosha, and the integrity of our body tissues. Further, ghee consumption prevents vata and pitta doshas from becoming unbalanced and releasing the catastrophic effects of nonstop motion and destructive heat. Ghee lubricates vata and cools pitta. Ghee makes for smoother passage of various substances inside our body's channels, the srotas. Ghee directly improves eyesight, memory, and the feel and texture of skin. It is a great antiwrinkle agent when it is consumed internally or massaged externally.

One of the reasons that ghee is so strongly lauded by Ayurveda has to do with the intense purification it goes through during the multiple-step process by which it is converted from milk into ghee. First, raw milk is boiled and then converted into yogurt. The churning of yogurt with the right quantity of water yields buttermilk. The butter derived from churning buttermilk is then further cooked on low heat until golden-colored fat (ghee) rises to the top, and the impurities settle below and are discarded. The pure fat is filtered and utilized as ghee.

What was originally heavy to digest, the whole milk, becomes lighter to digest due to undergoing multiple processes and the inducement of agni at each step from churning, boiling, and slow cooking. This transfer of heat potency in the ghee particles through the scientific production process (*samskaara*) is why Ayurveda says that ghee is the only fat that does not in some way compromise agni and, in fact, ignites it when consumed according to seasonal guidelines.

Because it is so very refined, ghee also adds directly to oja, increasing our immunity, and to *shukra* (sexual tissue), adding to our fertility. I speak more about ghee's effect on shukra in chapter 7. Now, I want to turn to an issue that, while it has been laid to rest in America, is of primary concern to many in India, where many have replaced ghee as the fat of choice with what I see as a villain fat—margarine!

In his article, "The Great Margarine Hoax," Dane Roubos references a study published in the *American Journal of Clinical Nutrition* that shows a dramatic difference between the heart-disease rates of populations in northern India (primarily meat eaters) and southern India (largely vegetarians).[8]

We might expect that the vegetarians would have the lower rate of heart disease, but in fact, the opposite was true. The vegetarians had fifteen times the rate of heart disease when compared to their meat-eating counterparts! The reason cited was that the southerners had replaced their traditional ghee with margarine and other refined polyunsaturated vegetable oils. Roubos further notes that twenty years later, a British medical journal, the *Lancet*, reports that in northern India, heart-attack deaths had also increased, and the reason was exactly the same: now, the northerners had largely replaced the ghee in their diets with margarine and refined vegetable oils.[9]

Here in America, I often find it difficult to convince my students that ghee is beneficial—and one of the main things they will say about it is that it must be fattening. This I know to be untrue. Let me tell you a little story about weight loss with ghee. My husband, son, and I often spend weekends at my cousin Rakesh's home, who, like us, lives in California's Bay Area. I naturally gravitate to the kitchen since we are in the habit of cooking fresh meals. During one particular visit, I learned that Rakesh wanted to lose some weight, and I was not surprised to find everything low-fat and low-sugar, and of course, olive oil instead of ghee.

Thankfully, my cousin is blessed with an open mind. After a few casual discussions on the virtues of ghee and the Ayurvedic perspective on weight loss through stimulation of the body's internal agni, Rakesh agreed that we could replace his entire and elaborate fats collection with only one product—ghee.

I told him to weigh himself daily during our "experiment" and that he should let me know if his weight began climbing. Well, it dropped. The moderate amounts of ghee he consumed with the light and easily digested diet that I recommended made his weight loss effortless, spontaneous, and a joy to watch happen in front of my eyes. Now Rakesh is ghee's greatest advocate.

Please do not construe my enthusiasm for ghee as permission to overindulge. Excessively fatty food is difficult to digest no matter what fat you use. Too much ghee will tax your agni instead of helping it. If you eat too much ghee, you will feel tired and gain weight.

You may need to vary the amount of ghee you consume according to the season and time of day, as these cause the strength of your agni to fluctuate. You can eat more lubricating foods in the daytime (as the agni is most efficient at noon), but you should eat more lightly in the evening (since the agni drops after sunset). In terms of the season, more lubricating foods are recommended in the seasons in which vata dosha peaks due to dryness (late summer or in the rainy season). However, these foods should be eaten sparingly in the spring, when kapha dosha peaks, and eaten only in moderate amounts in the fall, when pitta dosha peaks. In the winter months, when all doshas are balanced, you can eat ghee according to your individual agni. Winter is a great time to build the tissues and the physical strength that the quality of lubrication imparts. I increase my intake of nuts, dairy, and other such rich foods in winter—and only in the winter. See appendix 4 for seasonal recommendations.

A Sacred Food Philosophy

Regardless of religious beliefs, you can make your mealtimes sacred events by the gratitude and respect you bring to them. A deferential attitude will prevent any unconscious gulping down of food, any tendency to under- or overeat, any hoarding of food or carelessly discarding it. Most of all, it will stop you from mindlessly eating over the kitchen sink or in a daze in front of the television or some other electronic gadget in an attempt to escape from the present moment and from your awareness of the plate before you.

It is traditional to worship the food we eat—in Ayurveda, in the greater Vedic tradition, and in the four world religions it has spawned: Hinduism, Buddhism, Sikhism, and Jainism. It is my experience that most cultures throughout the world demonstrate a prayerful attitude toward food. Ayurveda, as world's first system of medicine, tells us that expressing our sacred intention toward a meal is part of what makes eating that meal a health-sustaining activity.

Over the years, I have taught many prayers and chants to my students. Before the food prepared at my school is consumed, it is first offered to the beautiful altar of Divine Mother, and everyone present joins in chanting a hymn of gratitude. The food that has been offered to God becomes *prasada*, a Sanskrit word meaning "divine grace." If you offer food before you eat it, then what you eat is divine grace.

The following mantra from the Bhagavad Gita has been chanted in my family since time immemorial.[10] Now it is chanted by my students, too.

Eating after chanting this mantra symbolizes a profound act of love and worship, which sustains the body so that we may further worship pure consciousness, the Ultimate Truth that is our foundation. There is also an implication that the eating of tasty, well-cooked, healing, and blessing

TABLE 27   Mantra from the Bhagavad Gita

Sanskrit Transliteration	Sounds Like
Brahmaarpanam brahma havir	Brahm-AAR-panam brahma hav-IRR
Brahmaagnau Brahmanahutam	Brahm-AAG-nou Brahma-NA-hu-TAM
Brahmaiva tena gantavyam	Brahm-AA-iva TENA GEN-tav-yum
Brahma karma samaadhiina	Brahma karmaa samaa-dhi-naa

sattvic food symbolizes the oblation of the individual Self to God, so that God may become a part of us by entering us through the food.

Meaning: The one who sees cosmic truth in action—through the food that is eaten, the eater, the act of eating, and the fire that has cooked the food—becomes one with this cosmic truth.

If you have prayers from your own tradition, or if you would prefer to write a prayer that feels appropriate to you, that would be lovely.

What matters most is that you recite the prayer aloud and feel each word in your heart.

What Ayurveda offers is nothing short of transformation at every level of our being. When right food is consciously cultivated, chosen for personal consumption with knowledge, cooked with love and right methods, and eaten with mindful reverence, our bodies—with their various problems and average life expectancies—can become superbodies with an enhanced life-span. We will manifest a quantum state of health that is vibrant with ease, with energy, and with a sense of flow. This is the promise of Ayurveda.

CHAPTER 7

Sleep, Sex, and Exercise

 One night I woke up suddenly to a lot of commotion and confusion. My mother had become sick due to the weak heart that she was born with. My sister was crying, our father looked worried, and though Baba was serene, he was meditating outside my parents' room, instead of his usual place in the family temple or outside under the courtyard tree. Mother looked like she was sleeping peacefully, but apparently she had fainted.

Then my aunt took my sister and me to her room and sang spiritual songs, appealing to the formless power behind all forms for my mother's recovery and, at the same time, soothing us with her melodious voice. My sister and I held each other tight for comfort and finally drifted back to sleep, with our heads in our aunt's lap.

Though the night ended with my mother getting better, still the disturbance and fear left lasting impressions on my young mind. I didn't appreciate this scary surprise at all. I simply wanted my mother to be her usual calm, strong and smiling, busy, bustling self at all times, as all eight-year-olds in this world want.

I developed a fear of the night. In daylight, all was well, but as night slowly approached and the sun began to set, I would feel a dread. "Will my mother fall sick again tonight?"

So many things that I knew by the light of the sun began to feel unfamiliar in the darkness of the night—the water drums that caught and stored rainwater; my Baba's hand-carved, wooden armchair; the empty cage of Mitthoo, the parrot we children had freed within hours after being given him because Baba told us we should never cage any living creature; and even my own beloved rope swing, which had been hung from the trees by my father. All of these household items and others, well-known by the day, took on menacing shapes and personalities in the dark of the night.

Many a night I would wake up and lie in my bed paralyzed with fear. Then, of course, it was harder to wake up in the morning for the walk to the river, and sometimes I would drag my feet while Baba's shakti carried me back and forth to the River Sarayu.

Baba, I know, was aware of all this, and one morning he looked me in the eyes and said, "You know, little Shunya, at night the sun never really goes away. It is only the revolving of the Earth that makes us have an experience of darkness. But this darkness never stays. The darkness is not real. Only light is the Truth. Light is always there, always present. Light is behind and beneath and through the darkness, so darkness does not stand a chance. It is only an appearance, a temporary reality, a passing phenomenon. Light is Truth. Light is the absolute, eternal, unchanging Ultimate Reality. Light always was, is, and will be."

As Baba talked on, I felt comforted. What my child's mind heard is that light, not darkness, is Truth. And I knew that this light dwelled in my heart and in mother's heart too. I knew that I was made up of light and that even sickness was a part of this light. The light is all things without itself being affected by any of its forms.

Baba's words conveyed his blessings to my heart, and slowly, the worries about my mother's health that I had internalized began to lift.

Baba asked my mother, who was now feeling much better, and my aunt to make sure that every evening I massaged my feet, my ears, and the top of my head with warm sesame oil, as he had taught me. So my mother and aunt sat beside my bed at night for several weeks so that I didn't rush through the practice but applied the oil slowly and deliberately. When I would begin this practice, I'd start feeling sleepy almost at once; my hands would feel heavy as the oil entered my body and calmed vata dosha and rajas, the mental quality of turbulence. This made room in me for sleep.

Also, my mother would chant many of my favorite bedtime mantras to me:

> Asto ma sad gamayah
> Tamso ma jyotir gamayah
> Mrityor ma amritam gamayah

Translated, this means:

> May I journey in consciousness from untruth to truth,
> from darkness to light, from fear of mortality of my body
> to recognizing my indestructible, immortal Self.

One night, when I was struggling a bit more than usual with falling asleep, Baba came to the room where my sister and I slept, and he chanted the greatest of Vedic mantras, the Gayatri mantra. Baba sang very softly, uttering each syllable with a power that landed in my heart like a million-volt electric charge. Then with great gentleness, he lightly touched the top of my head. I seemed to be suspended halfway between the waking word and the world of dreams. I experienced waves of comfort, reassurance, and a tremendous, inexplicable joy. Baba reminded me then that the Great Light of Atman, the Self, dwells inside me, right in my heart. "The Atman makes you all-powerful and truly invincible. Remember that," he said.

And I did.

Baba said, "Use this light to welcome the divine darkness of nighttime. Fear not the night. The goddess of sleep will nurture you carefully as you sleep, and then you can wake up with renewed energy to grow and serve the world. Rest now, so Mother Sleep can heal and rejuvenate you."

From that night onward, my fears were gone. The fears had fled, and I experienced the peace that is my natural state. I seemed to have become one with the Gayatri mantra. I became firm in the conviction that my true nature is greater than the darkness I could see at night—a darkness that is here to serve me, after all.

As for the monsters I saw in household items, the next time one of them stared at me through my bedroom window, I closed my eyes and focused on the light in my heart. I became so powerful and potent that the monsters revealed themselves in the light shining through my eyes to be no more than what they were. I felt that these "fearsome" water drums were actually rather lonely and were waiting out the night in anticipation of the morning, when I would come play hide and seek with my sister and my cousins around them once again.

Each evening, after my elders had chanted and left my room, I would gently await a different mother. Her name is Bhutadhatri, the Mother of the Universe, the Goddess of Sleep. She wears dark, flowing robes, soft and studded with infinite stars, and she holds us all like babies as we sleep. We are vulnerable then but filled with hope for a new morning. Because she is there with us, we are never alone. We can trust, and let go, let ourselves drop into sleep. My breathing would become very quiet with long pauses between each breath, and soon sleep would envelop me, ever so gently.

One night, between a breath in and a breath out, I observed my own true being. In this precious state, I could see that I was not even dependent on my body to experience my own light. This light is beyond the body. The light outlives the body. It is beyond day and night, beyond life and death. I could see then that my mother was not just her failing heart. Even mother's sickness was simply a temporary night in an eternal, unending, totally amazing light-filled reality. ✒

Thanks to my Baba, I sleep well to this day. When the first rays of light promise to scan the Earth, my slumbering body awakens naturally to welcome the dawning sun. To have such an awakening at the beginning of the day, it is vital that you have a good relationship with sleep. I share here some wisdom on how you can invite sleep into your life. Related to sleep are both sexual activity and physical exercise. These are the three topics of this final chapter.

In sleep we cultivate kapha dosha, while in exercise, through our movement, we reduce kapha and increase vata and pitta doshas. So exercise and sleep have an inverse relationship. In commonsense terms, it is critical that we do physical exercise daily, for if we don't, we won't be tired enough to fall asleep. When we are tired, natural tamas takes over to restore our equilibrium, and we doze off. On the other hand, if we exercise excessively, we do not have adequate kapha and tamas left to counteract the rajas generated by exercise. So, with too much exercise, we do not fall asleep with ease.

There is also a relationship between sex and sleep. Interestingly, a healthy sexual response in adults requires a healthy kapha dosha in our bodies, as does sleep. So, the foods and lifestyle choices that support sleep also promote sexual health, and vice versa.

We will begin with sleep.

An Invitation to Sleep

There is the morning, fresh and vivid. And then there is the night, dark and deep, bringing with it the opportunities for rest and rebirth. This rhythm provides a beautiful flow of life energy. We humans need sleep as much as any other living creature on our planet. The Charaka Samhita, an ancient text on internal medicine from the third to second centuries BCE that explores preventive medicine and promotes lifestyle measures at length, declares, "Our quota of happiness and unhappiness, nourishment and emaciation, strength and debility, sexual power and impotence, knowledge and ignorance, and in fact, life and death, are all dependent on sleep itself."[1] Sleep is that important.

Ayurveda's sleep wisdom can help you reunite with the mothering energy of sleep. It can guide you toward simplifying and harmonizing your life. Every night, sleep is made possible by the three gunas that we first explored in chapter 2. The list below describes the impact of tamas, rajas, and sattva on sleep.

Tamas: Tamas is the quality of dullness and inertia, a state of mind that is instrumental in falling asleep. In the right quantity, tamas creates sleep. In excess, tamas creates excessive sleepiness. When it is the dominant mode of mind for a period of time, tamas leads to depression, with its tendencies toward listlessness and apathy. Daydreaming, constant drowsiness, falling asleep at unexpected times, and remaining asleep even at the cost of life goals are all characteristics of tamas at pathological levels. Tamas is inherently related to kapha dosha in the body.

Rajas: Rajas supports activity—wakefulness, movement, actions, initiations, and speed. In excess, rajas creates an inability to fall asleep or to stay asleep. Other negative manifestations of excess rajas include agitation and relentless thoughts. Under the influence of heightened rajas, we can pursue goals to the detriment of our health and well-being with the result of interrupted sleep and insomnia. Rajas is inherently related to vata dosha in the body.

Sattva: Sattva is the quality of purity and balance—the perfect balance of rajas and tamas. Sattva makes for quality sleep, at the right time, and a happy awakening in the morning. It strikes a happy balance between restfulness and activity. Sattva quality is inherently related to pitta dosha in the body. However, excessively aggravated pitta will in turn also end up contributing towards rajas (not sattva).

In other words, when tamas increases in the mind, we automatically fall asleep. When rajas increases, it disturbs or even prevents sleep. And when sattva rises, we awaken naturally and cheerfully, and the mind becomes an agent of healing, clarity, knowledge, and purity. When sattva is dominant, we recover from all challenges of life with patience and self-assurance. When sattva is dominant, a healthy tamas operates at nighttime, and a healthy rajas operates in waking hours.[2]

Since tamas is the preferred mode of mind for sleep, its corresponding energy in the body, kapha, is the dosha that plays greatest role in a healthy sleep process. Along with tamas in the mind, we require kapha of the right quality and quantity in the body if we are to fall asleep and stay asleep.

In the modern world, however, our vata- and pitta-aggravating lifestyles (busy) and diets (low-fat or raw-food dominant) can deplete kapha dosha. We are often thin and overwrought at the cost of our sleep. For this reason, we need to consider how to promote healthy levels of kapha and tamas for the sake of good sleep.

Hearing this, some people may think that all they need to do to sleep is to burn themselves out, mentally or physically, or to promote excess kapha by ingesting a lot of alcohol. I promise you that while these may promote sleep, it is not a healthy, reinvigorating sleep, and that after such a sleep, you can wake up with a headache or a wooly mind, feeling even duller than you did when you went to bed.

I have found that getting a good night's sleep is both a vital issue and a challenge for many of my Ayurveda students. Nicole Matthiesen's journey demonstrates using Ayurveda's lifestyle wisdom to combat a chronic problem of insomnia. Here is her first-person account.

GETTING AWAY FROM OVERWHELM

My life used to revolve around my job. From the moment I woke up until I went back to bed at night, I was often working or thinking about work. My clients, mostly attorneys, expected me to work long hours driven by court-ordered deadlines. It was stressful, but I had convinced myself that constantly being on, overwhelmed, and busy was just my way of life. My daily routine was to roll out of bed about 7:00 a.m. and head straight to my home office computer to start my workday. I'd often be at my computer for hours before I took a moment to eat breakfast, take a shower, and get dressed. I would stay at my desk working sometimes until 7:00 p.m. or later.

Eventually, this lifestyle began to take a toll on me, particularly on my ability to sleep. Falling asleep was easy enough, but I'd wake up in the middle of the night and wouldn't get back to sleep for at least an hour, sometimes not at all. My mind would race. I'd think about what I needed to do the next day, what I had failed to do the day before, and how I could parse out my day to make sure everything got done. The next morning, I'd wake up groggy and exhausted. I wasn't a fan of sleeping pills, but sometimes I just had to get one night of good rest, and taking a pill was the only way I knew how to do it.

This lifestyle began to affect my well-being, and my disappointment with the Western pharmaceutical approach to health led me to explore Ayurveda. At Vedika Global, I began to take Ayurveda classes, consult the clinic, and eventually, attend classes where Acharya Shunya discusses the teachings of Vedas. Through all of these integrated teachings, I began to understand the far-reaching effects my lifestyle was having on my body, mind, and spirit—and that taking a pill is not the answer. I had more power than I ever dreamt of to heal myself by making some simple changes in my attitude, daily routine, and diet.

One of the first concepts I learned about from Acharya Shunya was the gunas. Understanding the nature of each of the gunas, or qualities, gave me a new framework to examine my life and, ultimately, helped me to acknowledge and change some of my harmful lifestyle patterns. In particular, it became clear to me that my busy work schedule was creating excessive rajas, which was at the root of my anxiety and sleeplessness. While quitting my job wasn't an immediate option, I did learn that I could introduce practices that would reduce rajas and bring me to a more balanced, sattvic state. I began to make some changes to my diet and lifestyle. Now, I rarely have a sleepless night.

The first of these practices was creating a dinacharya that changed how I approached the morning. Instead of jumping from bed to work, I started my day with more sattvic activities. I started getting up an hour earlier, so I could take a shower, dress in fresh clothes, and take thirty minutes to do some light yoga and a short meditation. I step outside to greet the sun and then make myself a warm breakfast, which I eat in silence—no TV, smartphone, or other device to distract me from enjoying my nourishing meal. Only after I finish breakfast do I turn on my phone or computer.

This routine means that I am not starting my days in a state of rajas. Now I find that I'm able to handle whatever comes up during my day with more ease and patience. And when my days started going more smoothly, so did my nights. I began to feel less anxious overall, and I'm now able to sleep soundly through the night much more often.

Another practice I found effective in relieving insomnia is drinking warm spiced milk before bed. Rather than checking messages on my phone before I turned out the light, I started turning off all devices and preparing this sattvic drink. This ritual set the tone for slowing down my evening. And drinking the spiced milk has had an incredibly calming and grounding effect on me before I go to bed. I have found that it is particularly helpful in reducing insomnia on days when I spend more hours than usual at the computer.

These practices sound simple, but living them has truly turned around my health and my outlook on life. Feeling constantly overwhelmed and exhausted is a thing of the past. I am so grateful for this wisdom of the Ayurvedic tradition. It has helped me to realize that I have the power to create well-being in my health, mood, situation, and life by making choices that align me with sattva and my true nature.

I hope you, too, become inspired by my student Nicole's ability to give herself good sleep, with all its attendant health and well-being benefits.

Now, let's look at Ayurveda's recommendations for dealing with insomnia.

Ayurveda's Timeless Wisdom to Promote Sleep

When any of my clients or students are faced with insomnia—which is a difficulty in falling or staying asleep—I usually find that there is a simple cause and a way to remedy the problem. The most common difficulties, I find, are psychological stress, too much stimulation right before bedtime, and an inconsistent sleep schedule.

Here are recommendations that are nothing more or less than Ayurveda's timeless wisdom to promote healthful sleep.

Fix Your Times to Wake and Sleep

As I discussed in chapter 2, it is vitally important to get up in the morning at a fixed time—at or before 6:00 a.m.—no matter how sleep deprived you may be. This is difficult in the beginning, I understand, but do your best. And try to go to bed at or before 10:00 p.m. Gradually, this steadiness, in and of itself, will adjust your sleep cycle.

Let me warn you that once the clock strikes ten, you might get a second wind from rising pitta in the cosmos. You might start thinking about unpaid bills, unanswered e-mails, or the closet that still needs to be reorganized. Creative and imaginative ideas may come to you too. These inspirations are great in the daytime, but at night, they simply make it harder to fall asleep. So as a precaution, I recommend that you take my advice and prepare to go to bed by 9:30 p.m. so that you are well asleep by 10:00 p.m.

It's important to establish and maintain this sleeping schedule. Go to bed at an exact time. There may be an exceptional day, or couple of days, when you cannot go to bed by this time, but let those be the exception, not the norm.

This is especially true if you are working to regulate your sleep and wake cycle. Remember that your inner clock has no concept of "sleeping in" or "making up sleep" by sleeping excessively long on weekends. Also try to have a gap of at least three hours between dinner and bedtime.

Enhance Kapha Dosha at Bedtime

An application of oil to the body pacifies vata and instantly adds kapha. So one important lifestyle recommendation is that you apply warm oil to the soles of your feet, your ear lobes, and if possible, the crown of your head. You can use a dry or warm and slightly wet towel to wipe off any excess oil. (See chapter 5 for details on oil massage for sleep enhancement.)

Eat Sleep-Inducing Foods

In the evening, we want to enhance kapha and pacify vata and pitta. Hence, before bedtime, plan to increase your intake of moist and naturally fatty foods, like warmed cow's milk (which promotes kapha), and decrease your intake of dry and spicy foods, like chips and salsa (which would promote vata and pitta).

From the perspective of flavor, minimize pungent, bitter, and astringent tastes and maximize sweet with moderate amounts of sour and salty. A sweet taste is especially sleep inducing. So if you have more than an occasional problem of interrupted sleep, examine your food choices through the daytime and over the week and months. See if you have any patterns that need to be changed.

Give up all drying foods and embrace naturally oily foods. Dry chips, crackers, dehydrated breakfast cereals, and even salads and raw foods are vata aggravating. Avocado, banana, dairy, cane sugar, sweet fruits, squashes, nuts, fish, and goat meat contain natural oiliness. (See chapter 6 for more details on drying versus oily foods.) Give up pungent and spicy foods as well, and always cook your onions if you wish to increase sleep-inducing kapha.

The danger of eating an ultra-light diet, missing meals, excessive dieting, or consuming burning or sharp foods, like wasabi, or dehydrated foods is that vata and pitta will become overstimulated (along with corresponding rajas guna in your mind), and this will leave you struggling for sleep and also for control of an overactive mind and its worrisome contents.

In regard to sleep, dairy can be your friend. All dairy, however, is not equal. Fresh boiled and sweetened cow's milk and its products—sweet cream, fresh butter, and yogurt sweetened with jaggery or cane sugar—are preferred over cheese and buttermilk. Fresh butter is especially useful in combating insomnia, and you can drink warm, spiced milk before bed to induce sleep (see recipe in appendix 4, "The Ayurvedic Diet Resource Guide"). The best spices to add for sleep inducement are turmeric, cardamom, and nutmeg, along with cane sugar. For adults, the dosage of ground nutmeg should be ½ teaspoon with a glass of milk, and for young people under age sixteen, ⅛ to ¼ teaspoon. The milk must be drunk while it's still warm—and don't have a cookie or anything else to eat. Simply sip the milk slowly, enjoying every drop of it.

If you live in an area where water buffalo's milk is readily available, know that it is said to be especially effective in inducing sleep. While cow's milk is sattva dominant, buffalo milk is tamas dominant—so naturally, it is excellent for sleep inducement. Goat's milk is the runner-up. Almond, soy, and rice milks do not count as "milk" in Ayurveda, since milk refers not to the color of the liquid but to a liquid that has been expressed from mammary glands.

Sugarcane products are also recommended by Ayurveda for improving healthy kapha. So replace highly processed white sugar, as well as aspartame, saccharin, and other artificial sweeteners, with organic cane sugar. Jaggery, an unrefined sugar obtained from evaporating cane juice, is especially good for promoting sleep and can be obtained online or at health food stores. Simply use it in teas and milk as you would any sweetener.

Seafood soup is especially useful for sleep in Ayurveda. Mildly spiced fish and crab soup, in moderate quantity, along with cooked rice on the side, can be a great selection for lunch at least twice a week. Remember, do not cook milk and seafood together. Do add turmeric and cumin to all your soup recipes, for digestibility. Rock salt is the best salt for taste. Grass carp, which can be sourced from Asian grocery stores, is generally considered a great fish in Ayurveda. Try it. It is known as *rohu* in Ayurveda tradition.

Wines are preferred over hard alcohol for sleep. Ayurveda especially recommends rice wine, which is made from fermented rice starch that has been converted to sugars. The older the wine, the better. Rice wines are part of the gastronomical culture of India, China, Japan, Korea, and other South Asian countries. Remember, milk and all alcoholic preparations are incompatible food combinations. So if you plan to drink milk at bedtime, finish any wine early in the evening.

In many cultures, lentils or beans are eaten on a regular basis. While the mung bean is considered a superfood in Ayurveda due to its ability to detoxify, for the purpose of inducing sleep, black gram (also known as urad dal) is more helpful. It is heavier in quality and has much more kapha- and tamas-inducing properties than mung. If you enjoy lentil soup, then try black gram soup cooked with Ayurvedic spices. (See recipe in appendix 4, "The Ayurvedic Diet Resource Guide.")

Make Your Bedroom Conducive to Sleep

Your bedroom should be cozy, inviting, quiet, and suited to your personal taste. My bedroom is my soul's personal retreat, and I take care to keep it beautiful and well-organized. Each item in my bedroom is kept there with intention and has significance for me—no room for randomness or clutter here. I display sacred art and have naturally scented candles and other personal or natural items that evoke beauty or have a symbolic association with beauty, goodness, and god consciousness. All such possessions, intentionally arranged in my bedroom, evoke an inner presence within me.

Keep your bedroom at a temperature that is neither too hot nor too cold for your comfort. I often crack a window and prefer sleeping with natural air circulation, especially in summer. I have planted gardenias and jasmine in pots outside my window. I have water lilies and a lotus plant floating in a large tub, right outside the French doors. The lotus opens to the first morning rays and the lilies sleep beautifully in the moonlight as the moon rays, the all-important ingredient for good sleep, enter the room also.

Make your bedroom a special, restful space (with right intention and not necessarily a monetary investment) that simply invites sleep and calm and awakens you with equal radiance in the morning. How we arrange the space around us does matter: it impacts our gunas, making the bedroom stimulating (rajasic), depressing (tamasic), or calming and inspiring (sattvic).

Before bedtime, make sure the stage is set for sleep. The lights can be dimmed in advance, and you can light candles as you prepare for bed. I use flowers, statues of divine beauty and grace, and loving family photos that evoke content memories in my bedroom. If you have to have a desk in your bedroom, then as night approaches, tidy this area deliberately, close the lid of your computer and other gadgets, and calm this activity area. Shut off all electronic devices at bedtime.

The classic text Ashtanga Hridayam, from 550–600 CE, suggests pleasant sounds in the background such as soft music or wind chimes; pleasing smells emanating from the essential oils you have applied to your body or fragrant flowers in the room; a fresh, natural breeze; and an inviting, comfortable, well-draped bed in the room, which is essential for a good night's sleep.[3] Sage Sushruta also talks about the virtues of a cushioned and comfortable bed.[4]

Prepare Yourself Mentally for Sleep

The best mental preparation you can do to welcome sleep is to accept the fact that sleep is your best friend in your quest for health, fame, wealth, and relationships. It is not merely a necessary pause in your life. Sleep is a time for retreat, when you can let go of the world and deeply rest. Once you realize what an important role sleep plays in your physiological and psychological well-being, you will begin to welcome sleep every night.

A short meditation every night in bed helps settle rajas in the mind. Since the last thing we need is to excite vata in body and rajas in mind, avoid watching stimulating TV or videos, listening to loud music, or exercising right before bed (including yoga postures).

Yoga postures can help tremendously with calming rajas and counteracting insomnia—but not when they are done at bedtime. Yoga postures increase healthy rajas and sattva, and what we require for sleep is kapha and tamas. For this reason, only *savasana*, the corpse pose, is recommended at bedtime. It is relaxing rather than stimulating. (See the box, "How to Do Savasana" for instructions.) You can also do savasana in the morning, as well as *janu shirshasana* (head-to-knee pose) and *paschimottanasana* (seated forward-bend pose) to help restore a disturbed sleep cycle.

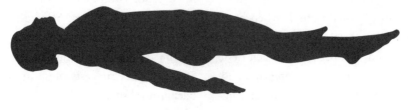

CORPSE POSE

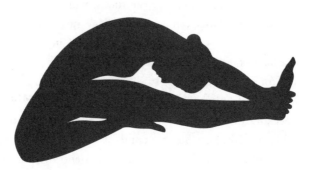

HEAD-TO-KNEE FORWARD BEND

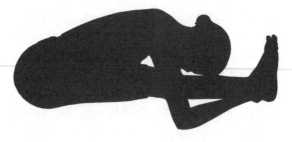

SEATED FORWARD BEND

How to Do Savasana

The benefits of a daily savasana practice are many: this pose is great for healing insomnia—it ushers in sound sleep; it is beneficial when the mind is especially gripped with fears, attachment, and other stresses; it benefits a scattered mind and calms free-floating anxiety; it makes possible a deep relaxation of the muscles, tendons, spine, and nervous system; and it increases the ability to adapt to the seasons and changes of life.

For those who are already calm, this pose is like a silent witnessing meditation, allowing separation from identification with the body and awareness of the witness consciousness principle.

Here are the steps of the savasana pose:

1. Lie flat on your back on your bed or on the floor, comfortably, with eyes closed and feet separated about a foot apart. Keep your arms out by your sides, with palms facing upward. Close your eyes. Mentally command your body to relax. You will feel your body relax into the floor or mat below. It happens naturally as soon as you say to yourself *I am relaxing . . . relaxing . . . relaxing.*

2. Now take your attention to different parts and functions of your body, one by one. First observe your breath as it enters and exits your body. Do this in a relaxed, natural way. Do not control your breath in any way; simply observe it. As you do this, your breath will relax into its natural rhythm, nice and slow.

3. Once the breath has become peaceful and relaxed, focus on your external body parts, one by one, from the toes to the top of the head. Begin with bringing your awareness to your right foot, stay here briefly, and then move on to your right knee and then to your right thigh. After this, move your attention to your left foot and so on, continuing upward to your belly, your chest, your hands and arms, slowly moving toward your head, relaxing each part of your body on the way. Once your awareness is on your head and face, you are done, and it is time to gently shift your focus inward.

4. Focus now on your internal organs (the heart, lungs, stomach, brain, kidneys, bladder, and colon) and relax each one to help purify each organ as a creation of a higher power within you. You don't have to know anatomy to do this. Simply imagine and pay inner attention. Maintain a peaceful breath.

5. Focus on each of the senses (taste, touch, smell, sound, sight), which will naturally become peaceful one by one.

6. Focus now on your mind, which has naturally become calm by this point. Simply watch it. Do not identify with the content of your mind.

7. Lie in this observer state of mind for a few minutes while this mindfulness feels effortless and flowing.

8. To exit from this deeply relaxing pose, simply begin to deepen your breath and direct your awareness back to your body, gently wiggling your fingers and toes. This helps reawaken your body from its restful state. Open your eyes and let your focus be soft. It is normal to yawn and stretch a little while you are still lying down. Now turn onto your right side and then slowly push yourself to an upright position using your right elbow.

9. You will experience renewal and deep relaxation. Practice savasana for five minutes for every thirty to forty-five minutes of yoga practice (or other forms of exercise) to become deeply relaxed. It is also fine to hold the pose longer—there is no time limit, as such—but be sure not to fall asleep. I recommend twenty minutes maximum.

Beware of Excessive Sleep

Excessive sleep, the opposite of insomnia, can also be a problem—and Ayurveda treats it in exactly the opposite manner. A sedentary lifestyle coupled with consumption of excessively oily and sweet, sour, and salty foods, like milk, ghee, and yogurt, will aggravate kapha. When kapha and tamas increase too much, and vata and pitta decrease excessively along with corresponding rajas and sattva guna, we sleep and sleep and sleep. We sleep too much.

To avoid the problem of excessive sleepiness, change your food focus from a kapha-increasing diet to a kapha-pacifying diet (see chapter 6). Here, I summarize some critical diet changes a person who sleeps too much should make:

- Drink Ayurvedic buttermilk (takra, recipe in appendix 4) and avoid yogurt, milk, and butter.

- Eat Ayurvedic khichadi (recipe in appendix 4) daily or as many times a week as possible.

- Embark on a course of physical detoxification (see appendix 4).

- Avoid curries and fried foods, eating instead boiled, steamed, light foods.

- Lean toward vegetarian options rather than meats in general.

- If you do eat meat, limit it to lunch and choose the easier-to-digest chicken, turkey, and rabbit meat rather than seafood, pork, or beef.

- Reduce the quantities you eat and drink and do more physical and mental work.

- Get physical exercise daily, following rules laid out in the upcoming section on exercise.

- Avoid sleeping in daytime, including naps right after eating.

The Daytime Nap

Daytime sleep, the cultural phenomenon known in some parts of the world as the siesta, is called *divaswapna* in Ayurveda tradition and is not advised for adults on regular basis, except in special cases.

We are to remain joyfully awake, along with the sky, which is full of sunlight all day long. Ayurveda reminds us that, as humans, we are programmed to move with the sun and, therefore, we must follow its course in knowing when to sleep and when to remain awake. As such, the urge to fall asleep during the daytime is not considered a natural urge for adults. In the cultures that have a siesta, people often eat their final meal very late in the evening and stay up very late indeed. Also, most of these cultures are in warm climates, where a daytime nap is considered helpful. For most of us, when the urge to sleep in the daytime comes, it's usually due to having eaten heavy meals, being bored, or having developed an unnatural habit. According to Ayurveda, the urge to sleep in the daytime must not be indulged.[5]

Here is what happens if we flout this universal rule and sleep in daytime. Since like increases like, kapha dosha with its tamas will build up in the body. Remember, tamas is the quality of inertia and dullness. This means that daytime sleep encourages oily, heavy, thick, and sticky qualities to alter and replace the quickness and concentration you need throughout the day. These qualities of kapha dosha may insulate you in the womb of sleep, but you will not wake up refreshed from this daytime sleep. Instead, you will wake up feeling heavy, tired, and maybe even depressed. And the longer you nap when the sun is shining, the more your digestion and elimination will also be filled with the sludge of kapha.

Who Should Nap in the Daytime?

There are, of course, exceptions to the rule against daytime napping, times when sleeping during the day is necessary for health. Here is a list of those who will benefit from a nap in the daytime:

- The very young (until age five)

- The elderly (above seventy)

- Any woman who is pregnant or lactating

- Anyone excessively tired from overwork or travel

- Anyone overcoming the effects of overdrinking or indigestion (including diarrhea)

- Anyone who is physically frail, whether from an accident or an illness

- Anyone who is having difficulty with a psychological condition such as excessive anger, fear, or grief

Also, as a general rule, daytime sleep as a lifestyle practice is recommended in hot, dry weather, as it builds kapha and helps counteract dryness.

If for any of these reasons, you choose to nap, be sure that your daytime sleep lasts no longer than forty-five minutes (thirty is better) and ideally is done at least one and a half hours after you have eaten lunch. It may also help to nap in a semi-reclined position.

Who Must Not Nap in the Daytime?

While daytime napping is discouraged for most people (exceptions noted above), there are some people in particular for whom it is especially important to not nap:

- Those who are obese or who eat a lot of fat (These people already have plenty of kapha dosha or kapha-related health challenges, including water retention, nausea, colds, and coughs)

- Those who believe they have food toxins (Sleeping in daytime suppresses the metabolism and encourages the spread of autotoxins; see chapter 6)

- Those whose appetite is not strong or whose digestion is slow (Sleeping in the daytime retards the digestive fire even further)

Healthy Sex with Ayurveda

The Ayurvedic tradition celebrates human sexuality not only because it enhances physical and sensual pleasure but also because it enhances emotional intimacy and mutual respect and can even, in the act of physical union, bring individuals to the experience of their own divinity.

One Sanskrit word for sexual intercourse is *sambhoga*, which brings together *samyaka* (a word that means "maintaining a balance") and *bhoga* (pleasure or sensual enjoyment). Thus, sexual intercourse in Ayurveda means that activity by which one maintains equilibrium and also acquires sexual gratification.

From time immemorial, human sexuality has been celebrated in India. The sages who gave us the holy Vedas were usually married and sexually active family men and women with spouses and children. The Hindu gods are likewise depicted to be enjoying conjugal bliss.

Though India also has a strong monastic tradition, there is no requirement that in order to know the Divine, a person must suppress natural, biologically rooted instincts. In ancient India, the souls who took a vow of sexual abstinence for spiritual purposes were few in number; they were the exception and not the rule. To be celibate was a voluntary choice and was never undertaken by the mainstream. The goal of the Vedas was certainly not to convert a human being into a sexless being in the name of spirituality. Rather, this tradition can help us appreciate the power of our inherent sexuality and—something much needed in today's world—to temper this sexuality with wisdom and moderation.

One word that is often identified with celibacy in India is the Sanskrit term *brahmacharya*. Translated literally this means "quest for the Ultimate Reality, Brahman." Within Vedic culture, brahmacharya represents chastity during a time of spiritual studentship. In this sense, it is celibacy but for a limited time and for a specific purpose. In an Ayurvedic context, brahmacharya also connotes the voluntary regulation of sexual energy and desires. In this context, brahmacharya means fidelity in marriage or sexual partnership; it means the monogamous, balanced, and healthy expression of sexuality between committed partners and lovers.

In Ayurveda, brahmacharya is often adopted as a way of life and refers to our acceptance of ourselves as more than just beasts under the control of a frenzied sex drive. Instead, we are asked to celebrate our sexuality and at the same time accept the responsibility to understand and regulate our sexual drive. We accept that our sexuality itself is God-given. Thus, the word *brahmacharya* beautifully brings together the opposites of sexual indulgence and sexual restraint. The Ashtanga Hridayam puts it this way: "From a disciplined indulgence in sex through brahmacharya, one gains memory, intelligence, health, nourishment, sharpness of sense organs, reputation, strength, and long life."[6]

The Vedic sages were farsighted, indeed, when they conceived of a society that holds its collective sexual energy with transparency, accountability, respect, sensitivity, and care. Human pleasures, such as singing, dancing, playing, enjoying material wealth, and sexual gratification,[7] are seen by the sages as pursuits that play an important role in the overall health and well-being of an individual and a society. In fact, the Ayurvedic sages go so far as saying that if the sexual instinct is forcefully suppressed, it leads to mental perversions and countless physical diseases.

Sexuality (*kama*) is, thus, recognized as a valid and legitimate human goal by Ayurveda. To aid the realization of this goal, several texts called *Kama Sutra* were compiled that serve as manuals for engaging in fulfilling sex. The *Kama Sutra* written by Sage Vatsyayana is one such example.

In the context of Ayurveda, our sexual desires along with all of our other personal wants and desires are seen in relation to the whole of dharma.

This context and sexual education within a larger framework of values and ethics gives our sexual desires a healthy outlet and prevents sexual perversions, addictions, and compulsions. Our preferences are not needs; our wants are not gut-wrenching cravings. Established in the spiritual Self, auspicious in its intent, universal in its character, abundant in its means, the embodied spirit is encouraged to play out its earthbound desires with its fellow beings and express itself through the joy of sex. Remember, cosmic ecstasy is a natural aspect of our divine nature.

To the one awakened to exercising choice, sex is like a magic tool, an inborn cosmic expectation of pleasure, a passion so pure, a permission to play with life and fondle and enjoy this world in which we have chosen to journey. It is, however, quite significant how we choose to indulge our sexuality.

When kama, or desire, becomes a dominant force, hiding our own higher purpose from us, then the potential to suffer emotionally increases. Lurid craving, restlessness, emptiness, and bondage to obsessions can descend on us as if from nowhere. A simple sexual desire and its pursuit can take us literally to heaven or hell in a single moment, and all within the hallowed cave of the mind. In the end, it is we who have to decide if kama or sex rules us, or if we rule kama.

The Ayurvedic sage Vagabhata described sex as a pleasure of two kinds: instant and delayed. Instant gratification is the happiness that is changeable and is related to the material world. Here is the kind of sexual gratification associated with one-night stands and pleasure with no commitment. Such sex may feel deliciously indulgent, but it is riddled with risks.

Delayed pleasure, on the other hand, implies accumulated happiness through self-control, self-respect, and the exercise of restraint and discernment. What one "discerns" is the difference between immediate sense gratification and the actions that lead to ultimate freedom, or moksha. This is the mindful path, the path of balance and moderation.

The art and science of divine lovemaking is an important facet of health in the Ayurvedic tradition, and a full treatment of this subject is not within the scope of this book. What I would like to do, instead, is to communicate some fundamental principles that you can incorporate in your daily life.

Choice of a Partner

In this modern age, sexuality is treated casually by many, and this casual approach to such a powerful act as sex is not what the sages of Ayurveda ever had in mind. Sex should be consummated with a partner you like and of whom you approve of mentally—someone who engages in respectful speech, who lives by ethical values, and who honors healthy boundaries. This ensures a healthy state of mind and emotions for both partners. Respect and affection are an important part of sexual consummation, and the ancient sages definitely recognized this. An ancient Ayurvedic text promises that after an "ethical" sex engagement, a person will enjoy "happiness, longevity, renewed youthfulness, improved luster, improved physique, and improved mental and physical strength."[8]

Without question, sex is to be performed with a person you know and love, beloved partners, spouses, and consenting adults with underlying honorable terms of engagement. Ayurvedic texts also stress the importance of not engaging sexually with a child, with someone who is married to another, with someone in your family of birth, with your guru or your guru's spouse, or with

someone who has excessive libido or is sexually demanding. And once the partner has been responsibly selected, Ayurveda recommends enhancing sexual anticipation with the use of fragrances (special desire-arousing perfumes), flowers, special beds, and cosmetics.[9]

The various guidelines I outline below will be considered a boon to anyone who is in a long-term, committed sexual relationship. These are rules that will allow you to maintain a sexual relationship without depleting yourselves. For those who have just embarked on a sexual relationship, it's probably difficult to imagine following rules of any kind in this moment. For you, I suggest that you eat the right foods to support your sexuality and take good care of yourself. You can come back to this full discussion at a later time.

The commonsense controls I go into are a strong protection against the loss of something precious: shukra.

The Presence of Shukra

One of the most important Ayurvedic concepts regarding sex involves *shukra*, a Sanskrit term that denotes not only the human sperm, ovum, and hormones regulating sexuality, but something more—a matter-based and intelligent potency that is located in every cell. It is because of the presence of the shukra that each and every cell can regenerate itself again and again.

It is important to note that shukra is not merely energy, like the Chinese concept of chi or the yogic concept of *prana shakti*. Shukra is formed from food that has undergone several levels of metabolic transformation. It is an extraordinary tissue. Inwardly it explodes as creativity in all that we think and do, and outwardly it can create an entire human being!

While shukra's presence in our reproductive organs becomes the cause of procreation, shukra's presence in the rest of the body is the basis for sexual attraction, beauty, and magnetism. Shukra is the generative tissue, and it has the power to create a human being and to endow that being with the capacity for pleasure, happiness, strength, and courage. Shukra's presence in our minds ties imagination, memory, creativity, and inspiration together into a bouquet of inexplicable enthusiasm and joy.

Shukra is present in our cells from birth, and from puberty onward, it becomes a potent force in the body, manifesting through the development of secondary sexual characteristics. The power of shukra peaks in our youth, and then, from middle age onward, its potency begins to decrease with the natural result of a decline in libido, fertility, and alas, youthful beauty, with progressing age.

Ayurveda addresses this issue head-on by slowing down loss of shukra, by following a regimen that directly protects shukra. Through activities like intercourse and masturbation, shukra is lost. Through activities like eating special foods and restoring the body between sexually active periods, shukra can be built up. By following certain rules regarding when to engage in sexual activity—the season, the time of day, the time in our own lives—we can protect ourselves from the unnecessary loss of shukra. This is, in essence, the sexual wisdom of Ayurveda.

Increasing age is a natural cause for shukra loss. But time is not in our control, so we need not fret. Fortunately, Nature does her job gently and gives us ample time to play and procreate if we wish. Shukra is also replenished naturally from time to time—by Nature in certain seasons and by ourselves by eating certain foods.

The most telling way to deplete shukra however is solely our own responsibility—and this is our choice to indulge in stress and in negativities like shame and self-pity.

Shukra, the sages declare, is the source of inexplicable joy and creativity, of skills and artistic talents, of cheer and poise in the face of life's challenges. If, however, our minds are especially negative or caught up in rajas and tamas modes of extreme passivity or extreme aggression, then the mind can have an unfortunate effect on shukra, destroying it, as if through emotional self-poisoning. It sounds harsh, but it's true.

Ayurveda taught the world's first holistic lesson on sexuality by identifying shukra's presence, not in the human genitals or organs of reproduction alone, but in each and every cell, as an inherent bridge to the mind. One significant way of seeing our sexuality, according to Ayurveda, is in its cycles.

A Cyclical Concept of Human Sexuality

I have great intellectual excitement about introducing you to Ayurveda's unique concept of cyclical sexuality. In Nature, there is a season to bloom and a season to be dormant. This is true for plants, of course, and it is also true for animals: there is a season of sexuality and then a season of rest. There are various natural checks and balances to ensure that animals do not mate constantly but follow a cosmic seasonal rhythm. Rta, which you will remember from chapter 1 as the intelligent rhythm controlling the swing of the seasons, is also the force that propels the recurrent cycles of birth, growth, and decay of all life forms. We have explored how Rta is the intelligent master rhythm that controls our lives—and now I want to add

TABLE 28   Human Sexuality and Seasonal Rhythm

	DECREASE SEXUAL ACTIVITY MOST → LEAST			INCREASE SEXUAL ACTIVITY LEAST → MOST		
Season	Spring	Summer	Late Summer/ Monsoon	Autumn	Early Winter	Late Winter
Health Status	Moderate health	Poor health	Poorest health	Moderate health	Healthiest two seasons of the year	
Frequency of Sex	Once to every 3 days	Once to every 2 weeks	Once to every 2 weeks	Once to every 3 days	Every day, if desire is supported by capacity	

that Rta also controls our sexuality. A great, indiscernible master clock is controlling countless physiological clocks, ticking at different beats in different bodies. This all-embracing natural order governs the physical and physiological universe—including, of course, the sexual behavior of all living creatures. It is Rta that maximizes shukra among the various animal species. In other words, human beings, too, are expected to be sexually active in certain seasons, ages, and stages of life.

From my research into human sexuality in Ayurvedic texts, I can see that the sages are making a case for cyclical human sexuality based on Nature's rhythms. This is especially relevant because we humans have exercised our choice away from any rhythm in general and indulge in extremes. We have sexual intercourse at odd times of day, we eat overly processed, chemical-laden foods, we sleep whenever we wish, and we have a proliferation of invasive surgical procedures—vasectomies, abortions—that can sometimes challenge our bodies. All of this

depletes our shukra, slowly but surely. It is no wonder that modern women have reduced fertility and premature, difficult menopause, and modern men suffer from erectile dysfunction at ever-younger ages. Our "improved" technology has not improved our sexuality; if anything, it has made us sexually inferior.

No medicine, no chemicals, and certainly no procedures can enhance shukra—though a life lived in appreciation of natural rhythms can. To lose shukra too fast is to lose our precious regenerative power. When our shukra levels drop, our mind-based symptoms range from a loss of enthusiasm and creativity to full-blown depression. Physical symptoms include decreased sex drive, pain in our reproductive organs (the penis, scrotum, and vagina), as well as a loss of sexual power—including premature erectile dysfunction, impotency, and sterility.

You may view what I am about to share with you as ancient wisdom of the East or as cutting-edge insights. Either way, I hope that if you are in need of this instruction, it convinces

TABLE 29   Human Sexuality and Diurnal Rhythm

	PITTA	VATA	KAPHA	PITTA	VATA	KAPHA
Time	10:00 a.m. to 2:00 p.m.	2:00 p.m. to 6:00 p.m.	6:00 p.m. to 10:00 p.m.	10:00 p.m. to 2:00 a.m.	2:00 a.m. to 6:00 a.m.	6:00 a.m. to 10:00 a.m.
Sexual Activity	Abstain	Abstain	Best time for sex	Abstain	Abstain	Second-best time for sex

you to begin leading a better life. The sages of Ayurveda taught that our sexual and reproductive powers are a sublime gift from this ever-creative universe. There is shukra everywhere, divine in its potency, divine in its capacity, and divine in its attributes.

We simply have to be willing to accept ourselves and our sexuality as part and parcel of Nature, and soon shukra will self-generate and blossom within our beings.

Seasonal Sex Cycle

To explore a cyclical approach to sexuality, we allow the seasons to guide our sexual behavior. The cool (and cooling) seasons are naturally endowed with kapha energy; this is the time when Nature is depositing shukra within our bodies.

Following this same logic, the warmer (and also warming) months have more vata (dry) and pitta (hot) energy, and so this is a time when our shukra must be protected by reducing sexual frequency. Also, since in these hotter and dryer months Nature is not adding shukra to our bodies through cosmic kapha, we must deliberately eat more kapha-increasing foods.

(See chapter 6.) This helps our bodies manufacture shukra on their own. In general, early and late winter are considered the healthiest seasons according Ayurveda. In spring and autumn, Ayurveda predicts that we will have moderate strength. Summer and late summer (the monsoon in some parts of United States and India) are the most difficult seasons in terms of extremely lowered body strength and agni.[10] Table 28 shows the effect of seasons on health and the consequent need to adjust the frequency of sexual activity during specific seasons. Excessive sex (in the wrong season) can potentially lead to loss of vital tissue (shukra) and consequent impairment of energy and vitality.

These guidelines may seem restrictive, given the spontaneous and passionate nature of the sex act, but the sages' insights into cyclical sexuality can be appreciated in light of the depletion and fatigue that can be experienced after sexual intercourse or symptoms such as erectile dysfunction. These recommendations have been adapted by several dozen couples through my school's clinics, and in each instance, we saw a turnaround in health and stamina and a revitalized enthusiasm and ability for sex.

TABLE 30   Sexuality and Aging Rhythm

	KAPHA	KAPHA/ PITTA	PITTA	PITTA/ VATA	VATA	VATA +
Age	Birth to eighteen	Eighteen to twenty-five	Twenty-five to forty	Forty to fifty-five	Fifty-five to seventy	Seventy and older
Sexual Activity	No sex	Highest frequency	Moderate frequency	Reduced frequency	Minimized frequency	Abstain

Diurnal Sex Cycle

The ideal time of day for sex is between two hours after dinner and before you fall asleep at 10:00 p.m. From the aspect of the doshas, sex at night is optimal as opposed to early morning sex, which is a second choice. Table 29 shows what the day looks like according to our natural sexual rhythms.

Human Sexuality Cycle by Age

Ayurveda recommends sexual activity from age eighteen to seventy. This means no sex before the age of eighteen. After the age of seventy, a person should engage in sex infrequently or—and this is ideal—not at all. These age restrictions prevent the loss of vital energy that is contained in sexual fluids. Table 30 shows ideal ages to initiate sexual activity, the time to begin tapering off the frequency of sex, and even the time to consider mindfully abstaining from sex (as a self-care practice). Of course, sexual intimacy is made possible by the presence of a partner and the right social situations, but the table can serve as a reminder that sexual frequency cannot and must not remain the same throughout our

lifetimes. It is best to be realistic and to preserve the body's vital shukra, whose production peaks in youth and early adulthood and begins to taper off with increasing age.

Women's Sex Cycle

Ayurveda recommends not engaging in sex during an active menstrual cycle because this can cause dosha problems. This is a complex issue, which I will only summarize by saying that vata dosha can become aggravated in a woman if she regularly engages in sex during her menses. Low back pain, tendency toward miscarriage, and a host of other problems can result. Sex during pregnancy, how much, and when to stop, are questions that are also important, and Ayurveda texts have addressed such questions in detail. Table 31 summarizes appropriate sexual activity during the moon cycle as well as from conception through postdelivery.

Digestion-Related Cycle

Digestion is also a significant physiological cycle, and sexual activity is neither a substitute

TABLE 31 Human Sexuality and Female Physiology

	ACTIVE MENSTRUATION	PREGNANCY: FIRST TWO TRIMESTERS	PREGNANCY: LAST TRIMESTER	CHILDBIRTH: NATURAL	CHILDBIRTH: SURGICAL
Active Dosha	Pitta and vata	Kapha then pitta	Vata	Vata	Vata
Sexual Activity	Abstain from the day before period starts until bleeding stops completely.	Continue sexual intercourse carefully if pregnancy is normal. Minimize or abstain from sex in high-risk pregnancy or where tendency to miscarry is present.	Abstain.	Abstain for a minimum of 40 days to a maximum of 3 months postpartum.	Abstain for a minimum of 3 months postpartum.

for eating nor a suitable activity to immediately follow eating. The body needs energy for each. Table 32 shows appropriate times for sex in relation to when food was last eaten. Following the rules summarized in this table will prevent uncomfortable symptoms such as regurgitation of food, cramps, and fatigue. The key is to allow the digestion to be far enough along in the process so that the body has freed up energy for sex.

Guidelines for Mindful Sexual Engagement

From all of the tables here, we can see that Ayurveda does not ban or curb our sexuality as much as connect it to natural cycles. For centuries, Ayurveda has been concerned with how to prolong sexual pleasure and enhance human fertility. Ayurvedic sages found interesting connections between sexual health and the immunological capacity. Sexuality was also found to be important for mental well-being and to be connected to creativity. For all of these reasons, along with the all-important reproductive function, sexual health is paramount in Ayurveda. Fortunately, a few simple lifestyle rules pertaining to our sexual nature and foods that replenish sexual tissues can help to ensure our sexual health.

These rules, which I share below, are a fraction of Ayurveda's vast body of sex-related wisdom. Ayurveda cautions that, in ignorance, we can fritter away our shukra and lose our God-given

TABLE 32   Sexuality and Digestive Rhythm

	WHEN HUNGRY AND THIRSTY	IMMEDIATELY AFTER A MEAL	TWO HOURS AFTER A MEAL
Sexual Activity	Abstain from sex; Eat and drink instead	Abstain from sex	Engage in sex if you wish
Adverse Symptoms if Advice Not Followed	Dizziness, headache, bloating, tiredness, possible exhaustion during or after sex	Indigestion, heaviness in heart region, pain in chest, possible breathlessness during or after sex	No adverse symptoms related to digestion

natural sexuality, something that could have been prevented. Perhaps shukra is a prize that only the wise can claim, through lives lived in harmony with the material and spiritual laws of Nature. So for starters, Ayurveda recommends initiating the sex act only when we are truly engaged—mind, body, and soul—and a genuine interest in sex is present. This is a precondition for sexual engagement. There is no room for obliging another, for faking it, and pleasing another if our own Self is not pleased.

Immediately after copulation—I'd say within thirty minutes of an orgasm—Ayurveda recommends drinking warm cow's milk with added cane sugar. This is like a miracle food for shukra. This tip may appear like the stuff of sexual fantasy, but the sages predicted that when the body experiences depletion of precious shukra tissue, it immediately attempts to restore it if it has the right ingredients handy. Hence the warm, sweetened milk bypasses regular channels of digestion with much more speed and converts into shukra within minutes!

Many an aging couple who has sought help for post-intercourse exhaustion at our school's clinics now approach lovemaking with a flask of warm milk at their bedside—and they cannot thank Ayurveda enough. And since milk is a natural sleep aid, it also helps the couple fall asleep like babies, when it is time to sleep, augmenting lost kapha further through restful sleep.

After sex, whenever possible, take a warm shower or bath, put on fresh nightclothes, apply fresh essential oils or natural scents, and prepare yourself for bed. If it is warm, then a light breeze through an open window or a fan is great. Moonlight exposure on summer nights is especially beneficial, so sleep with curtains open or sleep near an open terrace or balcony. The sages, I find, are quite poetic about the healing effect of moonlight, known as *jyotsna*. One says, "It confers coolness, pacifies pitta as the moon rays enter the body through exposed skin, and relieves our being of sexual exhaustion, thirst, and any pending morbid thoughts."[11]

For the next few days after engaging in sex, it is recommended that you eat nutrient-dense, rich foods that replenish shukra: goat's meat; chicken soup; meat and seafood lightly sautéed in ghee; black gram (urad dal) with rice and ghee; recipes including some form of winter melon, pumpkin, okra, sweet potato, asparagus, and avocado; pure sugarcane-sweetened syrups and desserts (rice pudding with cane sugar, wheat pancakes with cane syrup or sugar-cane-based molasses); cow's milk and cream-based recipes; coconut water and coconut cream; unsalted butter; dried fruits, especially figs, raisins, and dates; and of course, seasonal sweet fruits, especially sweet mangoes, bananas, peaches, plums, and pears. A spice that purifies the genitourinary tract in males and the uterus in females is cumin. Use cumin along with turmeric (always a help in daily microquantities!) and rock salt (a salt that sweetly enhances libido for next time).

Foods and Factors That Deplete Shukra

A strong, vital body that is well-fed and well-rested is the foundation of healthy shukra. Make sure every meal counts and provides fuel to build kapha. Various eating and lifestyle choices are particularly detrimental to shukra. Here is a simple list of things to avoid—nutritional and otherwise—to prevent shukra depletion:

- Avoid excessive eating of pungent, astringent, bitter, salty, and sour foods.

- Avoid excessive intake of dry foods. (Fats and oils are required for manufacture of shukra.)

- While balanced exercise improves shukra production (so do not remain sedentary), excessive physical activity reduces the quantity of kapha, which is required to manufacture shukra. So watch out for excess!

- Injuries, especially to the genital organs, do not help shukra—be careful during sports.

- Do not consume empty calories, such as diet soda.

- Do not fast excessively.

- Do not indulge excessively in alcohol (though wine in regulated doses can act as an aphrodisiac).

- Avoid or minimize habitual ingestion of detrimental substances such as coffee, tea, and soda.

- Simply abstain from tobacco, marijuana, and other recreational drugs. These substances are anti-kapha, anti-health, and quickly destroy shukra.

- Don't stay up late regularly. Try your best to go to bed by 10:00 p.m.—a good night's sleep restores shukra.

Eating to Enhance Shukra

Shukra can be consciously cultivated and enhanced through foods that increase kapha, but we must also take into account our digestive capacity. Optimum digestion is our best ally here because shukra is the final and seventh tissue formed in the body from the food we eat. (The other tissues are, Ayurveda says, plasma, blood, muscle, fat, bone, and nerve tissues.) Shukra is the ultimate, refined finale of a healthy digestion.

If you want to build a healthy stock of shukra, take stock of your daily diet and assess if you are eating adequate kapha-promoting foods. Shukra requires foods that are more nurturing, heavy, moist, sweet, cooling, and fatty in nature. See the box, "Shukra-Enhancing Foods," and incorporate these dietary choices into your diet.

Next, consider your digestion. If it seems inadequate, then before you embark on shukra-building foods, turn to chapter 6 and follow the eating suggestions or undergo the detox regimen in appendix 4.

Also, consider your elimination. It is important not only to eat and digest shukra-building foods but also to properly eliminate the physical waste afterward. If you have any challenges in this regard, see chapter 3, which provides details on ensuring predictable bodily purification.

Now you are set. When shukra-enhancing food is digested well, with maximum efficiency and minimum toxic by-products, then the shukra produced will be high in quality and quantity. You will experience not only higher libido but also a greater sense of well-being.

Of course, if the food is laced with toxins, fillers, chemical additives, and pesticides; if the food is overly processed; or if the food has been genetically altered, then your shukra will also be affected. There is no circumventing this issue. I feel, in fact, that these problems with food shed light on why sexual disorders, immunological disorders, and birth defects are on the rise. Our polluted food has damaged our seed. So, for the sake of your own body and the sake of your offspring, I advise you to take any measure needed—even those requiring extraordinary effort—to obtain your food from fresh, organic, non-genetically modified sources. This is a part of showing due reverence for yourself and for Mother Earth.

The Importance of Sweet and Fat for Shukra

Shukra is best enhanced by eating naturally sweet-tasting foods like milk, sweet fruits, and even cane sugar, and also by eating fatty foods such as ghee or clarified butter. With the modern trend of valuing thinness at any cost, sweet and fatty foods like these are considered an anathema to good health. So I think it's important to mention the Ayurvedic perspective on sugarcane and ghee.

Sugarcane (*ikshu*) has been researched by the Ayurvedic tradition extensively in its numerous forms: fresh cane juice, treacle, molasses, jaggery, sugar crystals, and powdered sugar. All of these forms are shukra-enhancing. Obviously, there are health issues involved in eating too much sugar. If, however, entire generations of humanity were to reject sugar and ingest instead only artificial sweeteners or honey (which is anti-kapha), then our collective sexual and fertility principle (shukra) would be seriously compromised.

Ghee is also considered a major promoter of shukra and of the body's natural immune principle (oja). Ghee is cooling in its potency and sweet in its taste. Though there are many forms of ghee available in India, in the West what is found is predominantly cow's milk ghee, which is the strongest of all in promoting both shukra and oja.

Ayurveda does not leap to either "fat is bad" or "fat is great." Ayurveda prescribes the responsible use of fats, considering with awareness and caution our own dosha requirements and digestive limitations. From a commonsense perspective, it's better to eat rich, fatty foods earlier in the day rather than in the evening. The season as well comes into play. You can eat more ghee in winter, less in summer and fall, and the least (or even none at all) in the spring. If you suffer from the symptoms of indigestion

Shukra-Enhancing Foods

Ayurveda wants to ensure that depletion of sexual tissue through orgasm (in both males and females) is countered by the shukra-enhancing foods listed here.

Dairy: Milk, cane-sugar-sweetened yogurt, sweet cream, sweetened *lassi* (yogurt drink with cane sugar), ghee, sweet butter, fresh-made cheeses such as cottage cheese (*paneer*) and mozzarella

Sweeteners: Sugarcane and all its derivatives

Fruits: Sweet mangoes, peaches, plums, pears, fresh or dried figs, ripe bananas, Indian gooseberry preserves or jam (amalaki), pomegranates, sweet and ripe jackfruits, and musk melons

Vegetables: Garlic and onions cooked in ghee (never raw), eggplant (fried in ghee), beetroot, sweet potato, pumpkin, okra, yams, snake gourd, winter squash, climbing spinach or Malabar spinach, water chestnuts, asparagus, drumsticks (all vegetables are to be cooked in ghee)

Spices: Cloves, carom seed or ajwain, cumin seeds (all of these spices purify the shukra-carrying channels), turmeric (removes toxins from shukra), saffron (aphrodisiac)

Meats: Goat and chicken and mildly spiced curry, soups, and ghee-based stir-fry; also meat of sparrow, duck, partridge, deer, rabbit, pig, quail, and grass carp; crab (aphrodisiac)

Eggs: Chicken, duck, goose, quail, turkey, pheasant, ostrich

Dried fruits and nuts: Almonds, walnuts, pine nuts, raisins, dates, figs, sesame seeds, and apricots

Cereals: Rice, wheat

Beans: Black gram (urad dal)

or toxins, you should abstain from eating ghee or any other fat until you have undergone a physical detoxification.

Given all of these considerations, people who are healthy should eat the amount of ghee that helps them remain healthy, and those desiring shukra, after thinking seriously about their digestion, should eat foods cooked in ghee to the extent that they can. In other words, as many as possible.

Besides, ghee and sugar, there are other dietary considerations to enhancing shukra (see the list I've prepared in the box "Shukra-Enhancing Foods").

Exercise for Health

Ayurveda recommends undertaking judicious and deliberate physical movements that produce tiredness but ultimately impart firmness and strength to the body. This considered and methodical activity is called *vyayama*, which translates as "exercise."[12] Sage Charaka, who is known as the father of internal medicine in Ayurveda (third and second centuries BCE), describes exercise as a laborious activity taken up "voluntarily" to increase physical strength (bala), and to this he adds a caveat: "Exercise should be practiced moderately by keeping age, capacity, season, and state of hunger/digestion in mind."[13] Ayurveda does not, for instance, recommend strong exercise for the very young or the very old. These kinds of considerations, I believe, set Ayurveda's concept of exercise apart from many contemporary concepts of exercise done by anyone of any age, at any time, and at any level of intensity.

Right exercise balances all three doshas and restores a dull digestive fire. Ayurveda declares that such exercise is the best practice to enhance bodily strength and to boost immunity.[14] Right exercise also builds sattva, which means that such exercise helps shed sadness or depression and build enthusiasm. Sage Sushruta really goes all out in support of exercise. He comments that even incompatible foods (cooked or raw) get metabolized or digested in one who exercises regularly and do not drag the body down with toxic overload.[15] I suppose this is a testimony to the positive impact exercise has on agni and doshas. Indeed, Ayurveda tradition upholds regular exercise as the best measure against obesity, and it is the best antiaging measure that also promotes muscle tone, strength, and youthfulness.[16] For all of these reasons, judicious exercise is a mandatory aspect of a healthy Ayurveda lifestyle.

Ayurveda's core text Charaka Samhita summarizes the features of the right amount of exercise, which incidentally complements our modern understanding of exercise.[17] These features include the following:

- Enhanced sweating, perspiration

- Deep and long respiration

- Experience of lightness in body parts (during movement)

- Increased heart rate

The same text summarizes the benefits of daily exercise. These too are corroborated by exercise enthusiasts worldwide:[18]

- Increased stability

- Increased endurance

- Increased power of digestion and metabolism

- Increased ability to work (physically and mentally)

However, while eulogizing the benefits of exercise, the sages raise the all-important question of how much exercise you should have. Hence, the same text adds an umbrella caution: When you begin to experience a feeling of excessive inhibition or resistance in the heart and lungs (*hrudayadi uparodha*), then it may be time to stop exercising.[19]

Ayurveda has words on how much exercise is healthy as does some modern research. It seems that while moderate exercise supports the immune system, excessive exercise impairs it—and Ayurveda tells us that excess exercise erodes shukra (sexual tissue) and has adverse long-term effects on libido and fertility. Menstrual disturbances can also occur when exercise is not supplemented with a fatty and strengthening diet as well as periods of rest and recovery. The raw-food-loving exercise junkie is often on a fast track to emaciation, exhaustion, tremors, and vertigo. Over the years, I have counseled many such cases; excessive exercise is an unexamined lifestyle fad, fueled no doubt by the desire to be thin.

Excessive exercise can contribute to the following symptoms:

- Fatigue
- Emaciation
- Excessive thirst
- Nosebleeds
- Breathlessness
- Dry cough
- Fever

With today's long list of exercise extremes—from midnight running and twenty-four-hour gyms to triathlons and at-home workout centers—it seems that people nowadays are constantly overdoing it. It is so common to hear of exercise-induced injuries and chronic fatigue as well as exercise addiction. One of the most important exercise-related messages Ayurveda can offer is that we must learn to evaluate when enough is enough.

The concept "like increases like" comes into the picture yet again. Given that some sort of motion is inherent in any form of exercise, then beyond a certain point, exercise will increase vata dosha past a normal, healthy level. Too much exercise can increase aches and pains that were not previously present, and it can certainly disturb sleep. With excessive exercise, it is just a matter of time before vata builds up in the bowels (the seat of vata) and constipation sets in. Eating ghee will help balance vata dosha, of course, and self-massage with oil (see chapter 5) will also balance vata—but, beyond a certain point, it's important not to overexercise.

In my Ayurvedic practice, I have come across runners, gym trainers, and even yoga enthusiasts and teachers who demonstrated an excited vata dosha in all of its forms. Imagine how hard it is to break the news about how overexercise is the cause of their problems to a person who is beaming with satisfaction because they are meeting their self-imposed goals of daily exercise! "You will be so proud of me," they tell me just before they outline their (overambitious) exercise regime.

Yoga teachers are especially surprised when I ask them to reduce the volume, as well as intensity, of their practice. Of course, yoga postures are great for the body. Yoga is considered the sister science of Ayurveda, so how can yoga postures contribute to imbalance? The wonderfully time-tested science of yoga postures is certainly not the culprit; the problem is our human tendency to take something good and overdo it. Perhaps this tendency existed in ancient days when the source knowledge for the Ayurvedic texts was first being compiled. A verse in one of the important source texts of Ayurveda, the Ashtanga Hridayam, clearly states that "excess in performing yoga postures" will lead to *vata vriddhi*, or aggravation of vata dosha.[20] This can happen to anyone who begins heavy exercising: vata can become aggravated. Know that many aches and pains and even arthritis can begin at the gym! Your vata joints may not be able to handle the exertion.

Of course, this is not an excuse to lounge around. To the contrary, getting little or no exercise—leading a sedentary life—is never in our best interest. On this, Ayurveda is clear. A lack of exercise will increase tamas guna in mind and excess kapha dosha in body, dull our agni, and influence our digestion to underperform. Once our digestion is disturbed, sooner or later elimination will also be adversely influenced. And this, you will recall, is a recipe for toxins and disease.

You may be wondering what is too much exercise and what is too little. How can you determine Ayurveda's "safe zone" of daily exercise and not overdo it? Below, I condense hundreds of pages of guidelines on right exercise from the ancient texts into few simple points. For most readers, making just a few simple adjustments over the next couple of months will go a long way in keeping their doshas in check.

Food, Drinks, and Exercise

Do not eat while exercising. It seems such an obvious rule, yet I see so many yoga students eating between yoga postures, and countless people snack inside gyms and in parks, eating and drinking between laps or sessions of their chosen exercise or favorite sport. This should not be done. During exercise, our agni is naturally not optimum, and all blood and energy is being supplied to muscles to support our physical exertion. Vata dosha is activated throughout our muscles, limbs, and brain. Any food that you eat at such a time will become a toxin.

Modern thought warns of the dangers of dehydration and counsels constant water drinking to replace the moisture lost in perspiration; Ayurveda suggests exercising gently enough so that the heart rate does not ever go up (something also taught by its sister science, yoga). When you exercise in this way, there is never any danger of dehydration. Drinking small sips of water only to hydrate the mouth and lips (if needed) is usually enough.

I suggest eating at least two hours before becoming physically active and drinking a full cup of water at least half an hour ahead of your scheduled exercise time. This timing should work. Resuming meals half an hour to an hour after you have finished exercising is another good measure to take—and one that's easily done if you plan your day well.

Usually before breakfast or before dinner is a good time for exercise. Please don't exercise right after lunch (or worse, during lunch, just because your company is employee friendly and the gym is next to your desk). You could exercise before lunch as long as you don't overheat yourself. Give yourself some consideration, and take a real break to eat peacefully and mindfully.

TABLE 33 Exercise and Seasonal Rhythm

Moderate Immunity	Poor Immunity	Worst Immunity	Moderate Immunity	Excellent Immunity	Good Immunity
Spring	Summer	Late Summer/ Monsoon	Fall	Early Winter	Late Winter
Exercise well but watch what you eat.	Pace yourself; eat easily digested foods; don't exercise under a hot sun!	Be extra careful—do not tire yourself; eat easily digested foods.	Build up your pace but do not overheat; exercise only in morning and evening.	Exercise vigorously; eat Vata pacifying/ Kapha enhancing nutritious food to supplement loss of energy through excercise.	Exercise vigorously; eat Vata pacifying/ Kapha enhancing nutritious food to supplement loss of energy through excercise.

How Much Exercise and When

Ayurvedic sage Sushruta recommends exercising to half of your strength and not to your maximum capacity. This prevents body tissues (including shukra) from becoming depleted.[21] Signs of overexertion include the following:

- Needing to breathe through your mouth (excessively)

- Excessive perspiration on the nose, forehead, hands, and legs

- Excessive dryness of the mouth

- Severe constriction in heart region or lungs

The seasonal guidelines for exercise are shown in table 33.

When Not to Exercise

There are times and situations when no exercise is the best choice. A quick glance at the following list will reveal Ayurveda's commonsense approach in offering this cautionary advice:

- While talking or laughing with others (in person or on phone) since this promotes vata dosha. Exercise with pleasant-minded, quiet focus is best.

- While eating, immediately after eating, or when feeling intensely hungry or thirsty, since this disturbs agni. Attend to your food needs fully when they arise.

- Immediately after sex or during periods of increased sexual activity (during a honeymoon or when a new sexual relationship has been initiated).

- If emaciated or if there has been excessive weight loss. Rest is advised to build kapha, not movement, which decreases kapha and increases vata and pitta.

- After traveling long distances, such as driving or flying cross-country, since the movement of a vehicle also increases bodily vata and pitta doshas. Exercising on top of this would push vata over the top. It may be better to take rest, a short nap, or even a massage first.

- When bleeding, as any kind of tissue loss will be quickened by exercise. First, attend to the bleeding.

- After staying up all night since lack of sleep has already aggravated vata and pitta. It might be useful to simply skip a day or to go for a very light walk.

- During your menstrual cycle since this is a vata-pitta time of the month. This important caution is mostly overlooked nowadays, almost as an act of defiance. However, it is important that women rest and renew themselves inwardly during the moon cycle.

- If you are ill, such as suffering from chronic or acute digestive issues, fever, cough or another respiratory condition, or autoimmune conditions.

- Whenever you are emotionally upset, afflicted with grief or anger. Meditation and quiet contemplation may be a better first step, and exercise can follow thereafter.

Modifying Exercise Intensity

Intensive exercise regimens, such as weightlifting, cross-country skiing, and so on, need not be given up completely simply because you are following Ayurveda. What I suggest is that you have an openness to modifying your regimen based on the rules provided here.

To begin with, you may want to revisit the frequency of exercising. Perhaps you might go to the gym every other day or three times a week instead of daily. Some rest days may be better for your body after all. If your exercise affects your sleep or libido, this is a sign that you are overdoing it. It is paramount that you get good rest and adequate sleep. You could combine high-intensity exercising with days on which you do low-impact, stress-combating exercise, such as restorative yoga, qigong, or walking in a park or the woods (without timing yourself!).

Unless you are a professional or competitive athlete, taking a playtime approach to exercise rather than doing it as an intense workout can be reinvigorating to all of your senses at times. Such an approach would balance your overall prana (energy), shukra (sexual tissue), and nidra (sleep). As with everything else in Ayurveda, the key is moderation and judicious discernment. Don't get caught up in blindly following a prescription, least of all one that comes from a trainer or your gym cohorts—people who do not know your body and its healthy limits. Use your best judgment and enjoy good health.

One thing I always like to recommend as exercise is yoga.

Yoga

Yoga, also from India, is an ancient sister science of Ayurveda. Yoga is not only a form of physical exercise, but it is also a systematic spiritual path, encompassing a comprehensive quest toward the highest states of consciousness.

The word *yoga* itself comes from the oldest Vedic text, the *Rig-Veda*, and the root sound of the word *yoga* is *yuj* which means "to unite, yoke, or harness," referring to the connection of the individual consciousness with spiritual or universal consciousness, the Ultimate Reality.

As a mystical tradition, yoga has influenced all of the major religions emanating from the Indian subcontinent: Hinduism, Sikhism, Buddhism, and Jainism. Yoga incorporates many subpaths, including the yoga of knowledge (jnana yoga), the yoga of devotion (*bhakti* or *upasana* yoga), the yoga of selfless service (karma yoga), and the yoga of special energizing and consciousness-elevating techniques involving body postures, sense-control techniques, and mind-calming methods (raja yoga, also known as the royal path of yoga). It is raja yoga that enjoys so much popularity today, with its focus on physical postures (known as asanas) and that I speak of now. I use the generic word *yoga* to denote physical postures.

The Benefits of a Daily Yoga Regimen

In recent decades, the benefits of a yoga regimen in lowering your risk factors for heart disease, including high blood pressure, high blood sugar, and atherosclerosis, are well-known and clinically validated. Yoga's ability to alleviate depression, insomnia, and mood disorders has also been well documented. Enhanced physical energy, joint flexibility, improved muscle tone, and weight control are other popular benefits of a yoga practice.

I recommend to most of my students that they adopt a daily yoga practice for stress management and improved flexibility. Detailed teaching of yoga postures to build a personal regimen is not within the scope of this book, but fortunately, it is easy enough today to learn the basics of yoga.

Beware the Yoga of More

What I do want to address is a concern related to a popular approach to yoga today, which involves excessive intensity. This is a relatively new trend in yoga, and it's something to be wary of from the perspective of excessive exercise. These particular yoga classes are all about speed. Some popular yoga studios in the United States will present as many as seventy postures in an hour-long class. Let me assure you: this is excessive exercise.

In such a class, no sooner have students finished one posture than they are rushed into the next, and the next, and the next after that. The sequences are like a yoga train you have to run to catch. It's easy to leave such yoga studios feeling physically drained. This is not yoga. And from an Ayurvedic perspective, this kind of exercise is too much for the body; it causes serious vata imbalances in joints and muscles.

It may seem like all yoga teachers and students are intuitively connected with the Eastern wisdom of balance and moderation, but I can say for certain that this is not the case. Our clinics encounter sincere yoga enthusiasts with injuries and out-of-control vata conditions—insomnia, erectile dysfunction, and infertility—due to what I call "the yoga of more," a trend taking the Western world by storm.

To accomplish yogic dexterity, many of these would-be yogis push their bodies to the extreme. They neglect a foundational recommendation from the science of yoga: never tire your body while practicing yogic postures. Perspiration, increased heart rate, or labored breathing are all signs that you have tired your body with yoga. In fact, yoga is a special form of exercise that is accomplished more from mindfulness while performing a posture than from exerting more physical energy. Thus, it requires even more vigilance in asking the question: *How much is enough?*

One of my students learned yoga at a prestigious studio in San Francisco—and left each class with a pain in her lower back. She visited orthopedists and rheumatologists for years and kept hoping yoga would fix her body. She never dreamt that her excessive yoga regimen was the cause of her obstinate back pain. After she consulted me, I recommended that she oil her body (see chapter 5) and stop her hectic yoga routine of seventy postures in a sixty-minute class. I suggested instead that she practice, gently and slowly, just one posture for several months, the cobra pose. What a contrast, from seventy to one! Her pain lessened over time and then completely stopped. Her back was fully healed. She had needed only that simple correction.

Another student of mine told me that he had fallen in yoga class while pushing himself into a headstand he clearly wasn't ready for. He also sprained his ankle twice through his fun but hectic yoga routine.

When this man approached me to express his disappointment with his yoga adventures, I told him that it wasn't the great science of yoga that caused his injuries, it was the mania of "more is better" that was to blame. I then suggested that he stop all yoga asana practice, do some deep-breathing exercise (pranayama), gentle walking, and normal household activities for a full year. I had him focus his energy on oiling and resting his body and on eating ghee and a nourishing diet that included wheat, urad dal (black gram), boiled cow's milk with turmeric, nuts (in winter), and dried dates to build bone and muscle strength. In short, I had him live by Ayurveda's beautifully restorative principles.

This same student now enjoys good health and is in love with a slow and spiritualized yoga practice I imparted to him, a practice composed of four comfortable poses which bring him joy and keep his body free of pain and inflammation. Now, he has even begun running, and his ankles hold him up without fail!

There are so many stories like these that I could recount of people for whom this factor of excess blocks the healing they could have received from the practice of yoga. I think that perhaps this current exercise phenomenon we are seeing worldwide shouldn't be called yoga. It's more like yoga-inspired gymnastics or yogic-aerobic workouts! If they were called that, then those who have stamina for such things could choose this type of exercise—and others wouldn't be misled.

Fortunately, wise yoga teachers worldwide join me in also cautioning against the trend of the yoga of more. Let us truly experience yoga, enjoy it, celebrate it, and let go of the pressure of more, faster, better.

Introducing Yoga for Atmabodha

I am always glad to support a return to the way yoga was practiced by the sages by teaching what I learned from my Baba. He taught that any yoga practice should not only exercise your muscles and limbs but should also infuse your body with rejuvenating prana shakti and connect you with your higher Self, which is the source of spiritual power, abiding health, and inner peace.

Baba was a renowned yogi and had spent several years in the Himalayas perfecting his knowledge of all dimensions of yoga. He taught me to perform yoga postures in a deliberate, slow, and spiritually suffused practice. Today, I am a natural proponent of slow, spiritualized yoga—the opposite of the culture of speed, excess, and physicality that is eroding yoga today.

My students at Vedika Global are deeply receptive when I introduce them to my Vedic lineage's slow and spiritualized approach, which is called Yoga for Atmabodha.

As I have said, yoga is a spiritual philosophy that comes from the ancient Vedas, and *Atmabodha* means "awakening to the truth of our spiritual nature." Hence, Yoga for Atmabodha is a decisive return to the ancient roots of yoga.

In its beginnings, the practice of yoga, including the physical disciplines of asana and pranayama, was always taught within the context of healthy lifestyle practices—prayer, sun worship, meditation, contemplation, sattvic food choices, balanced sexuality, and sleep. I've introduced all of these practices in this book.

My extensive teachings on Yoga for Atmabodha will be the subject of another book, but for this explanation of Ayurveda's system of health and healing—of which Yoga for Atmabodha is clearly a part—I wish to address one of the factors that makes this yoga practice the ideal foundation for spiritual endeavor: its deliberate lack of speed.

A Slow, Spiritual Practice

I initiate my students into a slowed-down, conscious practice in which they perform no more than one to six yoga postures (asanas) per hour.

This includes fifteen minutes in the corpse posture (savasana, see the box "How to Do Savasana" on page 227 for instructions) at the end. Additionally, a yoga practice session usually begins and ends with transformative Vedic mantras, and it often leads into an Atmabodha Meditation practice (described in chapter 2).

A slow practice is less demanding on your body, and yet it is much more impactful because it calms your mind. With regular practice, you can enhance your memory and mental dexterity and improve your sleep. Regular practice also benefits your body, enhancing immunity, improving physical energy, and reducing allergies, pain, and inflammation.

The benefits of slow, awareness-based exercise, like gentle yoga, tai chi, and qigong are being acknowledged by an increasing number of experts in integrative medicine and pain management. An article published in the *Los Angeles Times* quotes Dr. Vernon Williams, director of sports neurology and pain management at Kerlan-Jobe Orthopaedic Clinic in Los Angeles: "There is some evidence that as you do regular breathing and slow the heart rate, you can calm or quiet the autonomic nervous system." In the same article, a professor of psychiatry and biobehavioral science at UCLA's medical school commented that slow, rhythmic breathing and movement "target the pathways by shutting off or diminishing the inflammatory response."[22]

What gives a yoga practice this kind of power, I believe, is the way we connect with ourselves through each posture, the way we relate the postures to our sense of Self, the way we treat ourselves in this process, the way we experience our bodies as sacred, and the way we relax into our true nature (Atmabodha).

A cardinal principle in Yoga for Atmabodha is that one posture held mindfully for at least a few minutes, along with accompanying breathing and spiritual, contemplative insight has greater success in altering mind-based consciousness than a lengthy practice of complex or demanding sequences. From an exercise perspective, one posture is often enough—especially since yoga moves prana subtly. And with one posture, this can happen without exhausting you.

In the same way, do not push yourself for perfection in yoga postures—just gently try your best at any given moment. I ask my students to not worry about whether they can turn their ankle out or stretch their muscles precisely. I encourage them to hold the thought that yoga practice is their time to learn the art of the body's beautiful prana and to embody that energy with pride. I encourage them to practice the postures that attract them and to ask themselves why they are so attracted. Then, to do one, two, or three postures daily, settling into a beautiful rhythm, is enough. More than the number of daily postures you do, it's the repeated spiritual practice (sadhana) and the quality of your thoughts during this practice that make a difference.

Isn't that liberating?

Yoga is, first and foremost, a spiritual quest. Yoga invites seekers to enter the field of the Spirit—a field of being and becoming, where anything is possible. My Baba used to say that after you've held a yoga posture for some time, check in with yourself: Are you connecting with your higher Self or not? This is the fundamental question. The sign of that connection with your higher Self is that you feel inexplicable peace, light, joy, relaxation, and energy spontaneously emerge from within, every time, without fail. If you are not experiencing this, then slow down even more. Hold your posture even longer.

Deeply relax into the posture, without hurrying to do the next posture or to go anywhere, physically or mentally.

The deeper and longer you hold each posture—with natural breathing and a meditative attentiveness to your own body—the more your body and mind will relax into a state of profound restfulness. This is the state of Yoga for Atmabodha, union with your higher Self. What follows is physical health and an uplifted—even enlightened—mind. This is not the short-lived satisfaction of perfecting a pose. It goes beyond the yoga mat, leaping into the *chitta bhumi*, the field of consciousness where anything and everything is possible.

Ten Tips to Embrace Slow, Spiritualized Yoga

Any practice of yoga can be infused with the wisdom of Yoga for Atmabodha by slowing it down and spiritualizing it. By making this effort, you will reap great mental, physical, and spiritual benefits. Here are my recommendations for how to do this.

1. Plan your practice at a nonrushed time. Either wake up early enough to make time at the beginning of your day (this is ideal) or carve out time before dinner. Either way, you should not be ravenously hungry nor should you have just eaten. Set aside at least thirty minutes for your practice. Stick to this routine long-term and protect this time as marked for your personal care and self-growth.

2. Always begin your practice with a couple of rounds of centering and calming pranayama, like brahmari pranayama,

or humming bee breathing (see chapter 2). Humming bee breathing settles your mind, imparting the same benefits as a seated meditation.

3. Next, chant OM at least three times and as many as nine, synchronizing the chant with your breath. If you know other Vedic mantras, such as the Gayatri mantra (see chapter 2), you can also chant these. All Vedic mantras elevate consciousness and prepare you for a spiritualized yogic encounter with your higher Self.

4. Resist rushing into poses immediately. Instead, focus first on making a spiritual decision (*sankalpa shakti*). You might think something like this: *I, Atman (Spirit), choose to mold my body, my instrument, into X posture.* Name and then imagine yourself doing the posture with ease. Then begin doing the postures physically.

5. At all times, be aware of what you're doing. Ask yourself: *Am I breathing? Am I (the Spirit) witnessing the details of this experience? Shall I slow down and deepen even more?*

6. If you feel out of breath, you are likely moving too quickly. Breathe slowly and steadily.

7. Before a yoga session, read and meditate on the benefits of each asana and then choose no more than six. You can even begin with just two or three. Repeat each asana three times in the same session. An exception is sun salutations, which include twelve postures per cycle, and the cycle is usually done one to three times. Awareness and proper breathing is enough—again, more is not better!

8. End with a nice, slow corpse pose (savasana) for deep relaxation (see the box "How to Do Savasana" on page 227 for instructions).

9. After corpse pose, sit up and place your palms together at your heart (*namaste mudra*). Chant OM three to nine times to end your session. If you have a guru, visualize him or her. Thank the parampara (tradition/lineage) that's given you this knowledge.

10. Sit for some time before leaping back into your life. Open your eyes very, very gently. Smile to acknowledge your gratitude, and part your lips gently in a deliberate smile (*hasa mudra*) before opening your eyes fully. Your session is complete.

I hope that if you already have a yoga practice or plan on starting one that you will experience the highest truth within your practice.

Celebrating the Path of Moderation

Sleep, sex, and exercise (including yoga) are facets of healthy living. Ayurveda teaches balance in each. *More* does not mean *better*. Ayurveda's spiritually grounded science understands the humdrum, old-fashioned idea of moderation. Yes, this idea doesn't spark imagination;

it certainly won't fund millions of dollars in research and clinical trials. Nor will it spawn a new industry of slick products and infomercials. Moderation is a choice that's ours to adopt. This self-born moderation that allows us to adapt to our own unique constitution is the scientific contribution Ayurveda first made to the world thousands of years ago. Those who follow the Ayurveda system of health and healing listen to the wisdom within and seek balance not only in sleep, sex, and exercise but in everything in their lives.

Releasing Healing Intentions into the Universe

 One fully bloomed, heavily scented red rose; two water lilies, one yellow, the other white; one shy marigold, still opening her orange-colored petals; and one splendid lotus, a vivid pink: I remember carrying these five flowers in my flower basket to River Sarayu accompanied by my guru Baba; I was almost twenty-four by then. It was the last autumn my teacher spent with me in his Earth body.

It was almost morning. A majestic October sun was about to rise and sprinkle its golden radiance on us. First we meditated next to the river as usual and then sat beside it silently, as if in communion with all of Nature and the hidden spiritual reality that expresses itself through all of us. Then I released the flowers, one by one, into the flowing river as Baba watched me silently with his compassionate, all-knowing eyes. Baba's body was older now, he was almost ninety, and I was the physically stronger one, taller than him, my legs withstanding the strong waves as I entered the river. Yet, my guru's presence was ageless.

River Sarayu seemed to simply grab the flowers with her immense armlike waves, as if she were waiting for them, and then equally suddenly, they disappeared into her watery deluge of eternity. After monsoons, the river appeared no less than a mighty ocean; her depth was incomprehensible, her intentions indiscernible, and her power immeasurable.

After I had released the flowers into the river, we chanted together, master and disciple, in one voice, an ancient mantra for the health and providence of all beings. We wanted our blessing to reach all beings in all types of bodies, visible and invisible to our human eyes, dwelling in all realms of existence.

OM Sarveshaam Svastir-Bhavatu
Sarveshaam Shaantir-Bhavatu
Sarveshaam Purnnam-Bhavatu
Sarveshaam Manggalam-Bhavatu
OM Shanti Shanti Shanti

May all beings have health and well-being;
May all beings enjoy peace and serenity;
May all beings experience fulfilment and contentment;
May all beings know divine auspiciousness;
OM peace, peace, peace.

The chant had ended, but it seemed to be echoed by the sky, the river, and the rising sun. My heart, body, and mind embraced complete stillness because I knew intuitively that today, after many days of silence, my teacher would reveal to me yet one more gem of wisdom that would change my life forever.

Baba spoke, very quietly, and I had to strain to hear him above the crashing waves of the river. He said, "Shunya, now these flowers will always be with you. Always. When we open our hearts and offer to the universe our noblest and purest of intentions for all beings, then these thoughts, magnified by the power of cosmic sound, gain an infinite momentum. They travel everywhere in this ever-expanding conscious universe and yet will somehow circle back to you and bless you again and again, ad infinitum."

That day, my guru Baba evoked my higher order of thinking to connect to a grand, interconnected reality of existence that I may not immediately perceive with my physical eyes but can conceive of under instruction of my guru.

Baba spoke as if directly to my soul this time, "Imagine your being, many decades hence, blessed by these flowers. They will come back to you in the form of true grace, knowledge, wisdom, a helping hand, or a kind eye in times of distress and uncertainty. These flowers shall set you free from your suffering, of body, mind, and soul. When you set into the universe blessing for all beings, the blessings shall come back to you many times more. ✎

Perhaps you, too, would like to set an intention at the conclusion of this book along with me. Whatever you set into universal motion, with compassion in your heart, will come back to you exponentially because spiritual oneness is the underlying reality of our physical existence.

May Ayurveda's lifestyle wisdom bless all beings with ever-increasing health, well-being, peace, fulfillment, and joy.

With infinite love,

Shunya

ACKNOWLEDGMENTS

I offer profound appreciation for all my students worldwide who laid their trust in my teachings of Ayurveda and undertook a special healing journey with me leading the way. Their restored health, happiness, and empowerment became the creative inspiration of this book and source of great shakti rising. I especially celebrate all the students whose real-life stories of awakened health have become case studies in this book.

Thanks to the brilliant team at Sounds True, especially publisher Tami Simon and acquiring editor Jennifer Brown. Your belief in this book has gestated it from inspiration to manifestation. Content editor Gretel Hakanson did a masterful job with my completed manuscript. She offered insightful suggestions and polished my writing to a higher level of clarity. And she did it with such sensitivity to my creative spirit. Sarah Gorecki, my production editor, misses nothing. Her astute suggestions left me truly impressed with the care put into each book. My salute to the entire team at Sounds True!

My literary agent, Stephany Evans, president of FinePrint Literary Management, is a truly expansive soul who believes in our right to health and spirituality. She resonated with this book from the first day she read it, and we know we will do many more books together. Stephany, thank you for championing *Ayurveda Lifestyle Wisdom*! Margaret Bendet, an independent editor, offered critical developmental editing at a stage when my book was still being churned out of my being in bursts of creativity. Thank you for being so honest! You were a great resource.

On top of the list of people I want to thank and bless is my graduate student Ananta Ripa Ajmera, who is also a passionate teacher of lifestyle medicine and Yoga for Atmabodha at my school. Right from the beginning of the book to its end, she was available at every step to help me with research, compiling sources, proofreading, making chai, or walking my dogs as I wrote, and all this while working on her own soulful book! Your dedication to your teacher's message moved me.

Everyone needs those special, reliable people whose opinions and support they can count on. I am grateful to my illustrious colleagues at Vedika Global Foundation, Hema Patankar, president of the board of trustees, and Vaidya Abhijit Jinde and Vaidya Mahesh Sabade, distinguished faculty members in the Department of Ayurveda. Your suggestions were deeply appreciated. Special acknowledgement to Vimala Leann Brady, director of Charitable Clinical Operations; Aparna Amy Lewis, dean of the Vedic Studies Program; and Alexandra Krasne for reading specific chapters in the raw stages and offering critical suggestions along with significant editing early in the process. The recipes in this book were tested and organized by associate faculty members Teresa Pragya Steininger (food) and Janya Tuere Anderson (skin care). Thank you both. The food recipes were inspired and first taught by Chef Sanjai, who is the ever-popular food and cooking teacher. I also thank and bless Ishani Lauren Naidu, Shivani Maheshwari, Tracy Cunningham, Ambika Suzanne Saucy, Shaaranya Geetanjali Chakraborty, and Siddhi Joanne Trasky for giving important feedback and providing varied assistance. I offer heartfelt gratitude to my loving older cousin Rakesh Pradhan for being my champion always, and recognize the contribution of kindred spirits Arvind Kansal and Kevin Peer, and sisterlike friends Suhasini Janet Dobrovolny and Yogacharya Ellen O'Brian, for believing in me and my intrinsic message as a world teacher of Vedic sciences. Your encouragement fuels my fire!

I cannot fail to thank the brightest light of Vedic sciences today, David Frawley (Vamadeva Shastri), who has not only contributed the foreword to my book, but who, from the first day I set foot in the United States, has supported my message and work. Likewise, I am grateful to the eminent personalities who have appreciated this book and ultimately, through their association with my message, endorsed Ayurveda's timeless teachings on lifestyle. Thank you!

I can't express in words, how much I felt supported each time I talked to my beloved father Daya Prakash Sinha, who lives in India. He is my hero. His words always encouraged me to keep writing my truth, in all my power, day after day. He is a much-celebrated Hindi playwright, so I suppose the creative genes are something to thank too! I have to say that the best days of writing were those when my son, Dhruv, and nephew Sharang visited our home from college. Their sunny presence and our playtime with our beloved dogs and enjoying Ayurvedic meals and talks together inspired me to write with even greater joy. I want to thank my husband, Sanjai, who looked after my body like a mother and father would, through the long days of writing and meeting deadlines. How lucky I am for your incredible support through the writing of this immense book. Thank you for your unending patience with my process and tender care of my being. You have been my anchor, in so many ways.

In the end, no words can express my gratefulness to my guru, Baba Ayodhya Nath, and my guru's guru, Paramatman Sadhu Shanti Prakash, all the way back to the Vedic sages. The divine consciousness of my spiritual master has enabled me to write this book, in the ultimate sense. Without my guru, I am no one and I know nothing.

Each one of you has shown up in your own unique way in my life to help me awaken health and consciousness, which is my life purpose as a teacher and healer.

Thank you for showing up.

APPENDIX I

List of Recipes

Food and Drinks

Detox Recipes

Skin, Hair, and Oral Health

Heathy Elimination Resource Guide

Food Wisdom for Constipation Prevention and Treatment

Before you reach for fiber or laxatives, did you know your kitchen likely contains a variety of items that can counteract constipation without causing dependency or side effects? Try the following ingredients from your own "kitchen pharmacy."

Bananas

Bananas are a mild natural laxative due to their heavy and oily attributes. They also provide soft, oily bulkiness for the body. Take one ripe yellow banana after meals. Split the banana in half and sprinkle cumin powder and rock salt on it. Do not combine bananas with milk or other forms of dairy (except Ayurvedic buttermilk). For kids especially, bananas work great, since kids love the taste of bananas. It gives maximum benefit by adding bulk to the stool and thereby relieving constipation.

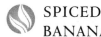 SPICED BANANA

Eating spiced banana generally guarantees a smoother motion the next morning, but it will not create loose stools.

INGREDIENTS

1	large or 2 medium ripe bananas
½	teaspoon ground cumin
¼	teaspoon rock salt
½	teaspoon lemon juice
1	teaspoon cilantro, minced

METHOD

1. Peel and dice banana(s) into bite-size pieces.
2. Sprinkle cumin, salt, and lemon juice over banana.
3. Toss and mix well. Garnish with minced cilantro.

Cow's Milk

To relieve constipation, boiled cow's milk is one of the best remedies, as cow's milk is a natural mild laxative.[1] Buffalo milk can also work well. Goat milk and sheep milk are highly nutritious but do not work as well in relieving constipation. Soy, almond, and rice milk also do not work for the purpose of relieving constipation. Vegans and those who are lactose intolerant need not drink cow's milk and can always choose from the other constipation-relieving foods.

Drink spiced milk at least three hours after dinner and no later than half an hour before going to bed.[2] This recipe is provided in appendix 4. I have found that this recipe is often tolerated by the "lactose intolerant" surprisingly well, especially if they introduce it into their diets gradually, in small doses, and drink it while still warm (without accompanying it with fresh or dried fruits, breakfast cereal, or other food).

Figs

Figs, whether fresh or dried, act as a wonderful natural laxative. When they're in season, you can simply eat two or three fresh figs daily, ideally in the morning at breakfast or as a midday snack. Before eating dried figs, presoak them overnight in water or cook them with cow's milk (2 figs in 8 ounces of milk) until soft. Or if you have strong teeth, try chewing two dry figs after each meal.

Unripe figs can also be cooked and eaten as part of a meal. To do so, cut the fruit into quarters and scrape some of the seeds out. The skin and fleshy interior can be parboiled and then either curried or mashed, as in the following recipe.

 SPICED MASHED FIGS

This mashed fig recipe has the exact ingredients that ignite digestive fire and support a good bowel movement. It does not require the use of milk, but it does use some ghee.

INGREDIENTS
- 2 cups ripened sweet figs, trimmed and chopped
- 1 tablespoon melted ghee
- 1 teaspoon lemon juice
- ½ teaspoon cumin powder
  Rock salt, to taste

METHOD
1. Boil figs in water till they become soft. Remove them from water and drain in a colander.
2. Mash the figs by hand or blend in a blender (do not add extra water). Add the other ingredients and mix well. Serve.

Grapes and Raisins

Grapes and raisins are great natural laxatives for everyone. Both the fresh and dried fruit counteract constipation. A handful of black raisins may be consumed at bedtime, or an hour after each meal. Another option is to soak twelve organic raisins in water overnight and eat them first thing in the morning on an empty stomach. If you sprinkle some rock salt on large raisins, they become an even more effective remedy for constipation. Raisins are the laxative of choice for young children, the elderly, and pregnant women.

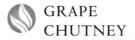

GRAPE CHUTNEY

This is an easy chutney recipe that you can make ahead of time. It can be left out at room temperature for at least a week (or more) in cooler temperatures.

INGREDIENTS

- 1   pound fresh grapes (any color)
- 4   cups water (or more for desired consistency)
- 1   tablespoon grated fresh ginger root
- 10 whole black peppercorns
     Rock salt, to taste
- 2   tablespoons cane sugar
- 1   teaspoon ground cumin
- 1   teaspoon ground fennel

METHOD

1. Chop grapes in half and remove seeds.
2. Bring water to a boil in a wide, heavy-bottomed sauce pan. Add all the ingredients and cook on low to medium heat until it comes to a boil. Reduce to a simmer.
3. Slowly reduce the mixture to the desired chutney consistency and simmer until the grapes are fully cooked. Add more water if it dries up too quickly. Eat as a relish when cooled to room temperature.

Lemons and Limes

Lemons and limes are effective remedies for constipation because they are a complete and potent package: they move impacted stools, remove toxins, clear a coated tongue, and remove bad taste from the mouth. Whether you have lemons or limes available, you can use them as a garnish on appropriate recipes, squeeze them into hot water, or lick a cut slice as an emergency nausea aid. These amazing little citrus fruits help your digestion in every way.

 VEDIKA LEMON SEMOLINA MEAL (*UPMA*)

This is excellent anytime as a snack or meal, depending on the quantity consumed. Wheat is an excellent source of soft bulk (natural soluble fiber) and an excellent food to consume when suffering from constipation (versus rice, for example).

INGREDIENTS

8 teaspoons ghee
8 fenugreek seeds
1 teaspoon black gram (urad dal)
½ teaspoon mustard seeds
½ teaspoon cumin seeds
5 curry leaves (optional)
Fresh ginger root, grated or minced, to taste
3 cups water
Rock salt, to taste
2 teaspoons ghee
1 cup wheat semolina (finely textured), dry roasted to avoid lumps
2 tablespoons lemon juice

METHOD

1. Heat a pan and add ghee. When ghee is hot, add fenugreek seeds and black gram. Sauté until the seeds start changing color, about 10 seconds.
2. Add mustard seeds and cumin seeds. Sauté until the seeds splutter and pop, about 10 seconds. Add curry leaves and ginger. Sauté 5 more minutes.
3. Add water and salt. Mix well. (If you add salt after the dish is prepared, it won't taste the same.)
4. When the water starts boiling, lower the heat to medium and add ghee to the boiling water.
5. Add the semolina, a very small amount at a time, mixing thoroughly until it is completely dissolved in the water. Only then add the next batch.
6. Cover and cook for 3 minutes. Remove the lid after 3 minutes and mix well.
7. Remove from heat and add lemon juice. Mix well and serve hot.

Mulberries

Mulberry is a well-loved fruit. While native to China and India, it grows all over the world today, including in the United States. Ayurvedic texts explicitly describe the unripe fruit as possessing a laxative quality.

The sweet fruit works well if you already have a decent digestive fire. With compromised digestion, the unripe sour fruit may be of greater assistance in relieving your symptoms.

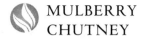

MULBERRY CHUTNEY

I typically recommend making a quick relish or dip from the unripe fruit; however, you can also use semiripe fruit. This chutney can be consumed as a relish along with regular meals. It rids the colon of impacted stools with ease every time.

INGREDIENTS

20	unripe mulberries (any variety)
	Rock salt, to taste
1	inch piece fresh ginger root, grated or minced
½	teaspoon cumin
	Few drops of lemon, lime, or tangerine juice (optional)

METHOD

1. Grind unripe mulberries in a blender or with mortar and pestle to the desired consistency. (You will likely not need to add water.)
2. Add salt, ginger, and cumin. Squeeze in a few drops of lemon, lime, or fresh tangerine juice for an extra-tart flavor.

Pears

Pears are *tri-doshic*, meaning they balance all three doshas upon digestion. On top of that, pears are easily digestible. Adding rock salt and black pepper to the cut fruit primes the digestion of the pear further. Finally, for all those fiber seekers out there, here is good news for you: pears are one of the leading fruit sources of fiber. A medium-size pear packs six grams of fiber, which equals about 24 percent of your daily requirement for fiber! The skin of the pear contains the majority of the fiber, so enjoy the skin for added flavor, texture, and nutrients!

 NECTAR FRUIT STIR-FRY

I remember my mother cooking this recipe every pear season. This dish is ideal for breakfast or lunch, but not dinner, especially if your evening meal will be eaten after sunset. Do not drink chilled beverages or dairy with this recipe; consume warm water instead.

MARINADE INGREDIENTS

- ¼ teaspoon ground turmeric
- 1/16 teaspoon asafoetida
- ¼ teaspoon ground cumin
- ¼ teaspoon rock salt

INGREDIENTS

- 2 medium-size ripe pears, sliced
- 1 heaping tablespoon ghee or clarified butter
- ¼ teaspoon cumin seeds
- ¼ teaspoon whole black peppercorns
- ½ teaspoon minced fresh garlic
- ½ teaspoon grated fresh ginger root
- 1 teaspoon ground coriander
- ½ teaspoon ground turmeric
  Rock salt to taste
- 1/16 teaspoon asafoetida
- 1 teaspoon minced cilantro

METHOD

1. Prior to cooking, pierce the pear slices with a fork and mix with the marinade ingredients. Marinate for 15 minutes.
2. Heat ghee in a pan. When ghee begins to shimmer, reduce heat to medium. Add cumin seeds and black peppercorns. Allow them to pop, about 10 to 15 seconds.
3. Add minced garlic and grated ginger and sauté for 20 seconds. Add pears.
4. Sprinkle coriander and turmeric over the pear slices. Add rock salt and asafoetida and stir the entire mixture. Turn heat to low and cover. Do not add extra water as the pear will cook in its own steam. Cook for about 15 minutes.
5. Occasionally remove the cover and stir gently to avoid burning or sticking on the bottom of the pan. After 15 minutes, turn off heat. Add cilantro as garnish. Serve hot. The pears can be served with Indian bread, pita bread, or quinoa.

Spinach

Spinach, when eaten raw, will aggravate vata. But when spinach is cooked in ghee with digestion-improving spices, its inherent sliminess and moistness become an aid in moving the stools effectively.

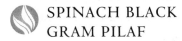

SPINACH BLACK GRAM PILAF

This recipe was a personal favorite of mine growing up. The black gram and spinach together create a creamy and unforgettable texture. Both spinach and black gram will induce a purging effect, along with specific spices that work to balance vata and cleanse the colon.

INGREDIENTS

½ cup split black gram (urad dal), soaked for 1 hour and drained well before cooking

1 cup water

Rock salt, to taste

½ teaspoon fresh turmeric

1 tablespoon ghee

½ teaspoon cumin seeds

½ teaspoon grated fresh ginger

⅛ teaspoon asafoetida

1 cup fresh spinach leaves, washed and finely chopped

1 tablespoon water

2 teaspoons lemon juice

METHOD

1. Combine black gram with water in a deep, heavy saucepan. Add salt and turmeric. Mix well and cook on medium heat for 10 to 12 minutes or until the water is mostly evaporated and the lentils are well cooked and soft (but retain their shape). Be careful not to overcook the lentils or mix with a heavy ladle, which will break up the lentils.

2. Heat ghee in a separate sauté pan. Add cumin seeds and sauté on a medium heat for a few seconds. Add ginger and asafoetida and sauté for 1 minute.

3. Add spinach. Mix well. Sprinkle with 1 tablespoon water and cook on medium heat for 1 minute, stirring occasionally. Add to the prepared lentils and stir well.

4. Garnish with lemon juice. Serve hot.

Tangerines

The Ayurvedic texts mention that the more sour (rather than sweet) tangerines can also effectively help with constipation as they are a natural laxative.[3] Follow guidelines on eating fruits and fruit-based recipes provided in appendix 4 or try the following recipe.

 ## SPICED TANGERINE AND BANANA DRINK

The banana adds bulk and the tangerine juice makes stools softer, both of which assist with elimination. The spices ensure that this recipe balances digestion and does not create the gas and discomfort that juices can often cause. This recipe is both medicinal and delicious at the same time. It should be consumed at room temperature. It is not a recipe for spring but is acceptable in all other seasons.

INGREDIENTS

- 1 medium or 3 miniature tangerines
- 1 banana
- ¼ inch piece fresh ginger root, grated
- ⅛ teaspoon ground cumin
- ⅛ teaspoon rock salt

METHOD

1. Peel and de-seed tangerines.
2. Blend tangerines, banana, ginger, cumin, and salt. Serve immediately.

Other Useful Food Items to Counteract Constipation

- *Aloe vera* gel: In the morning, before breakfast, swallow 1 tablesoon fresh expressed gel from a home-grown plant.

- Well-cooked black-eyed peas: Boil in water with added cumin seed powder and rock salt (to taste) or add cooked peas to other recipes of choice.

- Ripe guava: Sprinkle fresh cut slices with cumin powder.

- Sweet mango: Eat before sunset, and ideally as a meal unto itself.

- Ripe papaya: Sprinkle fresh cut slices with cumin powder.

- Wheat: Eat in variety of unfermented recipes, such as cream of wheat, wheat pasta, wheat chapatti, and wheat tortillas.

Note: Mango (fresh), figs (fresh and dry), and raisins (not grapes) are the three fruits that can be cooked in milk without concern of incompatibility. All other fruits are generally considered incompatible when cooked in milk or eaten along with milk. Eat fruit before sunset, ideally at breakfast or at midday, as a snack or a meal unto itself.

Yoga Postures to Relieve Constipation

- Boat pose
- Cobra pose
- Crocodile pose
- Rabbit pose
- Raised-legs pose

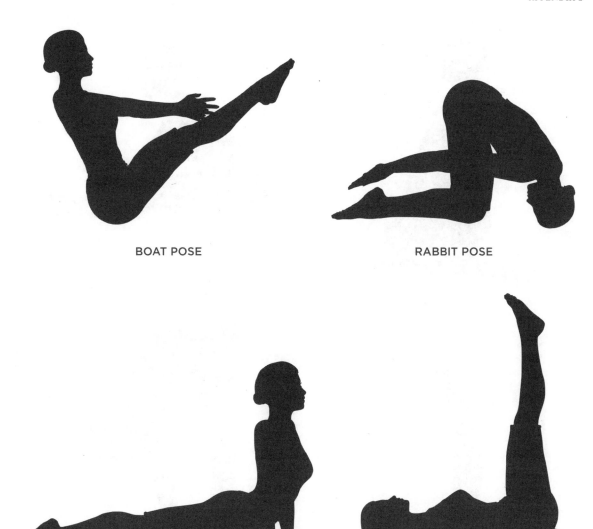

BOAT POSE

RABBIT POSE

COBRA POSE

RAISED LEG POSE

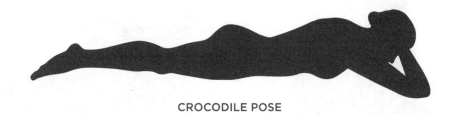

CROCODILE POSE

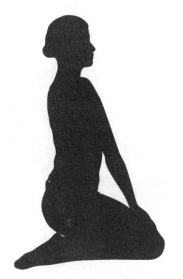

THUNDERBOLT POSE

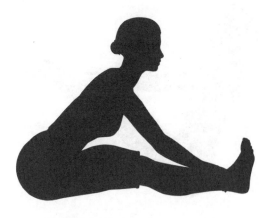

SEATED FORWARD-BEND POSE

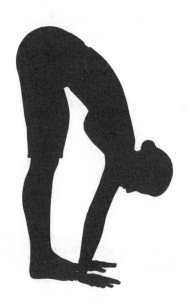

STANDING FORWARD-FOLD POSE

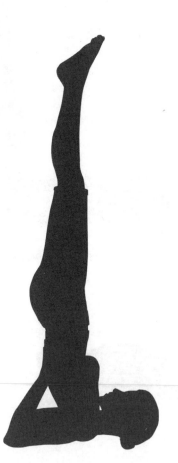

SHOULDER-STAND POSE

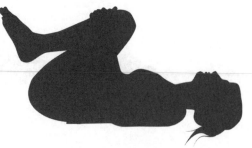

WIND-RELIEVING POSE

- Seated forward-bend pose
- Shoulder-stand pose
- Standing forward-fold pose
- Thunderbolt pose
- Wind-relieving pose

Breathing Practices to Relieve Constipation

- Alternate nostril breathing
- Bellows breath
- Skull-shining breathing

Food Wisdom for Diarrhea Prevention and Treatment

Use table 34 to better understand the foods and beverages that can best reduce or eliminate diarrhea. This list is by no means an exhaustive list, but it provides some guidance to help you make food choices.

Recipes to Counteract Diarrhea

The following recipes have been tried and tested in the Ayurveda tradition for several centuries. Regular inclusion of these recipes on a daily or weekly basis will help increase absorption, bind stools, and combat the tendency toward loose stools. Exclusively focusing on these recipes during an active episode of diarrhea will help ignite the all-important agni and help restore balance. (Also see the detox recipes in appendix 4, especially the gruels and khichadi recipes.)

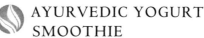 AYURVEDIC YOGURT SMOOTHIE

This recipe has a binding and drying effect on the stools. It can be consumed daily with meals and is especially useful in combating a tendency toward loose and frequent stools or even irritable bowel syndrome. It can be consumed in all seasons except spring, when yogurt is contraindicated. However, as an exception, it can consumed in spring during an episode of active diarrhea.

INGREDIENTS
1   part whole cow's milk yogurt
4   parts water

METHOD
1. Mix yogurt with water.
2. Blend in a blender or vigorously by hand for 3 to 4 minutes.

TABLE 34   Diet Recommendations for Diarrhea

Category	Always Include (*Pathya*)	Generally Avoid (*Apathya*)
Tastes	Astringent is best to reduce diarrhea; sour is okay in small amounts	Totally avoid the pungent and bitter tastes as well as excessively salty and sour foods
Qualities	Lighter foods that are warming in temperature and spices are preferred	Avoid excessively oily, cold, hot, and heavy qualities in food
Lentils	Mung beans, red lentils (masur), pigeon peas (arhar), preferably in soup form	Avoid black gram (urad), horse gram (chana), garbanzo beans, and frozen peas
Cereals	Cooked white rice	Barley, corn, couscous, quinoa, brown rice, wild rice, wheat
Water	Boiled; consume hot (adding spices like cumin, ginger, and nutmeg can help improve digestion)	Cold, iced, and excess water is contraindicated
Fat	Ghee (in traces)	Cheese, salted butter, sour cream, mayonnaise, coconut, and other oils
Vegetables	Snake gourd, winter melon, cilantro	Artichoke, cabbage, cucumber, Opo (white gourd), pumpkin, squash varieties including winter melon, all leafy vegetables
Tubers	Garlic and ginger (in traces only)	Beets, onion, sweet potato, white potato, radish, tapioca
Fruits	Unripe banana, pomegranate	Apples, avocados, ripe bananas, citrus fruits, mangos, pineapple, fresh sugarcane, watermelon
Meats	Chicken or goat meat soup in digestible doses; grilled meat or light soup of deer, partridge, or rabbit	Abstain from pork, beef, and seafood; minimize chicken, turkey
Dairy	Ayurvedic buttermilk is ideal; boiled milk of goat	Milk, butter, yogurt
Alcohol	Not recommended	Sour or carbonated alcohol is particularly not recommended

Category	Always Include (*Pathya*)	Generally Avoid (*Apathya*)
Drinks	Lentil soups, rice water, buttermilk, yogurt (according to digestive power)	Aerated drinks, smoothies, coconut water
Spices	Cumin, nutmeg, ground ginger	Overly hot and pungent spices

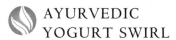 ## AYURVEDIC YOGURT SWIRL

This recipe is especially beneficial in diarrhea, igniting agni, mitigating vata dosha, and relieving hemorrhoids and tiredness. Eat it as a meal or as a snack.

INGREDIENTS
- 1 cup plain yogurt with natural cream
- ⅛ teaspoon cumin
- ⅛ teaspoon asafoetida
- ⅛ teaspoon rock salt

METHOD
1. Using a blender or handheld whisk, robustly churn the yogurt in a bowl (without the addition of water).
2. When it becomes frothy due to the churning, add cumin, asafoetida, and rock salt. Mix well.

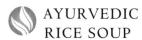 ## AYURVEDIC RICE SOUP

This recipe serves to rehydrate, rekindle digestive fire, remove pain in the abdomen, and purify the alimentary canal. Eat it warm as a meal. Do not reheat; it is not recommended to eat leftovers.

INGREDIENTS
- 1 part rice
- 14 parts water
- Rock salt, to taste

METHOD
1. Cook rice with water in an open pot, on low heat, until the rice grains are well cooked.
2. The finished product is rice that is integrated into the water to form a souplike consistency. You will find this recipe quite watery when done.
3. Add rock salt, to taste.

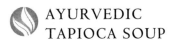 # AYURVEDIC TAPIOCA SOUP

Tapioca soaks up excess fluid and calms pitta. This recipe helps relieve weakness when ongoing or acute diarrhea has depleted bodily strength. This soup can be consumed during active diarrhea.

INGREDIENTS

- 1 tablespoon tapioca
- 1 cup water
- 1 teaspoon sugar

METHOD

1. Soak tapioca in plain water overnight.
2. The next morning, bring the tapioca and 1 cup of water to a boil. Add sugar.
3. Boil mixture until it thickens into a mushy consistency.
4. Eat only the thick liquid that rises to the top, while leaving behind the solid pieces that have settled at the bottom. The liquid is more easily absorbed than the actual tapioca beads, and it's nutritious too.

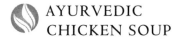 # AYURVEDIC CHICKEN SOUP

Begin eating this recipe only when you are feeling much better and active loose stools have stopped. This rebuilds bodily tissues and strength. Eat warm. Ideally, consume the soup more than the pieces of meat. Do not reheat; it is not recommended to eat leftovers.

INGREDIENTS

- ½ cup chopped chicken
- 4 cups water
- ½ teaspoon ground cumin
- 1 teaspoon ground coriander
  Rock salt, to taste

METHOD

1. Add chicken and water to a large pot.
2. Add cumin, coriander, and salt.
3. Cook slowly on low heat for about 30 minutes, until chicken is tender.
4. Remove the chicken pieces because they are heavy to digest. Consume the broth, which is full of nutrition and easy to digest.

Home Remedies to Counteract Diarrhea

- Mix ½ teaspoon ground nutmeg with ½ teaspoon ghee and ½ teaspoon sugar. Swallow at least three to four times a day with a small amount of lukewarm water.

- Lightly sauté ¼ teaspoon ground ginger with ¼ teaspoon aniseed in a small quantity of ghee. Consume this mixture with lukewarm water at least three times a day.

- Make a tea or decoction of equal amounts of ground ginger and ground coriander. Consume two tablespoons every few hours.

Yoga Postures to Prevent Diarrhea

Remember, exercise is contraindicated during active diarrhea, and even yoga postures must not be done during an active or acute bout of diarrhea. However, include the following poses in your usual morning routine when possible, since they especially help in igniting agni.

- Bridge pose
- Cobra pose
- Bow pose

Enjoy happy digestion and great bio-purification, nice and early, every morning!

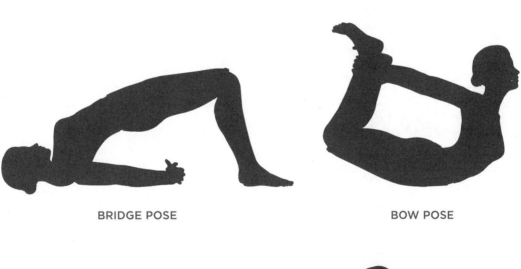

BRIDGE POSE   BOW POSE

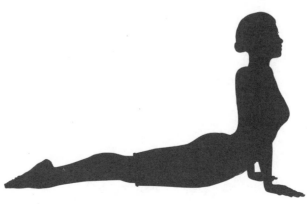

COBRA POSE

Oral Health Resource Guide

Highlighted Botanicals and Associated Recipes

Herbal tooth-cleaning powders can be used in conjunction with chew sticks (herbal twigs), as described in chapter 4, or they can be used in the absence of chew sticks with regular nylon toothbrushes. In Ayurveda, the texture of teeth cleaning substances is deliberately kept on the dry side to counteract the natural moistness of the oral cavity. Also, bitter- and pungent-tasting oral care products are preferred over other tastes, since these are antitoxic and antiseptic.[1]

I provide here a selection of easy-to-make recipes using a variety of natural ingredients. Try the recipes that appeal to you most or the ones with ingredients that you happen to have easy access to—in your own backyard, on your kitchen spice shelf, or at a local apothecary shop. Most of these ingredients are also available online.

I have made maximum effort to make recommendations for ingredients that are procurable with relative ease within the United States. Certain dental care botanicals such as turmeric and holy basil can even be grown in home gardens or planters, climate permitting.

Gifts from the Mystical Pomegranate Tree

Ayurvedic tradition utilizes the astringent nature of the flower, bark, and fruit rind of pomegranate (*Punica granatum*) for dental health.

Numerous studies and clinical trials are being conducted by modern Ayurveda researchers to look at pomegranate's healing properties. In one study, pomegranate mouthwash used twice daily for fifteen days resulted in a more efficient reduction of gingivitis and bleeding gums when compared to chlorhexidine.[2] And in another, a gel containing the extracts of pomegranate fruit peel applied to patients with candidiasis (thrush) proved an effective antifungal agent.[3]

Pomegranate peel: Save the peel and dry by exposing it to indirect sun for several days. Grind in a coffee grinder to a slightly gritty texture. The astringency of the powder helps arrest bleeding and tightens loose gums.

Pomegranate blossoms: Mix dried pomegranate flower blossoms with equal amounts of rose petals and marigold petals. Dry the blossoms in shade. When petals are dry, grind to a fine powder. Brushing with this powder prevents bleeding gums and eliminates foul breath.

Pomegranate leaves: Dry two dozen fresh leaves. Grind to a fine powder. Use the powder to brush your teeth, especially if your gums are infected, weak, or unable to provide a solid support to your teeth. Prevents tooth loss.

Pomegranate combo: Mix 1 cup each of dried pomegranate peel powder and neem powder.

Add ½ teaspoon of ground turmeric and ½ teaspoon of rock salt. Use this power-packed combination for toothbrushing every morning.

Turmeric Blessings

Ayurveda uses popular spice turmeric (*Curcuma longa*) for dental applications in the form of mouthwash and throat gargle.[4] Turmeric's anti-inflammatory properties help significantly with oral care. For centuries, Ayurvedic medicine has used turmeric in almost all of its pain and inflammation management, either by itself or in combination with other agents.[5]

Mouthwash for pain relief and cavity prevention: Boil 3 small turmeric roots or 1 tablespoon ground turmeric, 2 cloves (*Syzygium aromaticum*), and 2 dried guava leaves or 1 teaspoon ground guava leaves in 2 cups water to make a mouth wash. Boil down to 1 cup. Strain. Rinse with this daily or at least weekly for long-term protection from cavities and oral cancer.

Daily gargle for germ protection: Add ½ teaspoon of ground turmeric to 1 cup warm water. Gargle with this water after every meal or at least once before bedtime.

Daily tooth tonic: Mix equal amounts of ground turmeric with ground tulsi, or holy basil leaf. Use this combination to massage teeth and gums daily.

Daily tooth powder: Mix 1 part neem, 1 part ground turmeric, and 4 parts ground guava leaf. Use this combination to brush your teeth daily.

Relief for toothache: Combine equal quantities of asafoetida to ground turmeric. Sprinkle a few drops of water to make a paste-like consistency. Roll this paste into a tiny ball with your index fingers, and keep this ball on the painful tooth for pain relief.

Gingivitis treatment: Mix 1 teaspoon ground turmeric powder with ¼ teaspoon rock salt. Add ¼ to ½ teaspoon mustard oil to form a paste-like consistency. This paste can be rubbed on gums to counteract irritated, red, swollen gums.

The Amazing Acacia Tree

The acacia is a thorny tree common throughout India and grows in warm climates, such as Hawaii, Mexico, and the southwestern United States. Acacia seedpods are considered food by many communities worldwide, eaten raw or cooked in curries. Acacia's beautiful yellow and white blossoms are used for perfume and to flavor desserts and liquors.

Acacia bark, twigs, and leaves, according to Ayurveda, are mainly astringent in taste, making it a significant herb for balancing kapha and pitta doshas.[6] It is an antitoxic agent, alleviates skin diseases, and is widely used for a variety of conditions. A decoction (instructions follow) made from acacia bark mixed with rock salt in micro quantities can be used as a gargle for treating tonsillitis. In recent studies, gel and powder from *Acacia arabica* showed significant clinical improvement in gingivitis, plaque reduction, and gum tone.[7]

Chewing gum alternative: If you are in the habit of chewing gum after meals for oral health, then you may want to order an all-natural chewing gum manufactured from the acacia tree. Whole gum mixtures of acacia have been shown to inhibit the growth of oral bacteria and prevent gingivitis.[8]

Tooth powder for toothache: Make a tooth-brushing powder with the burnt ash of acacia seedpods. Simply char fresh or dried seedpods in a barbecue pit or the open flames of your kitchen stove. They will become quite blackened and brittle. Now grind the charred pods into a fine powder using a coffee grinder or mortar and pestle. This ash has medicinal value. It effectively relieves toothaches and also tightens the gum pockets around your teeth. This is especially beneficial if you have a loose tooth.

Antiplaque tooth powder: Seedpod ash can also be added to any home recipe for tooth powders, as it imparts wonderful astringent and antitoxic qualities that will prevent plaque buildup. Combine the burnt ash of seedpods with ash from burnt almond shells; pulverize them well into a fine powder. Add $\frac{1}{16}$ part rock salt, $\frac{1}{16}$ part ground black sesame seeds, and $\frac{1}{4}$ part ground guava leaf.

Chew sticks and brushes: The soft twigs of the acacia tree can be used as chew sticks. They are especially useful if your gums get easily infected or you have spongy gums that bleed easily. For added efficacy, you can also apply honey and turmeric to the twig before using. Many studies have shown that honey has antibacterial properties. Research has also indicated that honey may possess anti-inflammatory properties and stimulate immune responses. It can also be used in the treatment of various ulcerative oral conditions.[9]

Gargle for mouth ulcers: Tender leaves of the acacia tree can be boiled in water and then used as a gargle. Use about 20 leaves in 2 cups water. Bring to a full boil and then simmer for another 5 minutes. Use this as a gargle when it is lukewarm or at room temperature. It can even be made the night before. This gargle will help with mouth ulcers, bind teeth to gums (reduce looseness), and improve general oral health.

General tooth powder: Gather equal quantities of acacia bark, flowers, leaves, and pods and dry them in the sun. Grind them all and use this powder to brush your teeth. A dash of honey can be used to massage the gums and teeth. This powder will balance the ecosystem of your mouth and protect it from harmful microorganisms.

Gargle for sore throat and mouth ulcers: Make a decoction (see box "How to Make a Gargle" on page 281 for instructions) from dried bark powder or bark bits. Gargle with this decoction to keep your oral cavity healthy and prevent sore throats. Recurrent stomatitis, or mouth ulcers, can be quickly overcome with this gargle.

Strong teeth: The gum of the acacia tree is available in stores and online in the form of hardened, yellowish, translucent crystals of gum resin of varying sizes. You can lightly sautée the gum crystals in a tiny amount of ghee (enough to coat the bottom of the pan). The crystals pop within seconds, just like popcorn, and become crunchy. Be careful to not leave them in the hot pan too long as they will burn quickly. Mix 1 part popped gum crystals with 4 parts dry-roasted wheat flour, $\frac{1}{4}$ part chopped nuts such as walnuts and almonds, and organic raw sugar or rock candy crystals (to taste) to make a delicious snack. Simply eat a couple of teaspoons when you get the munchies. This recipe will not only satisfy your sweet taste, and please you with its nutty crunchiness, but the acacia gum will also nourish your bones and teeth. This recipe has been given to pregnant and lactating women in India for centuries to prevent osteoporosis or loss of dentine. The gum acts as a soothing analgesic and, together with wheat, helps in conditions of oral cavity lesions.

Canker sores and other oral lesions: The cooling styptic powder of acacia gum resin can also be applied directly to canker sores and other oral lesions to immediately arrest bleeding and reduce pain.

Sacred Song of the Holy Basil

The tulsi plant is a renowned herb that grows all over India. The word *tulsi* means "incomparable or matchless," an apt descriptor for its effectiveness for oral health. A triple-blind randomized controlled trial demonstrated that tulsi mouth rinse was equally effective in reducing plaque and gingivitis as chlorhexidine.[10]

Make it a habit to chew three to five fresh tulsi leaves a day or one or two tulsi leaves after every meal. This is the best way to protect your oral cavity (and overall health). Tulsi juice, which is hot in potency and penetrating, will effectively remove staleness and ensure that your mouth (gums and dental crevices) becomes a zone of perfect balance. The leaves are not bitter in taste; they are tolerably sharp in quality and quite likeable. In fact, even children chew on tulsi leaves in India. They freshen your entire oral cavity and wake up your senses if you overate at your last meal.

Toothpaste: Simply brush with dried tulsi leaf powder. Make a paste with water, and you are all set.

Toothache relief: Mix ½ teaspoon fresh tulsi leaf juice with 2 finely crushed black peppercorns and rub the juice on your aching tooth. Do this several times a day to relieve pain. You can also use this remedy for cavity prevention by applying tulsi juice to the gums at night before bed. This paste can also be used to fill an aching tooth cavity. Refresh cavity with new paste every few hours. In addition to providing relief from pain, the tulsi and black pepper are effective antibacterial agents.

Expressing juice from tulsi leaves is easy. Simply pound a handful of fresh leaves in a mortar and pestle. Then squeeze the pulp with your fingers and collect the expressed juice in a clean cup. You can refrigerate this juice in a covered jar if you like. It will stay good for at least a couple of days, but if you have the time, simply express the juice of 3 to 4 leaves as needed for your purposes. That is ideal.

Gargle: Mix equal parts fresh tulsi leaf juice with warm water to make a multipurpose gargle. It cures phlegm in the throat, improves your voice, and helps fight cavities. Massaging this onto gums helps overcome bleeding gums (gingivitis).

Amalaki (Phyllanthus emblica) the Wonder Fruit

Known as a *rasayana* in Sanskrit, amalaki is the fruit of a tropical and subtropical medium-sized tree that grows in dry areas. It is mainly a heart and brain restorative as well as a whole-body tonic, especially when consumed over an extended period of time. In fact, amalaki is considered Ayurveda's optimal rejuvenator: it balances all three doshas.

In oral health, amalaki is mainly utilized for tissue regeneration purposes, such as where gums or dental structure need to be nourished or simply strengthened against microorganisms.

Gargle: Amalaki powder (1 teaspoon) can be added to a glass of lukewarm water and used as a nourishing gargle to boost local immunity, voice, and gum strength.

Oral rinse for mouth sores: Amalaki also works especially well as an oral rinse in the case of mouth sores since it has cooling potency. It also promotes anticaries action, reduces plaque, and has an antibacterial effect.

Toothache relief: Squeeze leaves of amalaki to extract its juice and use for toothache relief.

Cloves, Love-Filled Buds

Cloves, known as *lavang* in Ayurveda tradition, are the dried flower buds of a small evergreen tree in the Myrtaceae family (*Syzygium aromaticum*). Throughout the year, this tree is dressed up with small, rosy buds and flowers. These buds are so beautiful that cloves are also called *devakusuma* in Sanskrit, which translates to "flowers of the divine." Clove mainly balances kapha and pitta doshas.[11]

Cloves are used for curing pathological thirst, reducing excessive sliminess in the oral cavity, and relieving bad breath. Clove is also a renowned pain relief agent for dental cavities. Every home should have clove oil handy in its first-aid box. Simply apply the oil to a swab and hold it close to your aching tooth or press an actual clove near the aching tooth. Some of the other benefits of clove include the following:

- Analgesic effects of the flower buds provide significant pain relief by acting through opioid receptors.[12]

- Eugenol extracts from clove have often been used with root canal therapy, temporary

fillings, and general gum pain. Eugenol and other components of clove combine to make clove a mild anesthetic as well as an antibacterial agent.[13]

- The germicidal properties of clove oil make it effective for relieving toothaches, sore gums, and mouth ulcers. Gargling with diluted clove oil helps in easing throat pain and irritation. The characteristic smell of clove oil also helps to eliminate bad breath.[14]

Other Medicinal Formulas

General antimicrobial formula: Mix equal amounts of the following three herbs in enough honey to make a paste-like consistency: neem, turmeric, and *guduchi* (*Tinaspora cordifolia*). This formula is packed with antimicrobial, antibiotic, and antifungal properties.

Painful and loose teeth formula: Mix equal parts ground cumin and Indian long pepper or *pippali* powder (*Piper nigrum*) with ¼ part rock salt. Use this powder to clean your teeth and also rub it on your gums. This combination is especially useful when gums are painful and teeth are loose.

Gingivitis formula: Mix equal amounts of ground ginger, ground black pepper, and ground long pepper (*Piper nigrum*) with ¼ part rock salt to make a powder for tooth cleaning. Use this daily, especially if you suffer from gingivitis.

Rotting teeth formula: Mix triphala powder with ½ part ground turmeric, ½ part ground ginger, and ¼ part rock salt. Use this combination to brush your teeth daily.

Swollen gums formula: Mix Indian madder or *majishtha* (*Rubia cordifolia*) powder with raw, unprocessed honey. Use this to massage your teeth and gums to overcome swollen or bleeding gums.

Tartar and foul-smell formula: Mix powder of licorice (*Glycyrrhiza glabra*) in honey and use this to brush your teeth. It is an effective anti-tartar agent.

Bleeding gums formula: Mix equal amounts of the following ingredients: ground clove, ground green cardamom, rock candy, and alum powder. This combination is especially useful to remove tartar buildup, counteract microorganisms, and prevent bleeding gums.

Eroding enamel formula: Mix equal amounts of the following powders: *musta* (*Cyperus rotundus*, also known as coco grass), rock salt, pomegranate, triphala, and ginger. Use this mixture to brush your teeth daily. All of these ingredients are available online or at specialty grocery and natural food stores.

More Home Remedies for Tooth Pain

- For pain in a tooth cavity, fill the cavity with the commonly available Indian spice asafoetida fried in ghee.

- Place a swab of cotton with pure edible camphor oil on the aching tooth.

- Fry 3 clove buds. Gently grind the buds into a powder with mortar and pestle (they will crumble easily), then mix with 1 teaspoon coconut oil. Apply on the aching tooth.

- Place a cotton swab mixed with oils of clove and cinnamon on the aching tooth.

- Mix a paste of fresh grated ginger with an equal amount of edible camphor powder and a small amount of rock salt. Apply this mixture to the aching tooth.

- Mix pippali powder with honey. Apply this paste to the aching tooth repeatedly.

- Mix ½ cup sesame oil, ⅛ cup licorice powder, ⅛ cup ground cloves, and ½ cup honey. Gargle with this mixture or hold it in your oral cavity for as long as you comfortably can, at least three times a day. This mixture will keep for several days on your kitchen counter (no need to refrigerate), as long as you keep it away from dust and water.

Kitchen and Garden Ingredients for Homemade Gargles

In the preceding sections, I have discussed many botanicals in-depth. They can be sourced to make oral gargles. Below are a few more important botanicals that you can use to make homemade gargles using the instructions in the box "How to Make a Gargle."

Aloe vera: The Aloe plant has several hundred varieties, and all of them demonstrate antibacterial, antifungal, and anti-inflammatory properties. In Ayurveda, it is known as *kumari* and is celebrated for its cooling, bitter, blood- and skin-purifying, and antimicrobial properties. It is a rasayana, an immunity-enhancing agent. Aloe is also used as an expectorant and an antitoxin.

Cinnamon: Known as *tvak* or *dalchini*, cinnamon is the dried inner bark of the middle-sized evergreen tree *Cinnamomum zeylanicum*. The bark is sweet and pungent in taste and warm in action. It has a cooling aftereffect in the mouth. This aromatic bark has demonstrated antimicrobial as well as antioxidant properties in studies. Cinnamon not only prevents cavities, but also eliminates bad breath.

Coriander: An aromatic herbaceous annual, coriander (*Corriandrum sativum*) is from the parsley family. Both the leaves and seeds are cooling in potency, and the herb itself balances all three doshas. A coriander gargle is great for counteracting chronic or acute stomatitis (mouth ulcers).

Corn mint: This is a special species of mint (*Mentha arvensis*), different from common grocery store varieties. Corn mint seeds are available online. A gargle made with fresh leaves is excellent for bad breath, as well as for preventing dental cavities.

False pepper: Vidanga (*Embelia ribes*) is a small-sized evergreen tree that grows in temperate forests. It is used in parasitical infestation. It is available online, as a powder, or as berries of *vidanga*, which is its Sanskrit name. As a gargle, it helps overcome dental infection as well as swelling and pain.

Fennel: *Foeniculum vulgare* is a glabrous biennial or perennial aromatic herb, known as *shatpushpa* in Sanskrit. The fruit is used as a mouth freshener. It is sweet in taste and semihot in potency. A gargle with fennel seeds acts as an anti-inflammatory and an antispasmodic agent, and is especially effective in sore throats and hoarseness.

How to Make a Gargle

Making your own all-natural gargle with any of the botanicals in this section is easy, and you can employ one of the two methods I suggest here: the steeping method (which is simpler and also quicker and works well when you are in a hurry) or the decoction method (which is a bit more time-consuming but creates a more potent formula).

Steeping method: Place 1 part herbs in a container and pour 4 parts boiling water over them. Cover the container and allow it to sit and cool naturally overnight. In the morning, strain and use. Remember to give a good shake daily.

Decoction method: Boil 1 part herbs to 8 parts water. Boil until water is reduced by half. Strain. Cool to desired temperature and use. The decoction method makes a stronger gargle than steeping, but the steeping process is less involved.

Additional Points to Remember

- Use only fresh, pure water. Never mix gargle ingredients in fruit juices or milk.

- Dried herbs generally need a heat source to bring out their qualities, so boiling is preferred over steeping when using dried herbs.

- Nonbotanical ingredients, such as rock salt or edible camphor, do not need to be heated; simply mix them to make a ready gargle.

- Essential oils should not be heated. Simply mix them into room temperature water.

Fenugreek: *Trigonella foenum-greacum* (known as *methica* in Sanskrit and *methi* in Hindi) is an annual aromatic prized for its seeds that are used both in cooking and medicine. The whole plant is pungent, hot, and drying. Gargling with an infusion of its fresh leaves a minimum of three times a day for a couple of days helps overcome gum infection and stomatitis (mouth ulcers).

Green cardamom: Known as *ela* in Sanskrit, green cardamom is an aromatic seedpod from an herbaceous perennial (*Elettaria cardamomum*). Its gargle is used mainly for correcting foul odor from teeth and/or rotting gums. Simply placing a pod directly in your mouth and sucking on it also helps. However, as a gargle, the herb reaches deep underneath the gum line.

Hibiscus: *Hibiscus rosa-sinensis*, known as *japakusum* in Sanskrit, is an evergreen shrub with ornamental flowers. A gargle made with these flowers or leaves, or both, is used for stomatitis (mouth ulcers) and mouth odor. Mixed with turmeric, it becomes an effective anti-infective as well as a soothing gargle.

Jasmine: *Jasminum grandiflorum* is a fragrant creeper with white flowers known as *sumana* in Sanskrit. It balances all three doshas, with special benefits for pitta and kapha doshas. Its leaf oil is a natural analgesic. A decoction of jasmine leaves (fresh or dried) cures boils in the mouth and fights periodontal disease. Its leaves can also be chewed directly.

Licorice: Known as *yashtimadhu* in Sanskrit, *Glycyrrhiza glabra* has been used successfully to alleviate vata and pitta doshas. As a mouthwash ingredient, it heals stomatitis (mouth ulcers). It also helps overcome dry mouth and bad taste on the tongue.

Mango: Grind the peel of ripe mango (known as *amra* in Sanskrit) along with fresh leaves from the mango tree (*Mangifera indica*) in equal amounts to make a fine paste. Mix this paste with water. Gargle with it to impart strength to your teeth and gums.

Marigold: *Tagetes erecta*, known as *zendu* in Sanskrit, is a flower that can be grown in most homes. A decoction made from leaves and petals (fresh or dried) of the marigold flower relieves toothache and helps overcome inflammation and stomatitis (mouth ulcers), since marigold is cooling in potency. Its leaf paste can also be applied directly to affected gums.

Homemade Breath Fresheners

Certain foods that we eat, or that get stuck in our teeth, can impart bad breath. According to Ayurveda, excess pitta dosha accumulated in the stomach can also cause a foul smell. Ayurveda has come up with the perfect all-natural solution for freshening the breath by suggesting sucking on spices or drinking teas that are not only aromatic, but also pacify pitta. Here is a list of few of them:

- Pop a whole green cardamom pod into your mouth and chew it. After a while, spit the empty pod out.

- Chew a whole clove; it burns in the beginning, but then it sweetens and cools the saliva and freshens the entire oral cavity (and makes it germ-free!).

- Chew ½ teaspoon dry-roasted fennel seeds after each meal. Simply pop them into your mouth and chew. They are sweet and tasty. You can also chew raw fennel seeds, but lightly roasted ones are crunchier.

- Dry roast equal amounts of fennel seeds, white sesame seeds, and split coriander seeds separately. Mix together and add rock salt and rock candy to taste. Chew this combination, about ½ teaspoon each time, after every meal.

- Drink a cup of mint tea at the end of your meal. Hold the tea in your mouth for a few seconds before swallowing. Mint will do the work!

The Ayurvedic Diet Resource Guide

Seasonal Food Recommendations

Ayurveda divides the year into six seasons (*ritu*). Doshas accumulate, peak, and subside in different seasons (macrocosm), influencing the doshas in our bodies (microcosm). It is therefore important to eat a diet that balances a peaking dosha in a given season (see table 35).

These recommendations are applicable for the northern hemisphere. Adjust calendar dates if you live in the southern hemisphere.

The recommendations provided below are timeless yet universal, and they are directly sourced from ancient texts. The diets also have been tested by me over the last three decades. My students and clients have affirmed the recommendations with great success in preventing disease and optimizing health and well-being.[1]

TABLE 35 **Season-Based Dosha Rhythm**

	LATE WINTER (Jan. 15–March 14)	SPRING (March 15–May 14)	EARLY SUMMER (May 15–July 14)	LATE SUMMER/ RAINY SEASON (July 15–Sept. 14)	AUTUMN (Sept. 15–Nov. 14)	EARLY WINTER (Nov. 15–Jan. 14)
Kapha	Kapha begins to accumulate	Kapha peaks	Kapha subsides			
Vata			Vata begins to accumulate	Vata peaks	Vata subsides	
Pitta				Pitta begins to accumulate	Pitta peaks	Pitta subsides

THE EARLY AND LATE WINTER SEASONS
November 15 to January 14 and January 15 to March 14

Nature: In general, Ayurveda declares winter as the healthiest season. However, the body's natural intelligence copes with the external cold by automatically increasing the agni in the belly (a physiological response), resulting in increased inner warmth. Naturally, appetite and hunger also increase in parallel. Hence, if we fast in this season or eat a lot of cold and light foods, like salads, vata dosha can go up due to increased quality of lightness and coldness (the principle of "like increases like" at work). So eating nutritious fatty food at the right time (in winter) is a precautionary measure.

Goal: We make the best use of a naturally increased agni in winter and make every meal count. We can eat nourishing foods (see "Preferred Winter Food List" that follows) to proactively build health and immunity for the entire year ahead.

Flavors: Increase intake of sweet, sour, and salty; reduce intake of sour, pungent, and bitter.

Qualities: Prefer heavy over light, and fatty over dry foods.

Specifics: Hearty meat and vegetable soups with added ghee fortify the body. A midday drink of Ayurvedic buttermilk is recommended every day (see recipe on page 313). Eat 1 tablespoon raw honey daily if possible (especially in the morning).

Preferred Winter Food List

Cereals: Unfermented wheat products (bran, cereal, chapatis, cookies, cream of wheat, crepes, dumplings, pudding, tortillas), white or brown rice, rice pudding. In moderation: quinoa, millet, oats.

Legumes and beans: Black gram, black beans, kidney beans, mung.

Vegetables: Asparagus, beets, cabbage, carrots, cilantro, eggplant, fennel root (anise), garlic, green beans, green peas, leeks, okra (in early winter only), onions (cooked), parsnips, pumpkin, radish, rutabaga, spaghetti squash, spinach, sweet potatoes, turnips, winter melon, winter squash.

Fruits: Amalaki (a nutritious fruit supplement; available online), almonds, apples, dates, figs, grapefruit, guavas, lemon, lime, mandarins, oranges, pears, plums, pomegranate, tangerines.

Meat: Chicken, deer, goat, pig, rabbit, seafood soup, turkey.

Alcohol: Aged wine is ideal.

Seeds: Sesame.

Dried fruits and nuts: Almonds, cashews, macadamia nuts, pecans, pine nuts, pistachios, raisins, walnuts.

Dairy: Sweet butter, Ayurvedic buttermilk (takra), sweet cream, milk (boiled), yogurt, (never frozen or with fruit, always eat with added raw honey or crushed back pepper).

Water: Drink boiled water reduced to warm, drinkable temperature.

Fat: Ghee is best; all other natural cooking oils are also fine (except mustard oil).

Other: Honey, *chyawanprash* (Ayurvedic supplement), vinegar in moderation.

Contraindicated in Winter

- Fasting and skipping meals
- Eating salads and raw foods
- Consuming chilled foods like ice cream, chilled water, frozen foods

THE SPRING SEASON
March 15 to May 14

Nature: Kapha dosha, which slowly built up or accumulated over winter, is said to peak in spring, dulling our agni. Due to the melting action of the increased heat in spring, excess kapha can result in allergies.

Goal: To follow a Kapha-balancing diet.

Flavors: Prefer bitter, astringent, and pungent over sweet, sour, and salty tastes.

Qualities: Prefer light-to-digest, drier, and warmer foods over cold, heavy, fatty, and liquid foods.

Specifics: Eat meat sparingly or avoid altogether. Use extra warming spices, eat smaller portions. Green gram, leafy greens, honey, and hot water plus a walking and exercise regimen is recommended.

Preferred Spring Food List

Lentils: Green gram is best.

Vegetables: Artichokes, arugula, bell peppers, bitter greens like kale and collard greens, bitter vegetables like bitter melon, broccoli, Brussels sprouts, cabbage, cauliflower, carrots, celery, curry leaves, daikon and daikon greens, dandelion greens, eggplant, green beans, leeks, neem leaves, raw onions, parsley, peppers, turnip greens, turnips, all varieties of gourds (especially pointed gourd).

Fruits: Minimize or completely abstain from fruit. Not many fruits ripen in spring anyway. Cherries and papaya along with rhubarb and plums are okay in moderation. Eat fruit only in the daytime, never in the evening.

Meat: Boil, bake, or roast all types of meats versus frying. Rabbit meat is best, followed by goat meat, chicken, and turkey. Add digestive spices and cook well.

Alcohol: Abstain from, or dilute in water.

Seeds: None recommended.

Dried fruits and nuts: None recommended.

Dairy: Diluted and boiled hot cow milk, goat milk, Ayurvedic buttermilk.

Water: Drink boiled water while still quite hot.

Fat: Minimize the amount of fat you use in daily cooking; ghee is best, can also use olive oil or mustard oil.

Other: Honey, as it is anti-kapha.

Contraindicated in Spring

- Overeating and snacking
- Late-night meals
- Most fruits, fruit juices, smoothies, excess drinking water
- Butter and cheese, cold milk, ice cream and cold desserts, chilled water, yogurt

EARLY SUMMER
May 15 to July 14

Nature: The increasing heat counteracts the cold quality of kapha from the previous season, which now begins to subside. The increasing dryness (from heat) causes vata dosha to accumulate. Because of the heat, pitta will begin accumulating in late summer and peak in autumn. So, all in all, both vata and some pitta need to be managed over the course of summer. Due to outer heat, the inner agni automatically retreats in terms of intensity—this is body's intelligence at work, so lighter foods must be consumed so they can digest with ease.

Goal: To balance both vata and pitta doshas with sweet taste, which pacifies both doshas.

Flavors: Prefer naturally occurring sweet taste in every meal. Minimize hot tastes (pungent, sour, salty) and drying tastes (astringent and bitter).

Qualities: Prefer moist over dry foods, less fatty over oily, light over hard to digest, cooling over hot foods, soupy or liquid over dense and hard food textures.

Specifics: Prefer yogurt smoothies (*lassi*) made with cane sugar, fresh squeezed sweet fruit juices, sweet lemonade, and coconut water, moist cooling vegetables like cucumber, squashes, and caramelized onions along with stir-fried vegetables and meats.

Preferred Early Summer Food List

Cereals: Rice (best), sweet corn, oats, wheat.

Lentils: Mung lentil.

Vegetables: Avocado, beets, carrots, cilantro, cucumber juice and soup, green beans, okra, white onions caramelized in ghee, opo squash, all squashes, snake gourd, summer squash, wax gourd, yam.

Fruits: Apricot, blackberry, cactus pear, cantaloupe, coconut (and coconut water), dates, honeydew, mango, melons, nectarines, oranges, peaches, plums, pomegranate, raisins, raspberries. **Note:** Do not eat if fruit is sour or unripe.

Meat: Seafood (best), chicken, or goat (soupy or mildly spiced curry recipes).

Alcohol: Minimize or dilute with water.

Seeds: Sunflower seeds.

Dried fruits: Raisins.

Dairy: All dairy: ghee, sweet butter, milk, yogurt with cane sugar (but not at night).

Water: Water cooled in clay pitchers.

Fat: Ghee (best), coconut oil, sunflower oil.

Other: Rose petal jam (an Ayurveda supplement called *gulkand*, available online), desserts made of milk and cane sugar.

Spices: Mainly cardamom, coriander, cumin, fennel, rock salt, mint, turmeric.

Specifics: Temperature-wise, food can be allowed to cool down a bit before consuming. Fermented and sprouted foods increase bodily heat; avoid them. Minimize salads; add a generous amount of oil or ghee if consumed.

Contraindicated in Early Summer
- Garlic and very spicy foods
- Salty chips, garam masala, raw onions, peanuts, salsa, sesame seeds, wasabi, and other such sharp, heating food
- Chilies, eggplant, mustard leaves, papaya, peppers, pickles, pineapple, red onions, tomato, and mustard seed oil, peanut oil, and sesame oil in cooking

LATE SUMMER
July 15 to September 14

Nature: Vata dosha peaks, pitta begins to accumulate, and agni weakens even further. This is the least healthy season of the year. Eat ultralight, easy-to-digest foods. This period requires two separate sets of diets:

- In areas such as California where I live, as well as in many parts of the United States, heat and dryness continue to build up in late summer. This requires one set of diet recommendations.

- In large areas of the southwestern United States and northwestern Mexico (and countries like India), this is the rainy season. The weather becomes wet in July and August, a contrast to the rather dry May and June. This is known as the North American monsoon or Arizona monsoon. It rains almost until mid-September when fall begins, which is drier and cooler (and quite cold on the East Coast).[2]

Diet for Dry and Hot Late Summer
Simply continue with the early summer recommendations given above.

Diet for Wet and Humid Late Summer

Goal: To continue eating foods that balance vata dosha since rains (monsoon) following a hot summer are said to aggravate all doshas, but especially the vata dosha. Since it is the season of poorest immunity and potential challenge to health, it is a good idea to eat measured quantities and ensure we are following the various food rules and not compromising our agni.

Flavors: Unlike early summer, when the sweet taste was maximally recommended, it is now time to add back the salty and sour tastes (while continuing with sweet taste) since salt and sour tastes additionally balance out the aggravated vata dosha. Also, continue avoiding the bitter, pungent, and astringent tastes.

Qualities: The key to cooking monsoon foods is preparing dishes that are light to digest, enhance digestion (via use of spices) and boost immunity (by using adequate ghee and turmeric). Use less (but adequate) fat in cooking overall so that the food is never a liability due to its oiliness.

Specifics: Essential ingredients include a moderate amount of ghee in cooking and spices such as black pepper, asafoetida, coriander, cumin powder, ginger, and turmeric. Enjoy seasonal fruits, but avoid raw foods and nuts as much as possible. Leafy vegetables must also be generally avoided in areas that get the late-summer monsoons.

Preferred Monsoon Food List

Cereals: Puffed rice, add a tiny amount of ground ginger to boiled rice for additional digestibility; eat wheat only in preparations where it is roasted with a minimal addition of fat; barley is also great during monsoon season.

Lentils: Green gram is best.

Dairy: Buttermilk with ground ginger, ghee, milk boiled with ground turmeric and ginger.

Vegetables: Eat more soups; avoid all raw vegetables. Choose mainly cluster beans, carrots, gourd family (snake gourd, pointed gourd, apple gourd, and bitter gourd), pumpkin, all squashes, yam.

Fruits: Lemon juice in hot water with added rock salt and ground cumin is helpful in aiding digestion. Blackberries, cherries, Indian plum (*jamun*), lychee, mulberry, peaches, plums, pineapple.

Meat: Easy-to-digest meats such as chicken, goat, rabbit, and turkey are preferred over heavy-to-digest meats, like beef and pork. Light soups are preferred over fried preparations.

Alcohol: Wine is okay; aged is better.

Seeds: Sunflower.

Dried fruits: Raisins mainly.

Water: Boiled; drink lukewarm.

Fat: Ghee; minimize quantity used to maximize digestibility.

Other: Eat 2 tablespoons raw honey first thing in morning during monsoons.

Spices: Must use black pepper, coriander, cumin, ground ginger, turmeric.

Contraindicated in Monsoon

- Astringent, bitter, pungent foods
- Heavy-to-digest foods including deep-fried foods, cream
- Cold milk, paneer and other cheese, yogurt
- Leafy vegetables
- Fish and other seafood

THE AUTUMN SEASON
September 15 to November 14

Nature: Pitta, which had been accumulating during the early and late summer/rainy season, accumulates enough to peak in autumn (even if the weather is apparently cooler). Pitta conditions, such as rashes, fever, diarrhea, acne, stomatitis, blisters, and heat rash proliferate. A dosha that builds up in a previous season is bound to peak the following season.

Goal: Ayurveda recommends consuming a pitta-balancing diet.

Flavors: Prefer sweet and slightly bitter and astringent over pungent, sour, salty foods.

Qualities: Prefer cooling over hot foods, light over heavy foods. Prefer sweet, light, cold, and slightly bitter foods.

Specifics: Pomegranate is the fruit of this season, to be consumed daily along with other sweet (not sour), well-ripened fruits.

Preferred Autumn Food List

Cereals: Barley, rice, wheat.

Lentils: Green gram.

Vegetables: Beans, bitter greens like kale, bitter vegetables like bitter melon, Brussels sprouts, cabbage, carrots, cauliflower, collard greens, dandelion greens, kohlrabi, leeks, lettuce, okra, cooked onions, parsnips, potatoes, pumpkin varieties, spinach, all squashes, sweet potatoes, yam varieties.

Fruits: Apples, berries, dates, grapes, nectarines, sweet oranges, peaches, pears, persimmons, plums, pomegranate, water chestnut.

Meat: Boil, bake, or roast meat of rabbit or deer versus frying or cooking in oil.

Alcohol: Abstain, minimize, or dilute in water; alcohol excites pitta so exercise caution.

Seeds: Sunflower seeds.

THE AUTUMN SEASON
September 15 to November 14 (continued)

Dried fruits: Raisins.

Dairy: Buttermilk with added cane sugar, sweet butter, ghee, cow milk, goat milk.

Water: Drink cool water in clay pitchers or by exposing to autumn moonlight.

Fat: Ghee, coconut oil, or sunflower oil.

Other: Cow milk, Indian gooseberry (amalaki) supplement (fruit, juice, or powder).

Contraindicated in Autumn

- Fermented, spicy, sharp foods
- Yogurt is prohibited
- All seafood

Notes on a Few Food Items

Honey: Ideally, honey should be local, raw, and unprocessed. Honey is never heated or cooked in Ayurveda, nor added to hot liquids or foods at any time. It can be eaten by itself or drizzled on room-temperature foods or on fresh or dried fruits.

Beans and lentils: *Dal* is a traditional term that refers to pulses, beans, lentils, and dried peas. It is also the name of a soup-like dish cooked with lentils. Mung dal (green gram) is considered the easiest to digest and great for all three doshas. Urad dal (black gram) is heaviest in quality and oiliest in nature (hence, ideal for vata dosha). Store dals for up to a year, away from direct sunlight. Dals always require presoaking.

The gourd family of vegetables: Also identified as squashes. I encourage exploring your local Asian or Indian grocery store for more exotic gourds. Here are the common Indian names for easier identification: bitter gourd (*karela*), pointed gourd (*parval*), winter gourd (*petha*), opo or bottle gourd (*doodhi*), ivy gourd (*kundru*), snake gourd (*chichinda*), ridge gourd (*torai*), and chayote (*tinda*). These gourds can be cooked like winter squash and zucchini.

Dosha-Balancing Diet Recommendations

As mentioned in chapter 6, a dosha-balancing diet is eaten for relatively short periods until dosha symptoms subside. For this purpose, eat mainly the foods in the following lists, based on which dosha needs balancing, and abstain from or minimize all other foods not listed. The following guidelines are specifically written with dosha pacification through food in mind. For instance, if you are noticing the symptoms of vata dosha aggravation (as described in Symptoms of Aggravated Vata Dosha on page 40), then you simply follow the vata dosha food guidelines below for a short while (say a few weeks or months) and notice the difference. At times, you may notice the symptoms of more than one dosha simultaneously. In such case, pacify the dosha that is maximally aggravated first through food choices.

Vata Guidelines

Regularity, predictability, and easy digestibility help counteract an overexpressed vata dosha. Follow these food guidelines to balance an over-expressed vata dosha. You do not have to eat exclusively from this list (although you could), but you can incorporate more foods from this list into your diet. Also, keep this list handy when you go grocery shopping:

- Prefer sweet, sour, and salty tastes over bitter, pungent, and astringent tastes.

- Eat hot versus cold foods (temperature- and quality-wise).

- Always cook foods in fats like ghee or vegetable oils.

- Use spices to help promote agni.

- Never eat raw foods (except fruits).

- Fix mealtimes and eat slowly.

Pitta Guidelines

Cooling, pleasing, digestive foods pacify pitta dosha. Follow these guidelines:

- Prefer sweet, bitter, and astringent foods over sour, salty, and pungent foods.

- Choose cooler foods over excessively hot foods (temperature- and quality-wise).

- Choose moderately oily foods (and not deep fried); prefer ghee as a cooking medium.

- Lightly spice your recipes versus overly spiced recipes.

- Always cook your foods; avoid raw.

Kapha Guidelines

The general rule to pacify kapha is to eat in moderation, never late at night, and stay active after eating. Follow these guidelines:

- Choose pungent, bitter, and astringent tasting foods over sweet, sour, and salty foods.

- Choose hot versus cold foods (temperature and quality-wise).

- Choose cooked versus raw foods for easy digestibility.

- Eat light-to-digest versus heavy-to-digest foods (keep dinner ultra-light).

- Eat less fatty foods versus heavy, oily, fried foods.

Stock Your Kitchen with Ayurvedic Spices

From time immemorial, Ayurvedic kitchen spices have served a dual function of protecting and optimizing the agni and imparting incredible flavor at the same time. Ayurvedic spices are easily procured online or at specialty grocery stores. Store them in a dry place away from direct sunlight. For maximum potency, plan to use within six to eight months of purchase. At a minimum, invest in rock salt, cumin seeds, ground turmeric, ground coriander, and asafoetida (*hing*), for daily use. In the following descriptions, I have listed both the Latin name (L) and the common Indian name (I) for easy identification.

Asafoetida

(L) *Ferula foetida* (I) *Heeng* or *Hing*

Qualities: Pungent, heating, sharp, subtle, light, oily; alleviates kapha and vata, but okay for pitta when cooked in ghee. Antiflatulent, digestive, anticolic, vermicide, stimulant.

Black Pepper

(L) *Piper nigrum* (I) *Kali Mirch*

Qualities: Pungent, heating, sharp, dry, light, alleviates kapha and vata, aggravates pitta. Appetizer, digestive, antitoxic, antipruritic, antiparasitic, great for respiratory health.

Cardamom, Black

(L) *Amomum subulatum* (I) *Badi Elaichi*

Qualities: Pungent, heating; mainly vata- and kapha-balancing. Can aggravate pitta in excess or when eaten in fall.

Cardamom, Green

(L) *Elettaria cardamomum* (I) *Elaichi*

Qualities: Pungent, yet cooling; vata- and kapha-balancing; does not aggravate pitta; appetizer, antiemetic, carminative, beneficial for hemorrhoids.

Carom Seed/Bishop's Weed

(L) *Carum roxburghianum* (I) *Ajwain*

Qualities: Pungent, sharp, heating, light, oily; kapha- and vata-alleviating, digestive, vermicide, antispasmodic, antiflatulent, antitoxin.

Cilantro/Coriander

(L) *Coriandrum sativum* (I) *Dhaniya*

Qualities: Bitter, astringent, heating; oily, light, alleviates all three doshas, appetizer, digestive, diuretic, stops burning sensation of urine, helps absorption.

Cinnamon Bark

(L) *Cinnamomum zeylanicum* (I) *Dalchini*

Qualities: Sweet, bitter, pungent, and heating. Mainly kapha- and vata-pacifying; helps regulate body's water content.

Clove

(L) *Caryophyllus aromaticus* (I) *Lavang*

Qualities: Pungent and bitter, cooling, but sharp, light, oily; alleviates kapha and pitta; appetizer, digestive, antitoxin, antiparasitic.

TABLE 36   Dosha-Balancing Food List

	VATA	PITTA	KAPHA
Cereals	Amaranth, cooked oats, rice, wheat, corn	Barley, buckwheat, corn, oats, rice, semolina, spelt, tapioca, wheat	Barley, millet, rice (mainly in summer or as utilized in Ayurveda recipes with spices), rye
Pulses	Black gram (best), mung beans, red lentils	Mung beans (best), red lentils, pinto beans	Mung beans with skin (best), horse gram (cow pea)
Vegetables	Asparagus, avocado, beets, carrots, daikon root and leaves, drumsticks (pods from the moringa tree; *sahjan*), eggplant, garlic, ginger, gourds (ash, ivy, pointed, snake), leeks, okra, onion, parsnip, pumpkin, radish, rutabaga, all varieties of squashes, sweet potato, turnips, winter melon, yam, zucchini	Asparagus, bitter gourd, bitter melon, broccoli, cabbage, celery, chayote, cucumber, daikon root and leaves, drumsticks (pods from the moringa tree; *sahjan*), gourds (apple, ash, ivy, pointed snake, ridge), green beans, leafy greens (except mustard and fenugreek greens), lotus tuber, onions (cooked), opo, parsnips, peas (sweet), potatoes (white and red), pumpkin, root vegetables, sweet potatoes, taro root (giant), water chestnut, watercress, wheat grass, zucchini	Asparagus, bell peppers, bitter gourd, broccoli, carrots, celery, chayote, chicory, daikon roots and leaves, drumsticks (pods from the moringa tree; *sahjan*), eggplant, endive, fennel, fenugreek, garlic, gourds (pointed and snake), green beans, leafy greens (including mustard, spinach), lettuce, onions (raw), radish

TABLE 36   Dosha-Balancing Food List (cont.)

	VATA	PITTA	KAPHA
Fruits	Almonds, apricots, bananas, berries, coconut, dates, figs, grapefruit, grapes, guava, jackfruit, lemon, lime, mango, nectarines, oranges, papaya, peaches, pears, persimmons, pineapple, plums, pomegranate	Amalaki (Indian gooseberry), apples, bananas, berries, coconut, dates, grapes, jackfruit, mango (sweet, in moderation), melons, nectarines (sweet), oranges (sweet), peaches (sweet), plums (sweet), pomegranate, raisins, water chestnut	Blackberries, blueberries, cranberries, figs, lemon and lime (in moderation), pears, pomegranate, prunes, raisins (in moderation), strawberries
Meats	Beef (in moderation, with spices), bison, buffalo, eggs (chicken and duck), fish and all seafood, goat meat is best	Ideal: goat, buffalo, and rabbit. Also eat freshwater or grass carp from ocean (in summer); chicken (more in winter); turkey; egg whites	In extreme moderation: chicken, goat, rabbit (eat roasted not fried)
Spices	All spices except red chili powder and flakes	Only use cardamom (green), cilantro, coriander, cumin, curry leaves, fennel seeds, neem (sweet), parsley, rock salt, saffron (only when cooked in milk), turmeric	All spices, including red chili powder and flakes in moderation
Dairy	All dairy (never cold) except cheese; yogurt (nonfrozen) eaten only in daytime, sprinkled with black pepper and rock salt to taste, or with added honey, or with green mung soup	All dairy except yogurt and cheese; never drink cold milk (fresh cottage cheese or mozzarella okay in moderation)	Ayurvedic buttermilk, best with added spices; goat or cow milk boiled with spices; avoid cheese and yogurt completely

	VATA	PITTA	KAPHA
Nuts and Seeds	All nuts and seeds	Charoli, coconut, pumpkin seeds, sunflower seeds	Pumpkin seeds, sunflower seeds
Fats	Ghee, avocado oil, flax oil, coconut oil, peanut oil, sesame oil, sunflower oil	Ghee, butter (sweet goat's or cow's milk), coconut oil, safflower oil, sunflower oil	Ghee, olive oil, mustard oil, sesame oil
Sweeteners	All sugarcane-based products (raw sugar, crystallized sugar, jaggery) and honey	Mainly sugarcane-based sweeteners (rock candy is best)	Mainly jaggery (in moderation), honey is great
Beverages	Licorice root tea, warm milk, warm water, Ayurvedic buttermilk with spices	Licorice root tea, warm milk with cane sugar, room-temperature water (cool during summer or fall), and Ayurvedic buttermilk with cane sugar	Licorice root tea, ginger tea, holy basil tea, peppermint tea, boiled goat milk with spices, warm/ hot water, Ayurvedic buttermilk with spices
Alcohol	Wine preferred over hard alcohol; aged wine preferred	Dilute, minimize, or completely abstain (until dosha returns to balance)	Minimize or completely abstain (until dosha returns to balance)

Cumin Seeds

(L) *Cuminum cyminum* (I) *Zeera*

Qualities: Pungent, heating, sharp, dry, light; promotes digestion, alleviates vata and kapha, increases pitta only slightly. Appetizer, antispasmodic, relieves diarrhea.

Fennel Seeds

(L) *Foeniculum vulgare* (I) *Saunf*

Qualities: Bitter, sweet, pungent, heating; light, oily, sharp; alleviates kapha and vata, does not increase pitta, improves agni; anti-inflammatory, diuretic, antiparasitic, antispasmodic, stimulant, digestive.

Fenugreek Seeds

(L) *Trigonella foenum-graecum* (I) *Methi*

Qualities: Bitter, heating; increases pitta, balances vata and kapha.

Garlic

(L) *Allium sativum* (I) *Lehsun*

Qualities: Possesses all five tastes except sour; heating, oily, sharp, heavy, slimy; alleviates kapha and vata; aggravates pitta. Laxative, aphrodisiac, rejuvenating, antitoxin, anticholesterol, antiobesity, antiparasitic.

Ginger, Dried

(L) *Zingiber officinale* (I) *Shunthi*

Qualities: Light yet oily, balances all three doshas, appetizer, antiflatulent, relieves constipation, aphrodisiac, aids recovery from coughs and colds, antitoxin.

Ginger, Fresh

(L) *Zingiber officinale* (I) *Adrak*

Qualities: Sharp, heavy, and hot; alleviates all three doshas; appetizer; antiflatulent; can increase pitta in excess.

Mustard Seeds

(L) *Brassica campestris* (I) *Sarson*

Qualities: Pungent, bitter, heating, sharp, heavy, oily; vata- and kapha-decreasing; pitta- and agni-increasing. Antiparasitic, antitoxic, antipruritic. The white variety is said to be superior to the red (or brown) variety of seeds.

Nutmeg

(L) *Myristica fragrans* (I) *Jaiphal*

Qualities: Pungent, bitter, astringent, hot, light, sharp, oily. Nutmeg mainly alleviates vata and kapha and acts as a digestive.

Rock Salt (Himalayan Pink Salt)

(L) *Sodium chloride* (I) *Sendha Namak*

Qualities: Salty-sweet (not salty alone), sharp, only semi-hot, penetrating, subtle, fluid but light (not heavy like other salts). While most salts maximally alleviate vata dosha, increase pitta dosha, and liquefy kapha dosha, rock salt pacifies all three doshas. Hence, it is the best salt in Ayurveda. It acts as mild laxative and mild sedative. It is an appetizer, beneficial for eyes (while most salts are harmful), and does not cause burning sensation in the digestive tract if consumed in excess (while all other salts do). It is an aphrodisiac, while other salts are not. See box, "Why Rock Salt?" to learn more.

Saffron

(L) *Crocus sativus* (I) *Kesar*

Qualities: Pungent, bitter, heating. Mainly vata- and kapha-pacifying, and pitta too, when cooked in ghee or milk. It is highly beneficial for skin.

Turmeric

(L) *Curcuma longa* (I) *Haldi*

Qualities: Bitter, pungent, heating; antidiabetic, hemopoietic, decreases kapha and pitta, also balances vata (when cooked in ghee, oil, or milk). Appetizer, antitoxic, anticarcinogenic, antiparasitic, antiseptic, antiobesity, antiacne. Purifies blood, improves skin, removes blemishes and imparts glow.

Commonly Recommended Pulses in Ayurveda

Pulses are a class of legumes including beans, peas, and lentils and have been used in Ayurveda cooking since ancient times. From

Why Rock Salt?

Rock salt, also known as Himalayan pink salt, has recently gained popularity in the United States. Ayurveda's textual as well as lived traditions greatly praise rock salt and suggest that it should be used (as required) by everyone, year-round, irrespective of dosha.[3] What makes rock salt so special?

Rock salt's story began more than 200 million years ago, when the Himalayas, earth's tallest (and youngest) mountain range, was still under water. Crystallized sea salt beds were covered with rich lava due to undersea volcanic explosions. Then, in the Ice Age that followed, this salt was enveloped in ice for millennia, during which time the qualities of coolness entered the salt crystals.

The ice also protected the salt, saturated with minerals, and locked in all its pristine goodness. Rock salt contains 84 of the 92 trace elements required by the body, including calcium, iron, zinc, potassium, magnesium, copper, and so on. An additional benefit is that because rock salt is less refined, we consume less sodium per serving than with regular table salt or sea salt.

Currently, the best rock salt is mined in the form of halite (colorless, cubic, mineralized crystals) from the mountains of the Himalayas, spanning across China, Nepal, Myanmar, Pakistan, Bhutan, Afghanistan, and of course, India. It isn't an exaggeration to say that among salts, rock salt is the purest and coolest salt on the planet today. This is why unlike the multiple other salts the Ayurveda texts mention (and also appreciate, such as sea salt, sulfur salt, and others), rock salt is mentioned with special reverence.

Rock salt is unique among salts in that it pacifies all three doshas. Its salty nature, heat, and oiliness perfectly pacifies vata dosha. Its extraordinary qualities of sweetness and coolness (imparted by geological forces) pacifies pitta dosha; and its lightness versus heaviness and its ability to evoke digestive fire and penetrate subtle channels helps pacify kapha dosha.

Note: Sea salt is superior to the ultra-processed common table salt, and it is also rich in minerals. It is, however, unlike rock salt, not three-dosha balancing (it increases kapha and pitta in excess), and it is also perhaps not as pristine as rock salt since our oceans are unfortunately more and more polluted today.

a modern nutritional perspective, legumes are a nutrient-dense plant protein as well as a great source of fiber, vitamins, and minerals, including folate, manganese, iron, potassium, magnesium, and copper. They are also economical and easy to store long-term and can be used in many dishes. Ayurveda texts examine the different pulses elaborately and make suggestions on how to benefit from them using Ayurveda principles.

Arhar Lentils

Arhar lentils, variously known as pigeon pea or tropical green pea (Ayurveda names: *toor, tuver*) is a beige-colored lentil with a yellow interior. The nutty-flavored dried and split peas are a favorite staple in everyday cooking and cooked as a soup called dal throughout India.

Culinary Varieties: Whole, split.

Ayurveda properties: Light, dry, cooling; sweet and astringent in taste.

Effect on doshas: Mainly pitta- and kapha-pacifying. Significantly increases vata (overcome by adding ghee, asafoetida, cumin, and even garlic during cooking; the sour taste in tamarind paste added during cooking or lemon juice sprinkled as garnish also balances out vata dosha). However, this lentil must be eaten with caution, especially if vata is already aggravated and during summers when vata dosha peaks in the macrocosm.

Digestibility index: Medium digestibility among lentils (lesser than mung and masoor).

Therapeutic points: Beneficial in skin rashes, and has a drying impact on stools (causes constipation), improves complexion.

TABLE 37   **How to Cook Arhar Lentils**

Type	Presoak	Stovetop	Pressure Cooker	Slow Cooker
Whole	Minimum 1 hour	30–40 minutes	6–8 minutes	Low, 5–6 hours
Split	Minimum 30 minutes	20 minutes	3–4 minutes	Low, 2–3 hours

Black-Eyed Peas/Azuki Beans

The black-eyed pea, also known as cow pea (Ayurveda name: *lobia*) is a small, polished white bean with a characteristic black eye. The red-colored pea of the same family is known as azuki bean (also known as red cow pea or *chori*).

Culinary varieties: Whole (black in color); whole, spilt, dehusked (white in color); dehusked, split.

Ayurveda properties: It is sweet and astringent, cooling, sweet postdigestion, and heavy. That which is biggest in size is considered best quality-wise.

Effect on doshas: Mainly balances pitta and kapha. Increases vata dosha.

Digestibility index: Hard to digest due to heavy quality hence contraindicated in dull agni or variable agni. Unless well-cooked with ghee and digestive spices (cumin, asafoetida, garlic, ginger, and so on) it tends to increase gas and distention in stomach during digestion.

Therapeutic points: Galactagogue (increases breast milk), helps improve taste. The biggest bean is best.

TABLE 38   How to Cook Black-Eyed Peas/Azuki Beans

Type	Presoak	Stovetop	Pressure Cooker	Slow Cooker
White black-eyed peas or red azuki beans	Minimum 8 hours, ideally overnight	60–90 minutes	15 minutes	20–30 minutes

Garbanzo Beans/Chickpeas

Garbanzo beans are the same as chickpeas or Bengal gram (Ayurveda names: *chanak*, *chana*, *chole*, *desi chana*, *kabuli chana*). They are available in two varieties, the smaller dark-skinned beans (chickpeas) and the larger white-skinned beans (garbanzo beans). The bean flour is also used in cooking as well as for body scrubs.

Culinary varieties: Whole, small (black-colored chickpeas); whole, big (white-colored garbanzo beans), small, dehusked, spilt to reveal yellow interior (known as yellow lentils or chana dal); powdered yellow lentil (besan).

Ayurveda properties: Dry, light, cooling.

Effect on doshas: Balances mainly pitta and kapha, increases vata dosha (fried in ghee after soaking helps counteract vata dosha).

Digestibility index: Medium digestibility.

Therapeutic points: Beneficial in blood disorders and fever, may cause constipation (for vata). Its soup can help with weight loss but in excess can cause tiredness (by aggravating vata).

TABLE 39   **How to Cook Garbanzo Beans/Chickpeas**

Type	Presoak	Stovetop	Pressure Cooker	Slow Cooker
Chickpeas, brown	Minimum 8 hours, ideally overnight	60–90 minutes	20–30 minutes	Low, 8–9 hours
Garbanzo, white, split	Minimum 8 hours, ideally overnight	60–90 minutes	20–30 minutes	Low, 8–9 hours
Garbanzo, split (yellow lentils or chana dal)	Minimum 2 hours	60–70 minutes	15 minutes	Low, 7–8 hours

Masoor Lentils

Masoor, or masur, is a brown-skinned lentil that is a bright orange when the outer skin is removed.

Culinary varieties: Whole with skin intact (brown-colored, sold as brown lentils), whole with outer skin removed (orange-colored, sold as red, orange, or pink lentils).

Ayurvedic properties: Sweet in taste and post-digestive effect, cooling and quite drying.

Effect on doshas: Mainly kapha- and pitta-balancing (hence must add ghee and cumin during cooking to overcome vata dosha).

Digestibility index: Easy enough to digest but may cause some dryness.

Therapeutic points: The soup (dal) is useful in overcoming fever, diarrhea (slightly constipating), blood disorders (purifying).

TABLE 40   How to Cook Masoor Lentils

Type	Presoak	Stovetop	Pressure Cooker	Slow Cooker
Whole	Minimum 2 hours	40–45 minutes	8–10 minutes	Low, 7–8 hours
Dehusked	Minimum 1.5 hours	20 minutes	3–4 minutes	Low, 2–3 hours

Mung Lentils

Mung lentils, also known as mung beans or green gram (Ayurveda names: *moong, mung*) are seeds with hard green husks and soft yellow insides.

Culinary varieties: Whole, split with the skins intact, split with the skins removed, sprouted.

Ayurveda properties: Dry, cooling, water absorbent, light, soft. Sweet and astringent in taste and sweet postdigestion also.

Effect on doshas: Mainly pitta- and kapha-pacifying. Only slightly increases vata (overcome by adding ghee and cumin during cooking).

This is considered the healthiest pulse that can be eaten by all doshas, in all seasons, by all ages, healthy or sick. Steamed, boiled, fried, or savory snacks made from mung are recommended for daily consumption.

Digestibility index: Maximum or easiest digestibility among lentils and can be digested with ease even by chronically dull agni.

Therapeutic points: Useful for detoxification, weight loss, and in acidity skin problems like eczema, heartburn and acidity, ulcers, poor vision, and fever.

TABLE 41   **How to Cook Mung Beans**

Type	Presoak	Stovetop	Pressure Cooker	Slow Cooker
Whole	Minimum 3 hours or overnight	60 minutes	8–10 minutes	Low, 5–6 hours
Whole, split	Minimum 2–3 hours	20–30 minutes	5–6 minutes	Low, 3–4 hours
Dehusked, split	Minimum 30 minutes	20 minutes	3–4 minutes	Low, 2–3 hours

Urad Lentils

Urad, also known as black gram or black lentil, is a little black seed husk with a white interior. It is similar to a mung bean in size and shape but tastes much more nutty or earthy and when cooked takes on a creamy texture which is highly prized.

Culinary varieties: Whole (black in color); whole, split (black outside, white inside), dehusked (white in color).

Ayurveda properties: Heavy, hot, oily, appetizing.

Effect on doshas: Pacifies vata dosha and increases pitta and kapha doshas.

Digestibility index: It is the hardest to digest and must be consumed only by those who have decent agni strength. It is ideally eaten in daytime versus nighttime and in winters more than any other season to maximize agni strength naturally.

Therapeutic points: Urad is the most nourishing lentil; hence, it is great if you want to put on weight and build muscles and strength. It is also a galactagogue, hence great for lactating mothers. The natural oil content provides laxative qualities and increases semen (shukra). Urad is especially beneficial in Ayurveda tradition for overcoming vata aggravation, which is responsible for hemorrhoids, Bell's palsy, and other neurological conditions. In all these cases, Urad prevents the condition, as well as supports recovery, by keeping vata dosha in check.

TABLE 42 **How to Cook Urad Lentils**

Type	Presoak	Stovetop	Pressure Cooker	Slow Cooker
Whole	Minimum 6 hours, ideally overnight	60–90 minutes	10–15 minutes	Low, 5–6 hours
Whole, split	Minimum 3 hours	40–60 minutes	8–10 minutes	Low, 4–5 hours
Dehusked, split	Minimum 1 hour	30–60 minutes	4–6 minutes	Low, 3–4 hours

Preparing Dal (Soup)

Standard dal (soup) recipes begin with pre-soaking in water to soften the hard, dry seeds, draining the water, and then boiling in an amount of water that is two to three times the volume of the beans, along with turmeric and rock salt to taste.

In some recipes (especially if the lentil has a dry quality), a dash of tamarind pulp or unripe mango slices are added to the cooking process, imparting a slightly tart or sour flavor. Chopped tomatoes can also be added, either during cooking or later, as a garnish, especially in summer when they are in season.

Adding a fried garnish of ghee and spices at the end of the cooking process is routine. This involves lightly sautéing spices (typically cumin and asafoetida) in a small amount of ghee for a few seconds on medium-low heat.

Sometimes the fried garnish is more elaborate, and ginger, garlic, and chopped onions (and sometimes tomatoes, too) are sautéed for 5 to 7 minutes on medium-high heat. After the onions turn golden brown, the garnish is poured over the cooked dal soup.

Sample recipes with dal include the Hearty Mung Soup recipe on page 321 and a traditional urad dal recipe that I call Spinach Black Gram Pilaf on page 265.

Ayurvedic Recipes
from My Home and Gurukulam

SPICED MILK

This is excellent as an everyday, anytime snack, before bed, or even as a complete meal by itself. The spice mix combination can be changed according to the season and your constitution. The process of cooking milk with spices and water renders the milk easier to digest, making it consumable even for those with compromised digestion. Drink at least three hours after dinner and no later than half an hour before bed.

INGREDIENTS

1	cup whole milk
4	cups water
2–3	green cardamom pods, crushed
2–6	saffron threads
¼	teaspoon ground turmeric
¼	teaspoon ground black pepper
⅛	teaspoon ground cinnamon powder
	Sugar, to taste (1–3 teaspoons)

METHOD

1. Combine milk and water in a medium saucepan. Add all the spices (but not the sugar).
2. Heat on high, stirring occasionally until the mixture begins to boil.
3. Quickly reduce heat to medium-low and stir occasionally, ensuring the mixture does not boil over. Cook until the added water has evaporated (20–25 minutes).
4. Once the liquid has been reduced down to 1 cup (approximately), remove from heat and strain, discarding any pods or spices left at the bottom.
5. Add sugar to taste. Drink hot or warm.

SEASONAL FINE-TUNING

- In spring, do not consume this recipe at bedtime.
- In summer and fall, only use cardamom and turmeric.

RICE AND MUNG BEAN PORRIDGE (KHICHADI)

Rice and lentil porridge is known as khichadi in the Ayurveda tradition. It imparts strength and balances all three doshas upon digestion. This recipe is very easy to digest and detoxifies the entire system. Regular consumption ensures optimum weight. It is considered a sattvic, or mind-calming and balancing recipe.

INGREDIENTS FOR PORRIDGE

- ½ cup basmati rice
- 1 cup yellow mung or split green mung
- 3 cups water
- ⅛ teaspoon asafoetida powder
- ½ inch piece fresh ginger root, grated or minced
  Rock salt, to taste (½–1 teaspoon)

INGREDIENTS FOR GARNISH

- 2 teaspoons ghee
- ¼ teaspoon cumin seeds
- ⅛ teaspoon asafoetida
- 1 tablespoon minced cilantro

METHOD FOR PORRIDGE

1. Wash and soak rice and mung lentils in water together in a bowl overnight (or for at least 3 hours before cooking).
2. Drain the rice and mung lentils and place in a medium saucepan. Add 3 cups water, asafoetida, ginger, and rock salt. The water level should be half an inch above the rice and mung bean mixture. If needed, add more water.
3. Cook on medium-high heat until the mixture comes to a boil.
4. Simmer on low heat, partly covered, until texture becomes soft, almost mushy, 20–25 minutes, adding more water if all water is absorbed before it is soft.
5. Turn off heat and set aside. Prepare the garnish.

METHOD FOR GARNISH

1. Heat ghee in a small frying pan. When hot (begins to shimmer, which will be almost immediately), add cumin seeds and sprinkle in the asafoetida.
2. Heat until cumin crackles slightly, about 10–15 seconds (any longer and the cumin will turn black and burn).
3. Add ghee mixture on top of the cooked porridge. It will make a sizzling sound.
4. Stir porridge; then garnish with cilantro. Eat and enjoy.

SEASONAL FINE-TUNING

- Add seasonal vegetables, in any combination, if you wish.
- In winter, you can use half black gram (urad dal) and half part green gram (mung lentils).
- Be liberal with ghee in the winter if required and if you can digest it.
- In summer and fall, omit the ginger.

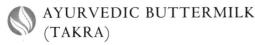 AYURVEDIC BUTTERMILK (TAKRA)

Ayurvedic buttermilk is known as takra. It is hot in potency and sour in taste but becomes sweet postdigestion. It is also light and drying. It is greatly vata- and kapha-pacifying and great to pick up a dull agni. It heals symptoms of IBS and flatulence and detoxifies the colon. It should be consumed for breakfast and lunch, but never after sunset.

INGREDIENTS

- ¼ cup whole-milk yogurt, ideally at room temperature
- 1 cup pure, room-temperature water (preferably, use stovetop boiled water cooled to room temperature)
- ¼ teaspoon ground cumin
- ⅛ teaspoon asafoetida
- ⅛ teaspoon ground ginger
  Rock salt, to taste (about ¼ teaspoon)
- 1 teaspoon minced coriander

METHOD

1. Whisk yogurt with water for 4–5 minutes, until foamy. The longer you are able to whisk, the lighter and more digestible the drink becomes.
2. Add the spices on top of the foamy liquid, along with cilantro as garnish. It is ready be consumed. (You may also use a blender instead of whisking.)

SEASONAL FINE-TUNING

- In winter, takra should be consumed daily at lunchtime.
- In spring, drinking takra is prohibited (as are all other yogurt preparations).
- In early and late summer, instead of spices, simply add sugar (to taste) to water and yogurt mixture. You can also blend in five freshly plucked (pesticide-free) rose petals.
- In fall, do not add spices; instead, add cane sugar (to taste).

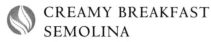 ## CREAMY BREAKFAST SEMOLINA

Ayurveda texts mention that depending on the methods of cooking wheat, it can be used to increase weight or to reduce and manage weight. In this recipe, semolina is first dry-roasted, which infuses the wheat with dry, hot qualities, rendering it easier to digest. This is a great breakfast item, especially for wintertime. If you have a sharp agni, you can eat it year-round. It is filling and satisfying. It also enhances sattva, or mind-calming, qualities.

INGREDIENTS

¼ cup wheat semolina
1 cup whole milk
1 tablespoon ghee (clarified butter)
¼ teaspoon ground cardamom
2–3 saffron threads (optional)
1 tablespoon slivered almonds (optional)
1 tablespoon raisins (optional)
Cane sugar, to taste (1–2 teaspoons)

METHOD

1. Dry roast the semolina in a pan until lightly toasted.
2. Slowly add milk to the pan, stirring constantly to avoid lump formation.
3. Add cardamom and saffron to the milk and wheat mixture. Bring it to a boil.
4. Reduce heat and simmer for 8–10 minutes until a thin porridge-like consistency is achieved. If too thick, add more water.
5. Add almonds and raisins.
6. Serve immediately. Eat hot.

SEASONAL FINE-TUNING

- In wintertime, you can garnish with chopped walnuts and almonds. You can also add a teaspoon of ghee on top.
- In spring, add ¼ teaspoon ground turmeric and ¼ teaspoon ground ginger. Keep sugar to a minimum or skip it. Do not add nuts or raisins. Replace cow's milk with goat's milk, if you wish.
- In summer and fall, abstain from nuts but be sure to add extra sugar or plenty of raisins.

WINTER MELON STIR-FRY

Winter melon, known as *kushmanda* or *petha* in Ayurveda tradition, is a pumpkin-like vegetable that pacifies imbalances in pitta, in vata, and also in blood since it is cooling in potency. It is deeply nourishing, and enhances fertility and libido (but is safe for children). Ayurveda sages also hail it as a great food for overall mind health.[4] Make it a weekly choice. Add to soups and pastas, or bake or grill it. Be sure to use ripe melon. You can also replace winter melon with butternut squash, which has somewhat similar qualities.

INGREDIENTS

1	pound winter melon/squash
1	tablespoon ghee
¼	teaspoon fennel seeds
¼	teaspoon ground turmeric
¼	teaspoon cumin seeds
	Rock salt, to taste (½–1 teaspoon)
	Minced cilantro for garnish

METHOD

1. Peel and dice melon.
2. In a sauté pan, heat the ghee and add fennel, turmeric, and cumin. Swirl until fragrant and the seeds pop.
3. Add the diced melon and salt to pan; mix well. Cover and cook on medium-low heat for about 15–20 minutes, stirring every 3–4 minutes so that it doesn't burn or stick to the bottom of the pan.
4. Garnish with cilantro.

SEASONAL FINE-TUNING

- In winter, toss in 1 tablespoon cashews while stir-frying, if you wish.
- In spring, add ⅛ teaspoon fenugreek seeds and ½ teaspoon grated fresh ginger root while stir-frying.
- Winter melon is an ideal vegetable for summer and fall. Consume it daily if you wish, in any cooked form.

⬡ OPO AND MILK PUDDING

This deliciously fragrant recipe is described in ancient texts of Ayurveda. The sweet and cold qualities of both milk and opo squash make for a highly sattvic combination, which is excellent for summer and fall too. It balances pitta and vata and builds healthy kapha. Kids love it. This pudding is great for breakfast and is a meal in itself. Opo squash can be easily found in Asian food markets. You can recognize it by its elongated bottle-like shape and pale-green color. In Indian grocery stores, it is known as *doodhi* or *lauki*. You can replace opo squash with zucchini in this recipe. This pudding should always be eaten pleasantly warm, never chilled.

INGREDIENTS

2	tablespoons ghee
8–10	strands saffron
2	cups grated opo squash (about 1 medium squash)
4	cups whole milk
½	cup cane sugar
¼–½	teaspoon ground cardamom

METHOD

1. Heat ghee in a pan on medium heat. When ghee is hot, add saffron and grated opo and sauté for about 2–3 minutes, until opo becomes translucent.
2. Add milk and sugar and bring to a boil. Add cardamom, reduce flame to medium-low, and simmer until the opo blends/disintegrates into the milk (about 30 minutes), stirring frequently to avoid burning on the bottom.
3. Serve warm.

SEASONAL FINE-TUNING

- While this dish is great for winter, summer, and fall, it is contraindicated in spring.
- In winter, garnish it with slivered nuts, especially almonds and pistachios.
- In fall and summer, garnish with fresh rose or marigold petals.

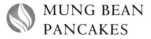

MUNG BEAN PANCAKES

Mung is mentioned as the best among beans in Ayurveda texts. This is my everyday breakfast. I make the batter ahead of time and make fresh pancakes for the entire family. This recipe is satiating but very light and works for everyone. Whether you are trying to lose weight or gain, mung supports a healthy metabolism.

INGREDIENTS

1	cup yellow mung beans (soaked 3 hours or overnight)
½	teaspoon ground, roasted cumin
½	teaspoon rock salt
¼	teaspoon ground turmeric
¼	teaspoon grated fresh ginger
⅛	teaspoon asafoetida
2	tablespoons ghee

METHOD

1. Drain soaking liquid from mung beans and place in a blender. Blend on high speed for about 1 minute, adding a small amount of water (about 2 tablespoons) until smooth.

2. Add cumin, salt, turmeric, ginger, and asafoetida and blend again briefly. Thin the mixture with enough water so that batter is a medium-thin consistency similar to wheat-flour pancake batter.

3. Heat a small amount of ghee (½–1 teaspoon) in a skillet or griddle on medium heat.

4. Drop a small ladle full of batter (¼ cup) onto griddle and spread in a circle. Cook on first side until edges start to brown and lift, about 5 minutes.

5. Flip pancake with spatula and cook on second side until golden brown, about 3–5 minutes.

6. Repeat steps 3 through 5 with the rest of the batter and ghee.

SEASONAL FINE-TUNING

- In winter, you can use equal quantities of black gram (urad dal) and green gram (mung) instead of mung exclusively.
- In spring, you can add finely diced greens like spinach, fenugreek, or kale to the batter.
- In summer, omit the use of ginger.
- In fall, omit ginger and asafoetida.

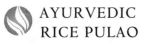

AYURVEDIC RICE PULAO

If you happen to have cooked rice, you can use it in step 4 below instead of 1 cup of raw rice. You'll need about 2 cups' worth. Omit the water, and cook 3–5 minutes until rice is heated through, and then proceed to step 5.

INGREDIENTS

- 2 teaspoons ghee
- ⅛ teaspoon asafoetida
- ¼ teaspoon ground black pepper
- ⅛ teaspoon fenugreek seeds
- ½ teaspoon cumin seeds
- ¼ teaspoon ground turmeric
- 1 teaspoon minced fresh ginger
- 1 cup chopped kale
- ½ cup diced carrots
- ½ cup green peas
  Rock salt, to taste
- 1 cup rice, presoaked in water for 30 minutes
- 1 cup water
- 2 tablespoon minced cilantro

METHOD

1. In a large saucepan, heat the ghee on medium-low heat. Add asafoetida, black pepper, fenugreek, and cumin. Cook 15–30 seconds, stirring frequently, until fragrant.
2. Add turmeric and ginger and cook for about 10–15 seconds.
3. Add kale, carrots, peas, and salt. Stir. Cover and reduce heat to medium-low. Cook for 3–4 minutes.
4. Add the rice, stir well, and add 1 cup water. Cover and cook 15–20 minutes, until rice is fully cooked. Stir.
5. Garnish with cilantro.

SEASONAL FINE-TUNING

- This recipe is great for winter and spring.
- In summer, replace kale with spinach, and peas with diced squash (any kind). Do not add black pepper.
- This recipe is not recommended for fall.

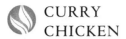 CURRY
CHICKEN

INGREDIENTS

4	teaspoons ghee
½	teaspoon cumin seeds
¼	teaspoon fennel seeds
1	medium-sized onion, diced
¼	teaspoon ground turmeric
½	teaspoon rock salt
1	pound chicken meat, cut into 1-inch cubes
½	teaspoon ground coriander
½	cup coconut milk (optional)
	Minced cilantro, for garnish

METHOD

1. Heat ghee in a pan on medium-low heat, add cumin and fennel, and cook for about 5–10 seconds, until fragrant.
2. Add onions, turmeric, coriander, and salt. Stir, and then cover and cook on medium-low heat for about 5 minutes or until onions are lightly transparent.
3. Add chicken and mix well. Cover and cook for about 10–12 minutes, until the chicken is fully cooked.
4. Add the coconut milk. Bring to a boil, and then cover and simmer on low heat for 2 minutes.
5. Garnish with cilantro.

Alternatively, to make dry/stir-fry chicken, do not use coconut milk. Grind cumin and fennel seeds into a powder and mix them with ground turmeric and coriander. Heat the ghee, sauté onions with salt, and then add chicken and the spice blend. Mix well and sauté until cooked through. Garnish with cilantro.

SEASONAL FINE-TUNING

- In spring, preferably go for the dry stir-fry recipe. Also, grind ¼ teaspoon each of black peppercorns and cloves to a powder. When the chicken is fully cooked, sprinkle this powder on top.
- Chicken is ideal for consumption in the cooler months of the year. If you wish, you can separately stir-fry 6–8 whole cashews to be used as garnish for the chicken.
- This recipe is great for summer.
- In fall, you can garnish the stir-fry recipe with fresh pomegranate seeds, if you wish.

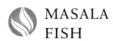 MASALA
FISH

INGREDIENTS

2	medium fish fillets
¼	teaspoon fenugreek seeds
½	teaspoon fennel seeds
¼	teaspoon ground turmeric
	Rock salt, to taste
2	teaspoons ghee
	Minced cilantro, for garnish

METHOD

1. Cut the fish fillets in half to make 4 pieces.
2. Combine fenugreek and fennel seeds in a mortar and pestle and grind to a powder. Add turmeric and salt to this powder.
3. Rub the spice mix on the fish and leave it in a bowl to marinate for about 15–20 minutes.
4. Heat a flat pan, and add ghee. Over medium heat, pan sear the fish, about 2–3 minutes on each side until golden.
5. Garnish with cilantro.

Alternatively, the fish can be baked after it has been marinated. Heat the oven to 375 degrees Fahrenheit, and put the fish in a baking tray. Melt ghee, lightly pour ghee over fish, and bake uncovered 15–20 minutes or until the fish flakes easily with a fork.

SEASONAL FINE-TUNING

- River water fish are ideal. Grass carp may be the best option.
- Fish is generally recommended in summer over all other seasons in Ayurveda due to its moisture-enhancing qualities. This recipe is, therefore, perfect for summer consumption.
- In spring, do not eat fish. If you do, eat it rarely and in the daytime only. The baked version is preferred over the pan-fried version.
- In winter, fish can be consumed, but meat from animals that live on land versus water (such as chicken or turkey) is preferred.
- In fall, seafood is contraindicated for pitta-disturbing qualities.

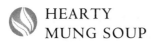

HEARTY MUNG SOUP

INGREDIENTS

- 1 cup green (split) mung dal
- 3–4 teaspoons ghee
- ½ teaspoon cumin seeds
- ¼ teaspoon ground turmeric
- 1 small onion, diced
- 2 cloves garlic, minced
  Rock salt, to taste
- ½ cup finely sliced carrots
- 1 cup chopped spinach
- ½ cup cubed winter melon or butternut squash
  Minced cilantro, for garnish

METHOD

1. Wash and soak 1 cup green split mung dal for about 3–4 hours or overnight; it will absorb water and yield about 2 cups of soaked mung dal.
2. Heat a large sauce pan on medium-low heat; add ghee and then cumin and turmeric. Cook until fragrant (about 5–10 seconds) and then add onion, garlic, and salt. Sauté for a few seconds. Then cover and cook for about 5 minutes.
3. Add the soaked mung dal and 2 cups water and bring to a boil over high heat. Then, lower the heat to medium-low, cover, and simmer for about 20–30 minutes.
4. When the dal is almost cooked, stir it vigorously so it becomes thick and the dal breaks down.
5. Add carrots, spinach, squash, and 1½ cups water. Cover and cook for another 8–10 minutes on medium-low heat.
6. Garnish with cilantro.

SEASONAL FINE-TUNING

- This recipe is great for winter and summer.
- In spring, remove onions and replace the squash with diced eggplant or green peas, or add both.
- In fall, do not add garlic.

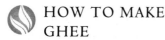

HOW TO MAKE GHEE

INGREDIENTS

2   pounds unsalted organic butter

METHOD

1. Put butter in a medium saucepan (2.5–3 quart capacity) and heat over high heat, stirring frequently until butter is melted and begins to boil. There will be a thick layer of foam on the surface.

2. Turn down heat to medium and continue cooking. The butter will bubble and boil as the water evaporates. After about 20 minutes, the foam will begin to subside, and the butter will begin to look clear. Solids will begin to settle on the bottom of the pan. Stir occasionally, scraping the bottom of the pan, so the solids do not burn.

3. Continue cooking for 15–20 minutes, keeping a close watch. When ghee is ready, it is golden colored with slightly browned solids at the bottom of the pan. There may be some slightly crusty bubbles on the top.

4. The ghee can be tested for the absence of water by dipping a piece of paper in the ghee and setting fire to the end. Properly cooked ghee will burn cleanly, with no sputtering.

5. Cool slightly (3–5 min); then filter through a mesh strainer lined with cheesecloth into a heatproof container (a 1-quart glass measuring pitcher is ideal for this). Then pour into clean glass containers (either one quart jar or two pint jars). Screw lids on loosely and allow to cool and solidify at room temperature. Discard the leftover milk solids that settle at the bottom of the pan.

6. The clarified liquid, Ghee, is shelf-stable and needs no refrigeration. The solidity of the ghee may vary with different butters and climates and may range from solid to a more runny, oily consistency.

Note: Ghee can be made in smaller or larger quantities, although smaller quantities are more easily overcooked and should be cooked on low heat during the last stage.

Shunya's Detox Protocol

Since toxins can be generated for a variety of reasons, including emotional and seasonal variability, at least once a year, I recommend that everyone eat a detox diet. Shared below is the detox protocol I have created and used successfully over many years.

Symptoms of Toxicity

- Feelings of heaviness, stiffness, lassitude

- Acute or chronic indigestion

- Expectoration of phlegm

- Coated tongue and tastelessness

- Abdominal bloating

- Nausea with increasing stomach discomfort

- Dull headache and general body aches

- Constipation or diarrhea

- Stools with more odor than usual

- Urine and menstrual blood with more odor than usual

- Excessive yawning, increased sleepiness, or exhaustion

- Excessive thirst

- Low-grade fever

- Loss of energy and physical strength

The Basic Concept

Ayurveda's word for detox is *langhanam*, which literally means "mindfully making light" by reducing the quantity or changing the quality of foods eaten. It does not mean complete abstinence. Foods must digest quickly so as not to cause indigestion or increase body weight. Thus, the qualities we prefer in detox foods are light, hot, dry, cooked, fresh, natural, and measured in quantity, and we control the use of oiliness.

Detox when you are home and able to follow a nonstressful, unhurried routine. Plan a minimum of three days. Season-wise, the first two weeks of spring are ideal, so plan ahead. You can also embark on detox other times throughout the year if you have more than a few symptoms of toxins present. However, detox is prohibited in both early and late winter. It is also prohibited during pregnancy, lactation, and menstruation. Here are some general recommendations:

- Cook each meal fresh. Always eat the detox meals warm.

- Eat breakfast at 8:00 a.m., lunch at noon, and dinner at 5:00 p.m. or by 7:00 p.m. at the latest.

- Go to bed by 10:00 p.m. and try your best to wake up before 6:00 a.m. Do not nap in the daytime.

- Walk one hundred steps after eating every meal.

- Gentle walking can be helpful, but do not overtire yourself, or you will crave rich foods.

- Do not do oil massage during detox; dry powder massage is preferred. (See chapter 5.)

- Spice formula: mix equal quantities of ground turmeric, ground ginger, and ground cumin and take ¼ teaspoon with warm water after every meal throughout the duration of detox.

- Continue taking your Ayurvedic herbs (if advised by a qualified practitioner) and medical prescriptions.

What to Eat

You will have to stop eating your routine foods, including coffee and tea, if possible. Eat specified recipes only. Slow down your chewing and eat mindfully. Throughout the detox, drink only hot water. Drink as is or add a pinch of bishop's weed seeds to the water. Only drink when thirsty. The following recipes will yield enough for one adult for all three meals (for average appetite), but you can cook a second time if you do not have enough left for your dinner.

 ## DETOX DAY 1: RICE SOUP

The best food to eat on the first day is rice soup. You will eat this at every meal, so prepare a fresh batch early in the morning. Ideally, presoak the rice the night before.

INGREDIENTS

2	cups rice
1	teaspoon ghee
12	cups water
1	teaspoon ground black pepper
1	teaspoon ground cumin
½	teaspoon ground ginger
1	teaspoon rock salt (plus more, to taste)
2	teaspoons minced cilantro

METHOD

1. Wash rice and soak in 4 cups water for at least 3 hours or overnight.
2. Heat a large stock pot on low to medium heat and add ghee. Drain the presoaked rice and sauté in ghee until rice turns a slight golden color and becomes fragrant (2–3 minutes).
3. Add 12 cups water and bring to a boil on high heat. When water begins to boil, reduce heat to low and simmer uncovered for another 15–20 minutes.
4. Continue cooking until rice is completely broken down and has acquired a porridge-like consistency.
5. Add black pepper, cumin, ginger, and salt.
6. Garnish with cilantro. Eat the rice soup warm.

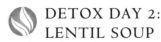 DETOX DAY 2:
LENTIL SOUP

On the second day of the detox, eat only this recipe for each meal. You'll likely want to presoak the mung beans the night before.

INGREDIENTS

1	tablespoon ghee
2	cups whole mung beans, soaked in 4 cups water for at least 3 hours or overnight
12	cups water
½	teaspoon ground black pepper
½	teaspoon ground ginger
½	teaspoon ground cumin seed
¼	teaspoon rock salt (plus more, to taste)
1	teaspoon lime juice (optional)
2	teaspoons minced cilantro

METHOD

1. Heat a large stock pot on medium-high heat, add ghee, and then add the presoaked and drained mung dal. Sauté until the lentils are slightly brown and mildly aromatic.
2. Add 12 cups water and boil until the lentils are fully cooked and individual grains of lentils begin to lose integrity, 30–40 minutes, or longer if required.
3. Add black pepper, ginger, cumin, and salt. Use a ladle to mash the lentils fully to get a porridge-like consistency.
4. Add lime juice and garnish with cilantro. Eat while hot.

 DETOX DAY 3:
RICE AND LENTIL STEW

On the third day of the detox, eat only this recipe for each meal. You'll likely want to presoak the rice and lentils the night before.

INGREDIENTS

1	tablespoon ghee
½	teaspoon cumin seed
⅛	teaspoon asafoetida
½	teaspoon ground turmeric
1	cup whole mung lentils, soaked in 2 cups water for at least 3 hours or overnight
1	cup rice, soaked in 2 cups water for at least 3 hours or overnight
6	cups water
½	teaspoon rock salt (plus more, to taste)

METHOD

1. Heat a large stock pot over medium heat and add ghee. When ghee is shimmering, add cumin, asafoetida, and turmeric (you may want to turn heat to low as you add the spices so that they do not burn but get only lightly browned).
2. Drain the presoaked lentils and rice and add them to the pan. Sauté for 5 minutes on medium heat until the mixture becomes golden and aromatic.
3. Add 6 cups water and salt. Cover and cook on low heat 25–30 minutes. You will know the porridge is ready when the rice and lentils become soft and mushy.
4. Eat while hot. Eat two or three times a day based on actual hunger.

Note: This preparation is the heaviest to digest in the series of advanced antitoxic recipes, but only when compared to the recipes preceding it. In itself, it is still superlight to digest, and it will be lighter than recipes containing ingredients such as wheat, vegetables, meats, oils, cheese, fruits, and nuts.

Detox Day 4 and Beyond: Khichadi

You can now introduce khichadi at every meal (see Rice and Mung Bean Porridge (Khichadi) recipe on page 312). You can also eat Hearty Mung Soup and Mung Bean Pancakes (see recipes on pages 321 and 317). You can drink Ayurvedic buttermilk at breakfast and lunch (see Ayurvedic Buttermilk (Takra) recipe on page 313). Continue with this less rigorous detox protocol for a minimum of three days (for a total detox period of six days) up to a maximum of seven days (for a total detox period of ten days), after which you can return to your normal diet. However, when you return to a normal diet, resume regular foods slowly and do not shock your system. Choose wisely.

Honey Support

If you get hungry at any stage of the detox protocol, instead of snacking, try swallowing 1 tablespoon of raw uncooked, unprocessed, pure honey. Do not mix it in hot water or tea. Simply place the honey directly on your tongue. You can have more than 1 tablespoon in the beginning, but never more than 6 tablespoons a day.

Sleep and Hunger Support

If honey is not enough, you can eat more of the same detox recipes between regularly scheduled mealtimes (up to six small meals a day) or even an hour before bedtime. In rare cases, if your sleep is disturbed during detox, then you can drink spiced milk at bedtime (see Spiced Milk recipe on page 311).

Herbal Tea

Boil 2 pods of cardamom with ¼ teaspoon coriander seeds and ¼ teaspoon fennel seeds in 2 cups of water. When only 1 cup of water remains, remove from heat and drink warm in small sips. You can drink this tea between detox meals as well as with the meals. This tea supports your digestion during the detox period and also keeps vata dosha in check.

Resuming Your Normal Diet

When you have completed a basic protocol of three to seven days, it is time to resume your normal diet. Return to normal foods gradually. Do not shock your system by suddenly stuffing it with chilled water or frozen and processed foods. Common experiences reported post-detox include the following:

- Improved (normalized) appetite
- Improved physical energy
- Improved mental clarity
- A light feeling
- Better-formed stools
- Less gas and bloating

For ongoing toxin management, take the following steps:

- Drink boiled water mainly.

- Eat ghee regularly with meals (though always in moderation).

- Incorporate Ayurvedic buttermilk.

- Use pungent and bitter spices daily especially turmeric, coriander, and cumin.

- Use rock salt only versus all other cooking salts.

- Eat special recipes: try to eat the detox recipes a few nights per month.

- Follow the dietary rules provided in chapter 6.

- Avoid incompatible food combinations.

APPENDIX 5

Glossary of Sanskrit Words

aama Toxin.

abhayanga Oil massage.

agni Digestive fire.

amalaki (also amla) Indian gooseberry.

asana Yoga posture.

Atmabodha Awakening to the truth of our spiritual nature.

Atman The eternal Self, transcending birth and death.

Ayodhya An ancient city, one of the seven sacred cities of the Hindus. It is situated on the banks of River Sarayu, some eighty-four miles east of Lucknow, the capital of the State of Uttar Pradesh in northern India.

Ayurveda The science of health and healing, also known as the science of life, from ancient India.

baba Elderly or holy person; also refers to author's grandfather (Ayodhya Nath), who was her Ayurveda guru.

bala Physical strength.

balya Strength-imparting.

brahma muhurta One-and-a-half hours before sunrise.

brahmacharya The quest for the Ultimate Reality; sexual fidelity in committed relationships.

Brahman The universal truth; refers to the Vedic concept of a formless Ultimate Reality.

chakra Refers to vortices or wheels of invisible spiritual energy said to be located in the energy body that lies within the physical body.

devas Gods.

devata God.

devi Goddess.

dhairyam Mental strength.

dharma Spiritual responsibility.

dhatu Tissue.

dinacharya Lifestyle practices prescribed by Ayurveda.

dosha   Three energies (known as vata, pitta, and kapha) believed to circulate in the body and govern physiological and psychological activity; their differing proportions determine individual temperament and physical constitution and (when unbalanced) cause a disposition to particular physical and mental disorders.

Gayatri mantra   A chant from the *Rig-Veda*.

ghee   Clarified butter.

guna   Quality.

guru   Spiritual teacher; the term also means "heavy."

gurukulam   A traditional Vedic school.

kapha   One of the three doshas, condensed from the elements water and earth. It is the principle of stabilizing energy, governs growth in the body and mind, is concerned with structure, stability, lubrication, and fluid balance.

khichadi   A dish made from boiling rice and legumes along with common Ayurveda spices. Alternate spellings include *khichdi, khichri, khichdee, khichuri, khichari, kitcheree, kitchree,* and many other variants.

krimi   Microorganisms.

krumi   Parasites.

loka   The universe.

manas   Mind.

manasika   Mental.

mantra   A spiritual chant in Sanskrit.

moksha   Spiritual freedom.

mudra   Yogic hand gesture.

nadis   The subtle and invisible channels through which, in Ayurveda and the spiritual science of yoga, the energies of the subtle body are said to flow. They connect at special points of intensity called chakras.

nidra   Sleep.

oja   Immunity principle.

OM   The supreme and most sacred syllable in Hinduism and Buddhism, consisting in Sanskrit of the three sounds |a|, |u|, and |m|, representing various fundamental triads and believed to be the spoken essence of the universe. It is uttered as a mantra and in affirmations and blessings.

parampara   Tradition; lineage.

pitta   One of three doshas; results from the combination of the elements fire and water. Pitta dosha regulates metabolism, heat, and body temperature.

Prakriti   Constitution; Mother Nature.

prana   Energy; also a synonym of vata dosha.

pranayama   Yogic breathing practices.

purusha   The individual; soul.

rajas   Dynamic or changeable quality of mind.

Rig-Veda   The most ancient scripture of the Hindus; the source of the Ayurvedic tradition.

rishi   Sage; wise man.

ritucharya   Seasonal regimen.

Rta   Rhythm.

sadhana   A disciplined spiritual practice.

Sanskrit   Ancient Indian language in which Vedic texts are composed, including Ayurvedic texts.

Sarayu (also Sarju)   River that flows through the Indian states of Uttarakhand and Uttar Pradesh. This river is of ancient significance, mentioned in the Vedas and the Ramayana. The author's hometown, Ayodhya, is situated on the banks of River Sarayu.

sattva, sattvic   Mental quality of balance of intelligence.

savasana   Also known as "corpse pose," it is a component of yoga practice that promotes a state of homeostasis, thus allowing the person to release emotional and physical tension; performed at the end of the entire asana practice.

shakti   Spiritual power.

shukra   Sexual tissue.

srota   Channels in the body through which doshas, nutrients, and wastes flow for body functions ranging from the gross to the imperceptible and classified by their origin and by the substances that they carry.

surya namaskar   A sequence of twelve yoga postures (asanas). Its origins lie in India where a large Hindu population worships Surya, the Hindu solar deity, daily. However, in modern times, this sequence is performed by non-Hindus, without any religious overtones, for its demonstrated health benefits.

Sushruta   An Indian physician who lived in the first and second centuries CE. He is the author of the treatise *Sushruta Samhita (The Compendium of Sushruta)*. This is one of the most important surviving ancient treatises on medicine. The treatise addresses all aspects of general medicine, but the translator G. D. Singhal dubs Sushruta "the father of surgery" because of the extraordinarily accurate and detailed accounts of surgery found in the work. He has also been called "the first plastic surgeon."

swastha   Health.

swasthavritta   Ayurveda's wholesome teachings to build and protect health.

swasthya   Healthy.

tamas, tamasic   Mental state of dullness, ignorance, or noncomprehension.

tila   Sesame.

tri-dosha, tri-doshic   Relating to the three doshas.

ubtan Bath scrub.

Upanishad The last section of the Vedas, known as Vedanta; contains the highest teachings on Ultimate Reality Brahman that transcend time, space, and change.

vaidya Physician. In India, generally refers to a person who practices the Ayurveda system of health and healing.

vata One of the three doshas; forms from the elements of air and space. It is the principle of kinetic energy in the body, is concerned with the nervous system and with circulation, movement, and pathology, and is eliminated from the body through defecation.

Vedas The most ancient Hindu scriptures; the philosophical bedrock of various religions from India and sciences of Ayurveda, yoga, and Vedanta.

Vedic Refers to an ancient period of Indian history when the Vedas were composed.

virya Courage.

yoga From the Sanskrit word *yuj*, which means "yoke" or "union." Traditionally, yoga is a methodology aimed toward joining the individual consciousness with the Ultimate Reality (universal consciousness). Hence, all yogic physical and mental exercises are ultimately designed to aid self-transcendence. On the physical level, yoga postures, called asanas, are designed to tone, strengthen, and align the body. On the mental level, yoga employs breathing techniques (pranayama) and meditation (dhyanam) to quiet, clarify, and discipline the mind. Yoga is not a religion, but a way of living with health and peace of mind as its goals.

NOTES

Preface

1. John Platt, "Ayurveda Out of Balance: 93 Percent of Medicinal Plants Threatened with Extinction," *Scientific American*, April 5, 2010, blogs.scientificamerican.com/extinction-countdown/ayurveda-out-of-balance-93-percent-of-medicinal-plants-threatened-with-extinction.

2. Dean Ornish, et al. "Changes in Prostate Gene Expression in Men Undergoing an Intensive Nutrition and Lifestyle Intervention," *Proceedings of the National Academy of Sciences* 105 no. 4 (June 2008): 8369–74, doi: 10.1073/pnas.0803080105.

3. Reuters, "Healthy Lifestyle Triggers Genetic Changes: Study," June 18, 2008, reuters.com/article/us-genes-lifestyle-idUSN1628897920080618.

Introduction

1. *Rig-Veda*, Book 1, Hymn 164, Verse 46.

2. Sushruta: Sushruta Samhita, Sutrasthanam-15, 41.

3. "WHO Definition of Health," World Health Organization, accessed July 11, 2016, who.int/about/definition/en/print.html.

Chapter 1

1. Charaka Samhita, Sutrasthanam-1, 44.

2. Sushruta Samhita, Sutrasthanam-15, 4.

3. Rishi Sushruta, Sushruta Samhita, Sutrasthanam-15, 41

4. Charaka Samhita, Sutrasthanam-16, 27. This concept, known as *swabhavo-paramvaad*, was first put forward by Sage Charaka between the third and second centuries BCE.

Chapter 2

1. Ashtanga Hridayam, Dinacharya Adhyaya-2, 1A.

2. Charaka Samhita, Sharirasthanam-5, 4.

3. Bhava Prakasha, Dinacharyadi Prakarana-5, 4–6.

4. Bhava Prakasha, Dinacharyadi Prakarana-5, 303–4.

5. The origin of this verse is unknown. It has been passed down orally in India over the last several thousand years. This verse has many variations, with "Gouri" in the last line sometimes being substituted with *Durga, Govinda, Govindam,* or *Brahma*.

6. The Savitri Gayatri Mantra, *Rig-Veda*, Book 3, Hymn 62, Verse 10.

Chapter 3

1. Bhava Prakasha, Purvakhanda, Dinacharyadi Prakarana-5, 17.

2. According to the science of Ayurvedic pharmacology, only black gram (*urad dal*) possesses the guru quality, or quality of heaviness (that is, it is harder to digest or takes longer time to digest), whereas all other lentils, such as mung lentils and so on, are considered *laghu*, or light to digest.

3. Charaka Samhita, Vimanasthanam-1, 24.

4. W. M. Sun, L. A. Houghton, N. W. Read, D. G. Grundy, and A. G. Johnson, "Effect of Meal Temperature on Gastric Emptying of Liquids in Man," *Gut* 29: no. 3 (1988): 302–5, ncbi.nlm.nih.gov/pmc/articles/PMC1433604/.

5. Ibid., 329–34.

6. Heinz Valtin, "'Drink at Least Eight Glasses of Water a Day.' Really? Is There Scientific Evidence for '8 x 8'?" *American Journal of Physiology: Regulatory, Integrative and Comparative Physiology* 283 (November 2002): R993–R1004, doi: 10.1152/ajpregu.00365.2002.

7. Rock salt, also known as Himalayan pink salt, is available online or in specialty grocery stores. Do not confuse rock salt with a type of blackish/dark pinkish sulfur salt known in Indian grocery stores as black salt or *kala namak*. Rock salt is more white than pink. It is never black or dark purple in color. And rock salt does not have a peculiar sulfuric smell.

8. Ashtanga Hridayam, Sutrasthanam-5, 13–18.

9. Bhava Prakasha, Purvakhanda, Varivarga, 79–81.

Chapter 4

1. National Research Council, "Neem: A Tree for Solving Global Problems," Report of an Ad Hoc Panel of the Board on Science and Technology for International Development (Washington, DC: National Academy Press, 1992), pdf.usaid.gov/pdf_docs/PNABN264.pdf.

2. D. P. Agrawal, "Medicinal Properties of Neem: New Findings," accessed November 10, 2014, infinityfoundation. com/mandala/t_es/t_es_agraw_neem.htm.

3. Harvard T. H. Chan School of Public Health, "Impact of Fluoride on Neurological Development in Children," accessed November 10, 2014, hsph.harvard.edu/news/features/fluoride-childrens-health-grandjean-choi/.

4. Deirdre Imus, "EPA Reverses Itself on Fluoride," Fox News Health, February 22, 2011, foxnews.com/health/2011/02/22/epa-reverses-fluoride/.

5. The "Section on Diagnostics" in the classical treatise by Sage Sushruta includes a description of the cavity syndrome caused by microorganisms including dull to severe toothache (*vedana*), sensitivity to hot and cold sensations (*dantaharsha*), back discoloration in the caries (*koth*), cracking of enamel (*kapalika*), loosening of tooth and consequent mobility (*chaladanta*), pus formation (*sravi*), and finally inflammation accompanied

by foul smell (*durgandha*). What is more, it appears that Sage Sushruta was merely taking forward early concepts on pathogens mentioned in the Vedas, where the term *krimi* has been used in broader sense—that is, it includes all pathogenic and nonpathogenic organisms covering a wide range of infection and infestation. These infectious diseases caused by krimi are explained under the title of "Communicable Diseases" (*oupasaigika rogas*), which spread through contact with patients and through other routes such as water, air, food, and so on.

6. Sushruta Samhita, Chikitsasthanam-24, 4; Charaka Samhita, Sutrasthana-5, 72–74; Bhava Prakasha, Dinacharyadi Prakarana-5, 14–29.

7. A. Hooda, M. Rathee, and J. Singh, "Chewing Sticks in the Era of Toothbrush: A Review," *The Internet Journal of Family Practice* 9, no. 2 (2009): ispub.com/IJFP/9/2/4968.

8. A. S. Malik, M. S. Shaukat, A. A. Qureshi, and R. Abdur, "Comparative Effectiveness of Chewing Stick and Toothbrush: A Randomized Clinical Trial," *North American Journal of Medical Sciences* 6, no. 7 (2014): 333–37, doi:10.4103/1947-2714.136916.

9. Ibid.

10. Bhava Prakasha, Dinacharyadi Prakarana-5, 27–28.

11. Bhava Prakasha, Dinacharyadi Prakarana-5, 29.

12. Sushruta Samhita, Chikitsasthanam-24, 8.

13. Note that the toothache tree, known as *tejovat* in Ayurveda and prized for its dental benefits on all varieties of oral diseases (*mukharoga*), was also known to Native American tribes and was prized for its ability to remedy toothaches. It is well known that Native Americans would chew on the bark or rub a paste of the bark on sore gums for relief from pain and swelling.

14. Bhava Prakasha, Dinacharyadi Prakarana-5, 30–33; Charaka Samhita, Sutrasthanam-5, 75.

15. M. I. Van der Sleen, D. E. Slot, E. Van Trijffel, E. G Winkel, and G. A. Van der Weijden, "Effectiveness of Mechanical Tongue Cleaning on Breath Odour and Tongue Coating: A Systematic Review," *International Journal of Dental Hygiene* 8, no. 4 (2010): 258–68, http://ebd.ada.org/en/evidence/evidence-by-topic/6585/effectiveness-of-mechanical-tongue-cleaning-on-breath-odour-and-tongue-coating-a-systematic-review.

16. Gordon Christensen, "Special Oral Hygiene and Preventive Care for Special Needs," *Journal of the American Dental Association* 136, (August 2005): 1141–43, doi: dx.doi.org/10.14219/jada.archive.2005.0319.

17. Charaka Samhita, Sutrasthanam-5, 74.

18. The practice of adding nano-doses of purified metals to herbal medicines, a prescription recommended in ancient Ayurvedic medicine, is done only in India and Southeast Asian countries such as Sri Lanka and Bangladesh. The United States and most European countries

prohibit any medicines that have metal as an active ingredient. It is vital for Ayurveda students and practitioners alike to respect these laws with no exceptions.

19. C. Norman Shealy, "Antiseptic Mouthwash Can Kill You," *Shealy Wellness* (blog), September 6, 2013, normshealy.com/antiseptic-mouthwash-can-kill-you/.

20. Ibid.

21. Pat Thomas, "Behind the Label: Listerine Teeth and Gum Defence," *Ecologist*, January 13, 2009, theecologist.org/green_green_living/behind_the_label/269558/behind_the_label_listerine_teeth_and_gum_defence.html.

22. Vikas Kapil, Syed M. A. Haydar, Vanessa Pearl, Jon O. Lundbergb, Eddie Weitzberg, and Amrita Ahluwalia, "Physiological Role for Nitrate-Reducing Oral Bacteria in Blood Pressure Control," *Free Radical Biology and Medicine* 55 (February 2013): 93–100, doi:10.1016/j.freeradbiomed.2012.11.013.

23. Charaka Samhita, Sutrasthanam-5, 78–80.

24. Bhava Prakasha, Purvakhanda, Taila Varga 1–23 Charaka Samhita, Sutrasthana-27, 286–88.

25. Bhava Prakasha, Dinacharyadi Prakarana-5, 34.

26. S. Asokan, P. Emmadi, and R. Chamundeswari, "Effect of Oil Pulling on Plaque Induced Gingivitis: A Randomized, Controlled, Triple-Blind Study," *Indian Journal of Dental Research* 20, no. 1 (January–March 2009): 47–51, ncbi.nlm.nih.gov/pubmed/19336860.

27. Sharath Asokan, T. K. Rathinasamy, N. Inbamani, Thangam Menon, S. Senthil Kumar, Pamela Emmadi, and R. Raghuraman, "Mechanism of Oil-Pulling Therapy—In Vitro Study," *Indian Journal of Dental Research* 22, no. 1 (2011): 34–37, ijdr.in/text.asp?2011/22/1/34/79971.

28. J. S. Tripathi and R. H. Singh, "The Concept and Practice of Immunomodulation in Ayurveda and the Role of Rasayanas as Immunomodulators," *Ancient Science of Life* 19, nos. 1–2 (1999): 59–63, ncbi.nlm.nih.gov/pmc/articles/PMC3336465/.

29. Charaka Samhita, Sutrasthanam-5, 78–80; Sushruta Samhita, Chikitsasthanam-24, 14; Bhava Prakasha, Dinacharyadi Prakarana-5, 32–36.

30. Bhaishajya Ratnavali-61, 20.

Chapter 5

1. Ram, or Rama, is the name of a Hindu god, considered an avatar of Lord Vishnu, the main protagonist of the Hindu epic Ramayana.

2. Here's what the chant sounds like in Awadhi, a dialect of Hindi spoken in the author's hometown: *Avadh Puri Mum Puri Suhavani, Uttar Disi bahi Saryu Pavani Ja majjan te binuhi prayasa, Mam sameep nar pavahi vasaa. (Shri Ram Charit Maanas.)* This is a verse from Ramcharitmanas, an epic poem written in the Awadhi dialect of Hindi, composed by the 16th-century Indian poet Goswami Tulsidas.

3. Here's what the chant sounds like in Sanskrit: *Gange cha Yamune chaiva Godavari Saraswati | Narmade Sindhu Kaveri jalesmin sannidhim kuru.*

4. Annetrin Jytte Basler, "Pilot Study Investigating the Effects of Ayurvedic Abhyanga Massage on Subjective Stress Experience," *The Journal of Alternative and Complementary Medicine* 17, no. 5 (May 2011): 435–440. doi:10.1089/ acm.2010.0281.

5. Charaka Samhita, Sutrasthanam-5, 81–92; Bhava Prakasha, Dinacharyadi Prakarana-5, 56–60; Ashtanga Hridayam, Sutrasthanam-2, 8–9; Sushruta Samhita, Chikitsasthanam-24, 25–26, 30–32.

6. Ashtanga Hridayam, Sutrasthanam-2, 9.

7. Sushruta Samhita, Chikitsasthanam-24, 25–26; Bhava Prakasha, Dinacharyadi Prakarana 60; Charaka Samhita, Sutrastahanam-5, 81–83.

8. Charaka Samhita, Sutrastahanam-5, 90–92; Bhava Praksha, Dinacharyadi Prakarana 61–62.

9. Bhava Prakasha, Dinacharyadi Prakarana 63–64; Charaka Samhita, Sutrastahanam-5, 84.

10. Sushruta Samhita, Chikitsasthanam-24, 35–37.

11. Sushruta Samhita, Chikitsasthanam-24, 42–43, 47–48.

12. Sushruta Samhita, Chikitsasthanam-24, 83; Dalhana's commentary on verse 83.

13. Ibid.

14. Bhava Prakasha, Dinacharyadi Prakarana-5, 71–78.

15. Bhava Prakasha, Dinacharyadi Prakarana-5, 65–66.

16. Bhava Prakasha, Dinacharyadi Prakarana-5, 76.

17. H. S. Datta, S. K. Mitra, and B. Patwardhan, "Wound Healing Activity of Topical Application Forms Based on Ayurveda," *Evidence-Based Complementary and Alternative Medicine* 2011 (2011): 134378. doi:10.1093/ ecam/nep015.

18. "Sodium Lauryl Sulfate: The Facts," SLS Free, accessed January 10, 2015, slsfree.net/.

19. The official website of the World Health Organzation's International Agency for Reserch on Cancer (iarc. fr/) has published several monographs on potential environmental and carcinogenic effects of coal tar and pitch; see specifically the monograph "Coal-Tar Pitch," accessed July 13, 2016, monographs.iarc.fr/ENG/Monographs/ vol100F/mono100F-17.pdf. Additionally, TOXNET, the National Institutes of Health's Toxocology Data Network (toxnet.nlm.nih.gov/cgi-bin/sis/search/ a?dbs+hsdb:@term+@DOCNO+5050), provides links to studies by the World Health Organization, International Agency for Research on Cancer, the EPA's Integrated Risk Information System, American Conference of Governmental Industrial Hygienists, National Toxicology Program; and many international organizations.

See also B. J. Mahler and P. C. Van Metre, "Coal-Tar-Based Pavement Sealcoat, Polycyclic Aromatic Hydrocarbons (PAHs), and Environmental Health: U.S. Geological Survey Fact Sheet 2011–3010," accessed January 10, 2015, pubs.usgs.gov/fs/2011/3010.

20. National Cancer Institute, "Formaldehyde and Cancer Risk," accessed January 10, 2015, cancer.gov/about-cancer/causes-prevention/risk/substances/coal-tar.

21. Madanphala Nighantu, Vatadivarga 80–81; Bhava Prakasha, Vatadivarga 39–40.

22. Indira P. Sarethyi, Niyanta Bhatia, and Nidhi Maheshwari, "Antibacterial Activity of Plant Biosurfatant Extract from *Sapindus mukorossi* and In Silico Evaluation of Its Bioactivity," *International Journal of Pharmacy and Pharmaceutical Sciences* 7, no. 10 (2015): innovareacademics.in/journals/index.php/ijpps/article/view/7263.

23. B. Seetha Lakshmi, "Bio Control of Phytopathogens by Soap Nuts *Sapindus emarginatus* L. Fruit Pulp," special issue, *Indian Journal of Research in Pharmacy and Biotechnology* 1 (December 2014): 109, ijrpb.com/specialissues/1/ijrpb%2022%20b%20seetha%20lakshmi%20109-111.pdf.

Chapter 6

1. Bhagavad Gita-17, 6–10.

2. This is based on the popularity of many spiritual paths (religions) that recommend a no-meat diet. However, Ayurveda takes a pragmatic approach that supports a light and easy-to-digest diet that is primarily lactovegetarian, but at the same time, it does not rule out consuming animal meats in moderation when cooked and consumed with a sattvic attitude.

3. Charaka Samhita, Sutrasthanam-27, 342.

4. Charaka Samhita, Sutrasthanam-1, 64–66.

5. Charaka Samhita, Chikitsasthanam-1, 4.

6. Charaka Samhita, Sutrasthanam-8, 20.

7. Charaka Samhita, Sutrasthanam-25, 40.

8. Dane A. Roubos, "The Great Margarine Hoax: The Deadly Truth about Dietary Oils," accessed July 13, 2016, rense.com/health/marg.htm.

9. Dane A. Roubos, "Margarine, Fatty Acids, and Your Health," *NEXUS Magazine* 4, no. 2 (1997).

10. Bhagavad Gita-4, 24.

Chapter 7

1. Charaka Samhita, Sutrasthanam-21, 36.

2. Sushruta Samhita, Sharirasthanam-4, 34, 35.

3. Ashtanga Hridayam, Sutrasthanam-7, 66–68.

4. Sushruta Samhita, Sharirasthanam-4, 45.

5. In Charaka Samhita, Sutrasthanam-8, 3–4, Charaka Samhita says that one should not suppress the thirteen natural urges relating to urine, feces, semen, flatus, vomiting, sneezing, burping, yawning,

hunger, thirst, tears, sleep, and breathing deeply after exertion. Sushruta Samhita echoes the same teaching (Uttar Tantra-55, 4). However, this rule pertains to the normal sleep cycle at nighttime, not in the daytime. If due to overwork, personal habit, or social activities we suppress sleep at nighttime, we can experience problems including heaviness and pain in the eyes and head, lack of enthusiasm, habitual insomnia, and agni disorders. The concept of irrepressible urges does not mean that we fall asleep at any time in any place when we want to, as when the "urge" to nap strikes us.

6. Ashtanga Hridayam, Sutrasthanam-7, 75.

7. These pleasures are collectively known as *kama purushartha* in Sanskrit.

8. Bhava Prakasha, Dinacharyadi Prakarana-5, 274.

9. Bhava Prakasha, Dinacharyadi Prakarana-5, 297.

10. Bhava Prakasha, Dinacharyadi Prakarana-5, 316–19.

11. Bhava Prakasha, Dinacharyadi Prakarana-5, 263.

12. Charaka Samhita, Sutrasthanam-7, 31.

13. Charaka Samhita, Sutrasthanam-7, 31–33.

14. The fact that right exercise leads to improved immunity is known as *vyayamaha sthairyakaaranam.*

15. Sushruta Samhita, Chiktsasthanam-24, 44.

16. Sushruta Samhita, Chiktsasthanam-24, 38–50.

17. Charaka Samhita, Sutrasthanam-7, 31–32.

18. Ibid; Sushruta Samhita, Chiktsasthanam-24, 39–42.

19. Charaka Samhita, Sutrasthanam-7, 34.

20. Ashtanga Hridayam, Nidanstthanam-1, 15.

21. Sushruta Samhita, Chiktsasthanam-24, 46.

22. Jeannine Stein, "Movement Therapies May Reduce Chronic Pain," *Los Angeles Times,* July 5, 2010, articles.latimes.com/2010/jul/05/health/la-he-pain-exercise-20100705.

Appendix 2

1. Bhava Prakasha, Purvakhanda, Dugdhavarga, 1–2.

2. Bhava Prakasha, Purvakhanda, Dugdhavarga, 24–28.

3. Bhava Prakasha, Purvakhanda, Phalavarga, 63–64.

Appendix 3

1. Refer to page 185 for a review of the six tastes and their impact on the body.

2. D. Prasad and R. Kunnaiah, "*Punica granatum*: A Review on Its Potential Role in Treating Periodontal Disease," *Journal of Indian Society of Periodontology* 18, no. 4 (2014): 428–32, doi:10.4103/0972-124X.138678.

3. S. Rajan, J. Ravi, A. Suresh, and S. Guru, "Hidden Secrets of *Punica granatum* Use and Its Effects on Oral Health: A Short Review," *Journal of Orofacial Research* 3, no. 1 (2013): 38–41, doi: 10.5005/jp-journals-10026-1061.

4. M. Nagpal and S. Sood, "Role of Curcumin in Systemic and Oral Health: An Overview," *Journal of Natural Science, Biology and Medicine* 4, no. 1 (2013): 3–7, ncbi.nlm.nih.gov/pubmed/23633828.

5. Bhava Prakasha, Purvakhanda, Haritakyadivarga, 196–97.

6. Bhava Prakasha, Purvakhanda, Vatadivarga, 36–37.

7. A. R. Pradeep, E. Agarwal, P. Bajaj, S. B. Naik, N. Shanbhag, and S. R. Uma, "Clinical and Microbiologic Effects of Commercially Available Gel and Powder Containing *Acacia arabica* on Gingivitis," *Australian Dental Journal* 57, no. 3 (2012): 312–18, onlinelibrary.wiley.com/ doi/10.1111/j.1834-7819.2012.01714.x/ abstract.

8. D. T. Clark, M. I. Gazi, S. W. Cox, B. M. Eley, and G. F. Tinsley, "The Effects of *Acacia arabica* Gum on the In Vitro Growth and Protease Activities of Periodontopathic Bacteria," *Journal of Clinical Periodontology* 20 (1993): 238–243, http://www.ncbi.nlm.nih.gov/ pubmed/8473532.

9. J. Ahmed, N. Shenoy, A. Binnal, L. P. Mallya, and A. Shenoy, "Herbal Oral Care: An Old Concept or a New Model?" *International Journal of Research in Medical Sciences* 2, no. 3 (2014): 818–21, imsear.li.mahidol. ac.th/bitstream/123456789/165296/1/ ijrms2014v2n3p818.pdf.

10. Devanand Gupta, Dara John Bhaskar, Rajendra Kumar Gupta, Bushra Karim, Ankita Jain, Rajeshwar Singh, and Wahaja Karim, "A Randomized Controlled Clinical Trial of *Ocimum sanctum* and Chlorhexidine Mouthwash on Dental Plaque and Gingival Inflammation," *Journal of Ayurveda and Integrative Medicine* 5, no. 2 (April–June 2014): 106–119, ncbi.nlm.nih.gov/pmc/ articles/PMC4061585/.

11. Bhava Prakasha, Purvakhanda, Karpuradivarga, 58–59.

12. S. Sateesh, S. Mathiazhagan, S. Anand, R. Parthiban, S. Suresh, B. Sankaranarayanan, R. Sandiya, and A. Kumar, "A Study on Analgesic Effect of *Caryophyllus aromaticus* by Formalin Test in Albino Rats," *International Journal of Pharmaceutical Science Invention* 2, no. 1 (January 2013): 28–35, ijpsi.org/ VOl(2)1/Version_3/F0212835.pdf.

13. S. Amruthesh, "Dentistry and Ayurveda V: An Evidence Based Approach," *International Journal of Clinical Dental Science* 19(1) (2008, Jan–Mar); 52-61, http://www.ncbi.nlm.nih.gov/ pubmed/18245925.

14. Ibid.

Appendix 4

1. These recommendations may read differently from other books on Ayurveda that describe seasons and related dietary dos and don'ts based on

authors' subjective opinions, but the suggestions provided here are based exclusively on the source texts.

2. "Monsoon," *Wikepedia*, accessed September 10, 2015, en.wikipedia.org/wiki/Monsoon.

3. Bhava Prakasha, Dinacharyadi Prakarana, Haritakyadivarga, 241.

4. Bhava Prakasha, Shakavarga, 53–55.

INDEX